Governors State University
Library
Hours:
Monday thru Thursday 8:30 to 10:30
Friday and Saturday 8:30 to 5:00
Sunday 1:00 to 5:00 (Fall and Winter Trimester Only)

DEMCO

GENES, ENVIRONMENT, AND PSYCHOPATHOLOGY

Genes, Environment, and Psychopathology

Understanding the Causes of Psychiatric and Substance Use Disorders

KENNETH S. KENDLER
CAROL A. PRESCOTT

THE GUILFORD PRESS
New York   London

©2006 The Guilford Press
A Division of Guilford Publications, Inc.
72 Spring Street, New York, NY 10012
www.guilford.com

Printed in the United States of America

This book is printed on acid-free paper.

Last digit is print number: 9 8 7 6 5 4 3 2 1

Library of Congress Cataloging-in-Publication Data
Kendler, Kenneth S., 1950–
   Genes, environment, and psychopathology: understanding the causes of
psychiatric and substance use disorders / Kenneth S. Kendler, Carol A. Prescott.
      p. ; cm.
   Includes bibliographical references and index.
   ISBN-10: 1-59385-316-5   ISBN-13: 978-1-59385-316-7 (cloth)
   1. Mental illness—Genetic aspects. 2. Mental illness—Environmental
aspects. 3. Psychiatric epidemiology. I. Prescott, Carol A. II. Title.
   [DNLM: 1. Mental Disorders—epidemiology. 2. Mental Disorders—
genetics—Statistics. 3. Risk Factors—Statistics. 4. Twin Studies—
Statistics. WM 140 K33g 2006]
   RC455.4.G4K46 2006
   616.89′042—dc22
                                                        2006017070

My parents, Howard and Tracy Kendler, were both academic psychologists in the neobehaviorist tradition. Together, they got their doctoral degrees in the early 1940s at the University of Iowa, where they studied under Kenneth Spence, after whom I was named. They gave me a loving and intellectually stimulating upbringing. I remember, as a child, long summer evenings when after dinner my mother would read books such as *Huckleberry Finn*, *The Last of the Mohicans*, and *The Red Pony* to me and my brother. When I was back in school, I would wait with anticipation for my father to come home and wrestle with me on the living room floor or play football in the backyard. My parents were always interested in and encouraged my academic achievements and provided ample emotional and financial support throughout college and medical school. Much of my curiosity and my drive to learn and achieve surely comes from the genes and the environment they provided for me. I dedicate this book to my father and the memory of my mother with deep love and gratitude.

—K. S. K.

I dedicate this book to my husband, Jack McArdle, who has been a source of strength, support, inspiration and fun throughout my years with the VATSPSUD. Writing with him in mind encourages me to aspire to his high standards of intellectual integrity and scientific excellence. Thank you, dear reader.

—C. A. P.

About the Authors

Kenneth S. Kendler, MD, is the Banks Distinguished Professor of Psychiatry and Professor of Human Genetics at the Medical College of Virginia, Virginia Commonwealth University. He received his medical and psychiatric training at Stanford University and Yale University, respectively. Since 1983, he has been engaged in studies of the genetics of psychiatric and substance use disorders, including schizophrenia, major depression, alcoholism, and nicotine dependence. Dr. Kendler has been the director of the Virginia Adult Twin Study of Psychiatric and Substance Use Disorders since its inception. His work has utilized the methods of both large-scale population-based twin studies and molecular genetics. He has published over 400 peer-reviewed articles, has received a number of national and international awards, is a member of the Institute of Medicine of the National Academy of Sciences, serves on several editorial boards, and is Editor of *Psychological Medicine*. Since 1996, Dr. Kendler has served as Director of the Virginia Institute for Psychiatric and Behavioral Genetics.

Carol A. Prescott, PhD, is Professor of Psychology at the University of Southern California and a practicing clinical psychologist. She received BA and MA degrees in experimental psychology from Johns Hopkins University and a PhD in clinical psychology from the University of Virginia. From 1992 to 2005, she was on the faculty of the Virginia Institute for Psychiatric and Behavioral Genetics of Virginia Commonwealth University, where she served as codirector of the Virginia Adult Twin Study of Psychiatric and Substance Use Disorders. Dr. Prescott has published extensively on genetic influences on alcoholism and other forms of psychopathology. She serves as Associate Editor for *Behavior Genetics* and *Alcoholism: Clinical and Experimental Research*. Her honors include election to membership in the Society for Multivariate Experimental Psychology and the Theodore Reich Prize from the International Society on Psychiatric Genetics.

Acknowledgments

This study has been like a long journey. Many have helped us along the way. Three individuals stand out who were vital to the overall success of the Virginia Adult Twin Study of Psychiatric and Substance Use Disorders (VATSPSUD). Lindon Eaves was, in many ways, the intellectual guiding force of this project. He was there at the very inception of this project, and many of the ideas that we sought to test in our study stemmed in one way or another from his ideas and work. Lindon's sparkling intellect was a source of continued inspiration.

Michael Neale was with the project nearly from its beginning. He played a key role as the "intellectual engine" for many of the developments in structural equation modeling that fill the pages of this book. His active participation in the project and his consistent willingness to engage in further model development to help us answer what we saw to be important questions contributed greatly to the success of this project.

Joel Silverman was Chair of the Department of Psychiatry at Virginia Commonwealth University (VCU) for nearly all the years during which this study was conducted and analyzed. We could not have had a more supportive chairman. Whenever he could, he provided us with the resources we needed and allowed us to do our work largely unencumbered by the worries so common in academic life.

Three other colleagues played critical roles in the early years of this project. Andrew Heath, along with Lindon Eaves and Kenneth S. Kendler, worked out the basic design of this project. Andrew also oversaw the first questionnaire assessment of the female–female twins. Nick Martin was also part of the team that launched the first wave of this study. Both Andrew and Nick made important contributions to the conceptualization of the project. Ron Kessler was a key addition to the collaborative group and, in the early years of the project, taught us much about measurement of both psychiatric disorders and epidemiological risk factors. He was a wonderful teacher and collaborator and to this day remains generous with his time if we have questions.

We acknowledge our gratitude to the U.S. National Institutes of Health, which provided much of the financial support for this project through Grant Nos. MH-

40828, AA-09095, and MH/AA/DA-49492. The Rachel Brown Banks endowment fund also helped support our work, as did the Department of Psychiatry at VCU.

We have, through the many phases of this project, been blessed with a talented and dedicated series of project coordinators—the ones who ran the project on a day-to-day basis. Patsy Waring, with great determination and organization, got this project off the ground and kept it running from its early to its middle years. Sarah Woltz (now Powers) assumed responsibility for the male–male/male–female project and saw the wave 2 study through to its completion with unfailing cheerfulness. The final wave of the female–female study was jointly managed by Barbara Brooke and Lisa Halberstadt, who nurtured it through our experiment with computer-assisted interviews. Frank Butera has served as our chief editor for many years, and we have relied completely on his sound judgment and eye for detail. The data quality was greatly improved by a cadre of dedicated editors armed with pencils and pink erasers, including Barbara Brooke, Fran Davis, Katherine Gagarin, Lisa Halberstadt, Karen Hough, Justine Jones, Tawna Koptis, Paige McCleary, Maureen Mullin, Bethany Patton, Martha Perry, Karen Petersen, Toni Phillips, Christy Shapard, and Ernie Wahrburg.

Over the years we were privileged to work with many fine interviewers. These individuals, often clinicians who were looking to try something different, lived and traveled all over Virginia, North Carolina, and Washington, DC. Many went to great lengths to find and interview twins, including leaving cookies on doorsteps, looking up tax records to find addresses, sweet-talking twins' mothers, visiting twins in prison, and getting up in the middle of the night to call twins stationed in the Middle East or Asia. In addition to our project managers and editors (most of whom previously conducted interviews), our interviewing staff included Elizabeth Achaval, Michelle Acree, Morgan Adams, Roberta Anderson, Cynthia Ayres, Joyce Barwick, Donna Bates, Mary Jane Bearman, Joseph Beaty, Brenda Berry, Melanie Berry, Mary Biddlestone, Arthur Bliss, Patricia Bolton, Carolyn Brankley, Ilze Brown, Stacia Carone, Edward Carpenter, Beverly Carter, Bronwen Cheek, Dale Clymer, Sally Conlon, Cathy Cooke, Marylin Copeland, Edwin Cotton, Kathryn Crone, Virginia Crone, Thomas Crooks, Puspa Das, Jennifer Davis, Judith (DeBusk) Davis, Jeanne Day, Cynthia Dougherty, Patricia Doyle, Loretta Dunn, Frances Easton, Shirley English, Linda Farris, Ellen Fay, Richard Firth, Elizabeth Fong, Marlene Fortenberry, Cheryl Fossum, Theresa Francisco, Marian Frenk, Nur Gangji, Cathy Garber, Mary Gillman, Linda Girdner, Teresa Gore, Calvin Graham, Suzanne Gregory-Coe, Michele Gunter-Thomas, Elaine Hailey, Susan Hall, Sandra Haney, James Harper, Johnnie Helms, Teresa Hill, Eddie Hoel, Constance Houchens, Rondi Hunt, Carol Hurst, Peggy Jerome, Elizabeth Johns, Enid Johns, Jill Johnson, Linda Johnson, Vera Johnson, Jones Jones, Diane Kane, Victoria Kavanaugh, Amy Kelly, Stephney Keyser, Carol Kinzer, Victoria Knox, Margaret Kraus, Barry Kuhlik, David Kyle, Linda Landry, Sarah Lawrence, Lori Lefter, Rosemary Lemon, John Lindeman, Sheila Lockmuller, Lois Lommel, Janice Lucero, John Ludgate, Steve MacGregor, Linda Matthews, Judith McGuire, Sheila Melville, Lori Mick, Sharon Miller, Catherine Moore, Janet Moncure, Stephanie Morrison, Karen Neary, Glenora Nelson, Terry Newman, Donna Nunnally, Marianne Orndoff, Elizabeth Owen, Dianna Parrish, Martha Peery, Toni Philips, Gwendolyn Pierce, Stephanie Porras, Vita Press, Paul Rosenfeld, Laura Rossi, Kathryn Sack, Gregory Schaller, Ann Schellhammer, Mary Lee Schuler, Sherlyn Shaughnessy, Thais Sikora, Leigh Simmons, Flora Smith, Helen Smith, Julia Spruell, Willis Suddith, Lydia Susnick, Anna Thomas, Michele Gunter Thomas, Elizabeth Tillett, Melinda Tilley, Julia Timberlake, Evelyn Tomaszewski, Mary Any Ullmer, Anne Van Nostrand, Pamela Vega, Eleanor Wabnitz,

Valinda Walker, Dee Watson, Gail Westpheling, Alison Wilkins, Susan Williams, Paula Wilson, Cynthia Wingate, and Joan Young. (We apologize to anyone we inadvertently omitted!)

During most of the years that this project was under way, we were blessed by the presence of a wonderful and devoted secretary, Becky Gander. She helped in innumerable ways for which we are deeply grateful. The administrator of our research unit, Stacey Garnett, oversaw the many fiscal and administrative aspects of this project with dedication and grace. Lou Hopkins for many years served as the project secretary helping to ensure that our interviewers had the materials they needed and got their reimbursements and pay on time. She was unfailingly pleasant even at the most stressful of times. We are also grateful to the other project staff who were with us for shorter periods, including Karen Brown-Davis, Margie Fanas, Joanne Vivas, John Waring, and Jackie Woodley.

To be used, data from interviews have to be entered into the computer. For many years, this has been the responsibility of Indrani Ray, who, with care and dedication, constructed the specialized screen-driven data entry system for each of our different interviews. Although a number of different individuals entered the data, much of the work was performed by Cheryl Smith with both great speed and precision.

Zygosity testing for the twins was conducted under the direction of our molecular genetics colleagues Richard Straub and, more recently, Brien Riley. They were assisted by a team of lab staff, particularly Brandon Wormley and Jen Vittum.

We are grateful to VCU President Eugene Trani for providing funding and space for the creation of the Virginia Institute for Psychiatric and Behavioral Genetics. Other colleagues at VCU who have provided helpful advice on the project management over the years include Mary Swartz, John Blatecky, Bob Cohen, and Jim Levinson.

Several generations of statistical analysts worked on this project and performed most of the analyses presented in this book and in the publications that emerged from this study. Leroy Thacker and Ellen Walters were in the first generation, and both were very productive and got the project off to a great start. John Myers has been with the project for the longest time, and throughout his many years, his work has always been characterized by great care and attention to detail. Many of the analyses that were specially performed for this book were conducted by John with his usual rigor. Laura Karkowski also made valuable contributions to the project in her analytic work. Charles Gardner has put in many years of dedicated, creative, and careful work and has also contributed by the introduction and development of new analytic methods. In addition to his work on longitudinal data analysis and measurement, Steven Aggen helped considerably with the substantial and essential task of database management. Jonathan Kuhn spent several years with the team and brought to us a high level of methodological sophistication.

A number of predoctoral students, postdoctoral fellows, and junior and senior faculty worked on this project, and many of their results are reflected in this book. We acknowledge the debt we owe to them, including Arpana Agrawal, Cynthia Bulik, Rebecca Cross, Ayman Fanous, Debra Foley, Rise Goldstein, Jack Hettema, Kristen Jacobson, Amir Khan, Hermine Maes, Tony O'Neill, Marc-Andre Roy, Eric Schmitt, Pak Sham, Judy Silberg, Patrick Sullivan, and Tracy Wade.

Kenneth S. Kendler's work on this book was greatly aided by a sabbatical year as the Fritz Redlich Fellow at the Center for Advanced Study in the Behavioral Sciences.

Our project would not have been possible without the tremendous amount of effort that went into the establishment of the Virginia Twin Registry and its maintenance. We are much indebted to Walter Nance, who began the registry, and to Linda Corey, who, for most of the years of this project, oversaw its updating and maintenance and its transition to becoming the Mid-Atlantic Twin Registry (MATR). In more recent years, Lenn Murrelle, Judy Silberg, and Lindon Eaves directed the MATR and were helpful with many aspects of the study. We are grateful to the MATR staff , particularly Carol Williams, who helped us identify and locate twins.

The quality of this book was greatly improved by the editorial expertise of Lisa Halberstadt and Becky Gander, who not only corrected our grammar but also provided many helpful substantive comments on the text. Lisa was also invaluable in helping prepare the figures and final text and was tireless in spending many hours with us proofing the final versions of the book and detecting numerous errors and other problems that escaped many attentive eyes. Our colleagues Alan Gruenberg and Jonathan Flint read over preliminary drafts of this book and provided helpful feedback. Barbara Herrmann spent long hours pulling everything together for the final version of the text, figures, and references. We are grateful to Barbara Watkins and Seymour Weingarten of The Guilford Press for their guidance and assistance in preparing this book for publication. Any errors that remain are our own.

Kenneth S. Kendler: Although I have always been devoted to my work, it is in fact my family that provides my world with structure and meaning. My three children, Jennifer, Seth, and Nathan, grew up during the years I worked on this project. From a young age, they knew my interest in twins and would be quick to point out a twin pair if we met them in a shopping mall or at a restaurant. They have enriched my life immeasurably. My wife, Susan Miller, has been a devoted and loving partner in raising a family and together pursuing our professional careers. It would not have been remotely possible for me to have done the work we describe in this book without her assistance and support. Susan also strongly encouraged me to take the sabbatical that gave me the time and quiet needed to get the bulk of my part of the book written.

Carol A. Prescott: I spent 10 years working nearly full time on the VATSPSUD. The project staff were unusually dedicated, wonderful people, and a number of them have become close friends. Thanks to all for your support, humor, and hallway gab sessions. My brother, Dan Jobe, an exceptional salesman and project manager, lived with me during the early years of the project and was a source of love and caring, as well as invaluable advice about subject recruitment and interviewer training.

Finally, our sincere thanks go to the twins of the Virginia Twin Registry and their family members. They welcomed us into their homes. They trusted us with their varied and sometimes difficult personal experiences. It was a privilege for us to be able work with these twins, who were overwhelmingly cordial and helpful. Like us, they believe in the tremendous value of twins in helping to expand our understanding of basic questions about the human condition. We are deeply in their debt.

List of Sidebars

List of Abbreviations

A, a	additive genetic component
AAD	alcohol abuse or dependence
AASB	adult antisocial behavior
ACE	basic twin model
AD	alcohol dependence
ASB	antisocial behavior
ASP	antisocial personality disorder
AUI	Alcohol Use Inventory
C, c	shared (common) environmental component
CCC	causal, contingent, common pathway
CD	conduct disorder
CI	confidence interval
CSA	childhood sexual abuse
DSM	*Diagnostic and Statistical Manual of Mental Disorders*
DZ	dizygotic (fraternal)
DZF	dizygotic female
DZM	dizygotic male
E, e	individual-specific (unique) environmental component
EEA	equal environment assumption
FD	family dysfunction
FF	female–female
FF1–FF4	waves 1–4 of FF twin study
FFP	female–female–parent study

FTND	Fagerstrom Test for Nicotine Dependence
FTQ	Fagerstrom Tolerance Questionnaire
GAD	generalized anxiety disorder
GAS	generalized anxiety syndrome
HR	hazard ratio
IV	interview
κ	kappa (chance corrected agreement)
LTCT	long-term contextual threat
MATR	Mid-Atlantic Twin Registry
MD	major depression
MF1–MF2	waves 1–2 of MM/MF twin study
MM/MF	male–male/male–female
MT	multiple threshold
MZ	monozygotic (identical)
MZF	monozygotic female
MZM	monozygotic male
N, n	number, sample size
N	neuroticism
NCS	National Comorbidity Survey
ND	nicotine dependence
NS	novelty seeking
OR	odds ratio
OS	opposite sex
PBI	Parental Bonding Instrument
r	correlation coefficient
SD	standard deviation
SEM	structural equation model
SLE	stressful life event
VATSPSUD	Virginia Adult Twin Study of Psychiatric and Substance Use Disorders
VTR	Virginia Twin Registry

Contents

Introduction

This is a book about the causes of psychiatric and substance use disorders. In it we describe the origins, methods, and results of one large-scale study that systematically addressed why some individuals are highly vulnerable and others are resilient to the development of these disorders. This study is the Virginia Adult Twin Study of Psychiatric and Substance Use Disorders. We refer to it by the admittedly cumbersome acronym VATSPSUD.

Although the study has limitations, it also has four noteworthy strengths unusual in research of this kind. First, we follow an unselected population of individuals through time. We do not study the correlates and causes of psychiatric disorders based on individuals who have received treatment and who may not be representative of the entire population of affected individuals.

Second, this study takes seriously the possible role of genetics in the etiology of psychiatric and substance use disorders. The participants in our investigation are twins. Twins are a valuable "experiment of nature," and studying them can teach us a great deal about how genes influence human behavior.

Third, this study also takes seriously the role of environmental risk factors in psychiatric and substance use disorders. We made a major effort to assess exposure to a wide array of potentially pathogenic environmental experiences, as well as factors that may help protect against the development of disorders.

Fourth, this study represents a serious effort to understand how genetic and environmental risk factors interrelate in the development of psychopathology. The title of this book was carefully chosen. We do not believe that the etiology of psychiatric disorders can be understood solely by examining genetic or environmental risk factors in isolation. Nor does it reflect a simple adding together of genetic and environmental risk. Rather, the underlying

1

process is almost certainly more subtle. Risk is likely to arise from an inter-weaving of genes and environment.

We use data to test systematically a range of hypotheses about the etiol-ogy of psychiatric and substance use disorders. Often, books in the mental health field have a high "speculation to fact ratio." We wanted to avoid that pattern. As a result, this book might be considered "data dense." To make it as accessible as possible, we have attempted to focus on our key findings and their implications for understanding the causes of mental disorders. We pro-vide only the details necessary to understand our conclusions and how we came to them. Readers interested in the more technical aspects of our mea-surements and analyses can refer to the original publications in which much of this work appeared.

We have three goals in this introduction. First, rather like an overture, we preview the major themes that are developed throughout the book. Second, we outline the structure of the book. Third, we offer a brief personal perspec-tive on the development of the VATSPSUD and the key contributions of its main developers (see Sidebar I.1).

OVERTURE

We suggest that readers be attuned to four major questions as they read this book.

1. *What can we learn about the role of genetic factors in the etiology of psychiatric and substance use disorders?* This question is answered by the results of the VATSPSUD and our reviews of other studies.
2. *Can we clarify the nature of the associations between key environ-mental factors and the risk for psychopathology?* Are environmental factors causal or only correlational?
3. *Can we begin to understand how genetic and environmental factors together contribute to risk for psychiatric and substance use disor-ders?* Do they simply add together, or might they interweave in more complex ways?
4. *How do genes and environments combine over development to influ-ence risk for psychiatric and substance use disorders?*

In our effort to address these major questions of the book, we also con-sider several narrower but related questions:

1. To what degree are the genetic and environmental risk factors for psy-chiatric and substance use disorders specific or nonspecific in their effects?
2. How important are shared or family environmental factors—those environments that affect the members of a twin pair in the same way?

SIDEBAR I.1. Collaborators in the Development of the Virginia Adult Twin Study of Psychiatric and Substance Use Disorders

Lindon Eaves completed his PhD in genetics at the University of Birmingham in 1970 with a thesis titled "Aspects of Human Behavior Genetics." After having achieved the height of success in British academic life—a faculty position at Oxford—he left in 1981 to move to Virginia Commonwealth University. The major focus of Dr. Eaves's career has been to further develop and apply the corpus of biometrical genetics to the problems of human behavior and psychopathology. This is no small task because all of the standard methods used in animal and plant genetics, such as controlled breeding and strict environment exposure, are not feasible in humans. As Lindon once said: "It just means that if you want to study humans, you have to be that much smarter." In many ways, Lindon Eaves can be viewed as the intellectual godfather of the VATSPSUD.

Andrew Heath studied with Lindon Eaves at the University of Birmingham. His early career was spent on methodological developments in biometrical genetics as applied to human phenotypes. Subsequently, he has become a preeminent researcher of genetic influences on alcoholism and other substance use disorders. He contributed to the VATSPSUD during his several years at VCU and afterward as a close collaborator on later waves of the female–female twin study and early phases of the male–male/male–female study.

Ronald Kessler trained in sociology at New York University and quickly entered the field of psychiatric epidemiology. When one of us (K.S.K.) realized that we needed someone on the project with skills in this area, he began asking his colleagues whom they considered to be the "best and brightest" young researcher in psychiatric epidemiology. After two trusted colleagues both named Ron Kessler, Kendler made a "cold call" to Ron—then an associate professor in the Department of Sociology and associate research scientist at the Survey Research Center at the University of Michigan. They ended up talking for over an hour. Ron enthusiastically accepted the invitation to collaborate, and throughout the project, especially in its early years, he provided invaluable advice on a range of issues, including interview instruments, the assessment of environmental risk factors, and the statistical methods of data analysis. Ron has since gone on to become a leading international figure in the field of psychiatric epidemiology.

Michael Neale joined the VCU group in 1986 following his doctoral studies in biometrical genetics and psychology. Soon after arriving, he became a close collaborator. He has, over many years, made numerous important intellectual contributions to the VATSPSUD. His structural modeling software program, Mx, was written to aid researchers conducting twin and family studies. Many of the advanced analyses we describe in this book would not have been possible without Mike's conceptual and statistical expertise. On a number of key occasions in the history of this project, we came to Mike with critical substantive questions and were able to work out together how to translate our often vague ideas into elegant analytic models.

We have highlighted these individuals because of their important roles in the early stages of the VATSPSUD. But the thousands of interviews completed as part of the VATSPSUD could not have been collected without the efforts of many talented and dedicated colleagues and project staff. And of course we are particularly indebted to the twins, who have been so generous with their time and willing to share their life experiences.

3. It would be nice to assume that we can measure the history of psychiatric and substance use disorders without error, but we cannot. How does unreliability of measurement alter the interpretation of our results?

4. Do men and women have the same or different genetic and environmental risk factors for psychiatric and substance use disorders?

5. How can we progress from initial findings that a risk factor and a disorder are correlated with each other to the much more difficult and important problem of clarifying whether the relationship between them is a causal one?

6. There is a large gap between genes and the clinical symptoms of psychiatric and substance use disorders. Can we develop indices of genetic risk and/or identify the "intervening" or "mediating" variables that sit in the pathway from genes (or environmental risk factors) to the outcome of illness?

7. Some disorders are best understood as a series of stages. For example, it is not possible to abuse a substance until you have used it. Do genetic and environmental risk factors differ across these stages?

8. The major focus of our study is on twins, who are always in the same generation. However, by studying twins and their parents, we can begin to ask what etiological factors are involved in the transmission of risk of illness from parents to their children. In particular, do parents convey risk to their children only through the genes they pass on to them or also through the environments they provide for them?

STRUCTURE

In Part I, "Background," Chapters 1 and 2 describe the scientific and social context of the study and its methodology. Chapter 3 provides a brief and (we hope) reader-friendly introduction to the statistical and conceptual tools that we utilize in the rest of the book. We have attempted to avoid overwhelming the reader with complex statistical models, but some basic knowledge about the methods will be very helpful in understanding the rest of the book. Therefore, we urge readers not to skip this part.

In Part II, "Genetic Risk," we put on the hats of *psychiatric geneticists* and examine the results of standard twin models applied to the large array of psychiatric and substance use disorders that we studied. After reviewing these results, we address the validity of the key assumptions of the twin model. We examine the plausibility of our results and the extent to which they might be distorted by possible biases in our methods.

In Part III, "Environmental Risk," we change hats and view our results from the perspective of *psychiatric epidemiologists*. We examine the effects of both temporally distal environmental risk factors (such as parent–child relationships) and temporally proximal environmental risk factors (particularly stressful life events).

In Part IV, "A Closer Look at Genetic and Environmental Influences," we explore a range of issues, including sex differences and the causes of stability and change in psychopathology. In this section, we also examine evidence for the specific versus general effects of genes and environments on different forms of psychopathology.

In Part V, "Bringing It All Together," we conclude by exploring our central theme: how genes and environment interweave in producing risk. This includes what we call genetic control of exposure to the environment and gene–environment interplay. We then present an integrative model for major depression and end with a summary of our major conclusions.

We use a lot of abbreviations in this book. While this saves space and can make for quicker reading, it can also sow confusion if readers forget what the abbreviations mean. Therefore, we include a list of abbreviations at the front of the book (pp. xiii–xiv).

THE DEVELOPMENT OF THE VATSPSUD

In this section, we describe our own motivations for undertaking this work and pay homage to those who have influenced our thinking and choices.

Kenneth S. Kendler: I concluded medical school with what many viewed as two contradictory impulses. I wanted to be a psychiatrist, and I wanted to be a rigorous scientific researcher. Although I found my psychiatric training to be very stimulating and personally rewarding, it was intellectually confused and confusing. During the course of my residency, I received supervision from a family therapist who was convinced that psychiatric disorders could be understood as arising from disturbed patterns of family interactions, from a social psychiatrist who believed that poverty was the most important risk factor for most psychopathology, from psychoanalysts who were convinced that nearly all psychiatric illness could be traced to deep intrapsychic causes that had their roots in early childhood, and from a biological psychiatrist who was solely interested in neurochemical molecular aspects of brain activity. I felt more as if I were in a medieval university, faced with competing theological positions, rather than in a modern medical setting. Surely, I kept thinking, it must be possible to use the methods of natural science to evaluate the validity of these varying positions.

In the fall of 1983, 3 years after the conclusion of my psychiatric training and after a brief career in neurochemistry, I moved to the Medical College of Virginia of Virginia Commonwealth University (VCU) to continue formal training in genetics with Professor Lindon Eaves and shortly afterward spent 4 months studying biometrical genetics at the feet of the masters in Birmingham,

England. Upon my return to VCU, the research team was expanded by the arrival of two of Dr. Eaves's very talented former doctoral students, Andrew Heath and Nick Martin. With a great deal of help from Eaves and Heath, I spent much of the next year analyzing questionnaire data collected by Martin on a large number of twin pairs from the Australian twin registry. In good English tradition, tea breaks were taken twice daily and provided the opportunity for many stimulating conversations. The standing joke in our group was that I was there as the "token" American.

Sometime in early 1984, discussions among Drs. Eaves, Martin, Heath, and myself began about a new kind of psychiatric twin study. Later that year, we began working on a grant application to the U.S. National Institute of Mental Health, requesting funds for such a study. We decided the grant should focus on depression and anxiety disorders because these were the most common disorders in the general population and had not been previously studied in twins. Because we knew that such disorders were more common in females than in males, we decided to study only female–female pairs. Evidence from other survey researchers suggested that women would be more cooperative than men with such a study. Based on the degree of familial resemblance for these disorders observed in other studies, we calculated how many twin pairs we would need to study to estimate genetic and environmental influences. Our estimate was about 1,100 twin pairs, which seemed to us an impossibly large number.

One problem remained. None of the members of our research team had primary expertise in psychiatric epidemiology. Several colleagues suggested that we contact Ronald Kessler. He enthusiastically agreed and contributed his substantial knowledge about recruiting and assessing people in the community and measures of the environment to our project.

The first phase of VATSPSUD, our study of female–female twin pairs, began when funds were formally awarded in February 1986. During this time we had the great fortune to have Michael Neale join our group at VCU. The second phase of the study began in 1992, when we obtained funding to begin studying twins from male–male and male–female pairs. It was at this point that Carol Prescott joined the research team.

Carol A. Prescott: My early training was in experimental psychopathology, a field that tries to discover the processes underlying the development of psychiatric disorders. Under the guidance of my mentors, Milton Strauss (at Johns Hopkins University) and Irving Gottesman (at the University of Virginia), I conducted research to find attentional deficits and personality features that could serve as markers of familial vulnerability to schizophrenia. During my internship in clinical psychology, I became impressed with the pervasiveness of substance abuse and its influence on the etiology and treatment of other psychiatric disorders. In 1991 I moved to the Department of Human Genetics at VCU for a postdoctoral fellowship in biometrical genetics as applied to alcohol use and alcoholism. A year later I had the opportunity to join the Department of Psychiatry and to begin working on the VATSPSUD.

I joined the group with some trepidation, rather in awe of the reputation and intellect of Drs. Kendler, Eaves, and their colleagues. Although I had some quantitative background and experience in twin studies, I had trained primarily as a clinician. I wondered whether I could hold my own in an environment of matrix algebra and challenging argument. Looking back, I can say that the VCU group functioned as a true meritocracy—my (then!) youth, gender, and background were never held against me. My work on the VATSPSUD has been very stimulating and rewarding, and I feel very fortunate to have had this experience.

The rest of the story of the VATSPSUD—how we actually conducted the study—is described in Chapters 1, 2, and 3. The remainder of the book details what we have learned about the etiology of psychiatric and substance use disorders.

PART I

BACKGROUND

CHAPTER ONE

The Scientific and Social Context of the Virginia Adult Twin Study of Psychiatric and Substance Use Disorders

The study described in this book reflects the integration of developments in three research areas: biometrical genetics, psychiatric twin studies, and psychiatric epidemiology. We review these briefly and then describe how they were integrated into the Virginia Adult Twin Study of Psychiatric and Substance Use Disorders (VATSPSUD). This chapter concludes with some other introductory thoughts about our approach to the subject matter and substance of this book.

BIOMETRICAL GENETICS

In its early years, the field of human genetics included two distinct and sometimes antagonistic approaches to the study of genetic variation: biometrical genetics and Mendelian genetics. Biometrical genetics focused on quantitative traits—ones that could be measured, quantified, and then put on a scale. Examples of such traits include height, blood pressure, and extroversion. In contrast, Mendelian genetics was concerned with qualitative traits, traits one either has or does not have. Examples of such traits include the color of peas in Mendel's famous experiments, human blood group, and classical human genetic disorders such as cystic fibrosis and Huntington's disease.

When studying humans, biometrical geneticists began by examining correlations of quantitative traits in different classes of relatives, such as among siblings or between parents and offspring. Mendelian geneticists, by contrast, collected pedigrees and looked at specific patterns of transmission, such as dominant, recessive, or sex-linked. For the first 20 years of the 20th century, advocates of biometrical and Mendelian genetics fought vigorously over the validity of the two approaches. It was the brilliant statistician Ronald Fisher who showed, in his epic paper "On the Correlation between Relatives on the Supposition of Mendelian Inheritance" (Fisher, 1918), that these two approaches were compatible. The inheritance patterns of quantitative traits could be explained by assuming the existence of multiple genes, each of small effect, that combine in the manner expected given Mendelian inheritance.

From the seminal work of Fisher and the earlier leader of the biometrical school, Karl Pearson, a large body of increasingly elegant biometrical genetics developed over the next 40 years. Although important work was done in the United States, the two world centers of statistical genetics during this time were both in the United Kingdom: Edinburgh and Birmingham. These centers examined the genetics of organisms such as fruit flies, plants, and livestock, which could be subject to experimentation. Driven in part by the practical needs of animal and plant breeders, these groups developed sophisticated statistical models for the different ways in which genes influence phenotypes (physical and behavioral outcomes) and are affected by different environmental conditions (Falconer, 1989; Lynch & Walsh, 1998; Mather & Jinks, 1982).

PSYCHIATRIC TWIN STUDIES

The first known description of the use of twins to study human differences was by Augustine of Hippo (354–430; De civitate Dei, Bk. 5). He observed that the lives of a set of twins turn out differently, and he used this as a way to falsify the accepted belief that the alignment of the stars at the time of one's birth determined destiny. The more formal scientific use of twins to study the origins of individual differences in humans did not begin until the last quarter of the 19th century. The English polymath Francis Galton wrote a monograph, "Hereditary Genius," which is probably the first systematic behavioral genetics study in humans. Galton published an essay in 1875 in *Fraser's Magazine* with the propitious title "The History of Twins as a Criterion of the Relative Powers of Nature and Nurture" (Galton, 1875). He was interested in using twins to evaluate the power of environmental experiences to make pairs similar or different. He did not then understand that twins could be divided into two groups: identical (monozygotic, or MZ) and fraternal (dizygotic, or DZ). This was not finally clarified until the 1920s.

The twin method as we now understand it consists of comparing the levels of similarity of MZ and DZ twin pairs. This method was described in 1924 by the American psychologist Curtis Merriman (1924) and the German dermatologist Hermann Siemens (1924). It did not take long for those working on the problems of psychiatric disorders to apply this new methodology. Four years later, Hans Luxenberger (1928) published the first systematic twin study of a psychiatric disorder. The following 50 years saw the completion and publication of more than a dozen major twin studies of psychiatric illness.

In its infancy, psychiatric genetics—under the leadership of Ernst Rüdin (whose critical contributions to the birth of this field were colored by his dealings, later in his life, with the Nazi party in Germany)—was at the forefront of the methodological developments of the emerging field of human genetics (Zerbin-Rüdin & Kendler, 1996). From the mid-1930s until the 1970s, however, there was almost no contact between these two fields, and the methodological sophistication of psychiatric genetics suffered substantially.

With rare exceptions, these traditional twin studies of psychopathology shared seven methodological limitations. First, they examined only severe forms of psychiatric illness, usually schizophrenia or bipolar disorder. Second, the twins were identified (ascertained) directly through hospitals or through registries that collected their information from hospitals. This meant that, in order to be included in these studies, twins had to be sufficiently ill to have been hospitalized. Third, the psychiatric diagnoses of both members of a twin pair were assigned by the same individual, typically on the basis of some kind of personal interview and/or a review of medical records. Fourth, psychiatric diagnoses were assigned by clinicians without the use of explicit diagnostic criteria such as those listed in the *Diagnostic and Statistical Manual of Mental Disorders* (DSM) of the American Psychiatric Association. Fifth, little effort was made to measure environmental risk factors, although some studies examined variables such as birth order, social class, age when the twins separated, or parental loss. Sixth, with a few notable exceptions (e.g., Kallmann, 1946; Kendler & Robinette, 1983), sample sizes were small and rarely included more than 100 twin pairs. Seventh, the statistical analyses of these studies were limited, usually consisting solely of determining whether the level of similarity (assessed as twin concordance, the proportion of pairs in which both twins are affected) was greater in MZ than in DZ pairs. As we describe in detail in Chapter 2, in the VATSPSUD we attempted to address all of these limitations.

PSYCHIATRIC EPIDEMIOLOGY

The discipline of psychiatric epidemiology examines the distribution of psychopathology within populations and the risk factors that influence that distribution. Dohrenwend (1995) has proposed a useful framework for understanding the historical evolution of psychiatric epidemiology from its origins

at the beginning of the 20th century until today. The first generation of studies, conducted between 1900 and World War II, relied almost exclusively on
reports from key informants and agency records for case detection. Rates of
illness were low (averaging under 4% in these studies) and were particularly
likely to underestimate conditions that did not lead to treatment or to contact
with the criminal justice system.

Second-generation studies, conducted between World War II and about
1980, relied largely on direct interviews with participants. Two different
approaches to these assessments dominated during this period. In most European studies, a single psychiatrist or a small group of clinicians personally
interviewed community residents. The interviews were "free form" and
unstructured, mimicking the standard clinical assessment. On this basis, the
clinicians would record their global psychiatric diagnoses. The second approach used a systematic approach to data collection that relied on brief questionnaires. The goal of using these instruments was not to obtain psychiatric
diagnoses but to produce a scaled score that reflected broad concepts such as
"mental illness," "emotional adjustment," or "symptoms of stress."

The third generation of psychiatric epidemiological studies began in the
early 1980s with the development of structured and semistructured psychiatric interviews that were closely linked to systems of "operationalized" diagnostic criteria. These interviews share two major characteristics. First, each
consists of a script of questions asked in a systematic order. Second, there are
formal algorithms for combining items to determine whether or not a respondent meets criteria for a range of psychiatric diagnoses. The United States has
seen two major third-generation studies of psychiatric epidemiology: the
Epidemiologic Catchment Area Study, which interviewed more than 19,000
individuals at five study sites during the late 1970s (Robins & Regier, 1991)
and the National Comorbidity Survey (Kessler et al., 1994), which studied
more than 8,000 individuals from a national probability sample in the 1990s.

In addition to improving the assessment of psychiatric illness, during the
past 20 years clinical and epidemiological researchers in psychiatry have made
important advances in the assessment of putative risk factors. Well-studied
and validated instruments have been developed for use with general population samples to assess key variables such as stressful life events, social support,
parent–child relationships, and childhood sexual abuse.

The use of structured interviews represented a substantial improvement
over previous methods of assessment. However, this approach is not without
its difficulties. Two are worth noting here (and others are described later in
the book). First, the diagnostic criteria are largely based on the experience of
clinicians working with patients in treatment settings; however, it remains to
be established that the patterns of symptoms seen in individuals in treatment
are the same as those for untreated individuals in the population. We know
that severity of illness tends to be milder in community than in clinical cases,
and there may be other important differences. A second limitation is that,
although the reliability of structured assessments exceeds that of the unstruc-

tured interviews performed in earlier studies, their reliability is far from perfect. This is a particularly critical issue in genetic studies because unreliability of measurement imposes an upper limit on the estimated impact of genetic and environmental factors.

A NEW PARADIGM FOR TWIN STUDIES

Sometime in early 1984, a new paradigm for psychiatric twin studies began to emerge out of discussions among Kendler, Eaves, Martin, and Heath (see the Introduction). These discussions led eventually to the development of the VATSPSUD. The new paradigm drew on the traditions of biometrical genetics, psychiatric twin studies, and psychiatric epidemiology, merging the strengths and attempting to address the limitations of each. We decided that our study would have six key features.

1. It would be population based. Instead of selecting twins through treatment facilities (with all the expected biases such as selection for severity and comorbidity), we wanted to study a representative sample of twins from the general population.

2. Our conceptual and analytic approach would be based on the rigorous methods of biometrical genetics. Our goal was to test explicit hypotheses about the role of genetic and environmental risk factors in the etiology of psychiatric and substance use disorders and to obtain statistical estimates of their importance.

3. We wanted to collect a sample large enough to obtain these estimates. Most prior twin studies of psychiatric illness had too few participants to resolve the question of whether familial resemblance was due to genetic or shared environmental influences. Although large twin studies had been conducted of psychological traits and symptoms of depression and anxiety using mailed questionnaires (Eaves et al., 1989; Jardine, Martin, & Henderson, 1984), this would be the first large-scale interview-based twin study of psychiatric illness.

4. Because such large numbers of twins would have to be assessed, we needed to borrow the methods that had been developed in psychiatric epidemiology to assess accurately the history of psychiatric illness in large numbers of individuals. The old model for twin studies—in which a single clinician spends a year or two driving around the countryside conducting interviews—was no longer feasible.

5. We wanted to take the environment seriously. It has sometimes been said that for a "real" geneticist, environment is just something that gets in the way of gene expression. That was not our view. We did not want to prejudge the outcome of our results, and so we decided to spend at least as much of our assessment evaluating environmental risk factors as we did in the assessment of psychiatric and substance use disorders.

6. The study would be longitudinal. By interviewing participants more than once, it becomes much easier to move from correlational observations (in which A and B tend to occur together) to more causal conclusions (A truly increases the risk for B). As is seen later in this book, multiple waves of measurement allowed us to address interesting questions that would not have been possible if the twins had been interviewed only once.

GENES

At this point we need to say a bit about "genes." Few concepts in biology have been so long debated (Carlson, 1966; Kendler, 2005a). The gene can be seen from a number of perspectives, particularly as the primary unit of evolution, a specific span of DNA, the source of information required for the production of a particular biological molecule, or a latent (or unobserved) entity that contributes to risk of illness. In this era of the sequencing of the human genome, the double helix has achieved the status of a cultural icon (Nelkin & Lindee, 1995).

The results reported in this book are not based on directly measuring individual genes, as might be done with the now powerful methods of human molecular genetics. Instead, by using information we obtain from twins (the details of which are described in Chapter 3), we indirectly assess or *infer* the impact of all of an individual's genes on the risk for a particular trait or disorder.

Why in the era of the human genome project would we pursue such an approach? Why did we not just measure everyone's genes and directly study the effects of each gene? Despite major advances in the science of human genetics, we are not even close to having the capacity to do anything like this. Indeed, only in the past few years have researchers begun to identify, in a way that can be replicated across laboratories, individual genes that influence the risk for psychiatric or substance use disorders. The human genome is extraordinarily complex, with some 20,000–25,000 different genes. Many of these genes are expressed in a variety of different forms in different tissues and at different times. The genome contains a wide range of new kinds of genetic elements (such as short-inhibitory RNA) that influence gene expression and function in ways we only dimly understand. Multiple control regions exist for many genes, often separated from the gene itself by very large distances. In addition to the problem of understanding the intricate biological aspects of genome function, understanding the conceptual and statistical issues surrounding the actions and interactions of these large numbers of genes and their effects on human behavior and disease is also an extraordinarily daunting task that currently lies far beyond our power.

It may be possible years in the future to measure directly all the genes in the human genome and, more important, to know what is being measured and how to analyze it. But we are not there yet, nor are we even close. At the end of this book, we return to the question of the relationship between twin studies and molecular genetics and show that these two scientific traditions are ultimately mutually complementary.

What, then, does it mean to "infer" the action of genes from twins? Can that be a very scientific way of doing things? Doesn't science always require that we measure things directly?

In fact, many scientific theories inferred the action of forces that could not be directly measured at the time the theory was developed. When Newton proposed his theory of gravitation, he inferred the action of this force from features of planetary motion. When the electron was first discovered by Thompson, it was not directly observed. Rather, its mass and electric charge were inferred from its behavior in a cathode ray tube. The initial theories about tectonic plates were proposed long before we had any idea of how the earth's crust could "float" over the earth's surface. So the method used in this book—to assess an underlying process indirectly though patterns of results seen in nature—has a long and distinguished history.

THE SOCIAL AND POLITICAL CONTEXT OF THE VATSPSUD

The question of the role of genetic factors in human behavior raises complex emotional, social, and political issues. Although we wish it were otherwise, medical genetic research has sometimes been applied to support particular political agendas and misused to justify the denial of human rights. This troubled history sometimes affects attitudes toward modern psychiatric genetics research and researchers. We address three related issues here.

First, we saw our task in the design and implementation of the VATSPSUD to be that of "basic scientists" trying to understand how the world works. We did not begin this study with a strong agenda to demonstrate that psychiatric and substance use disorders are strongly influenced by genetic factors. Similarly, we did not begin with a strong bias for or against specific environmental theories about the origins of these disorders. Our goal was to conduct the best study we could, incorporating as many of the risk factors we could and letting the data "speak for themselves." We are not naive in assuming that we have not shaped the results with our hypotheses. However, we have tried earnestly to be ecumenical in our approach.

Second, we do not agree with many of the biases that exist about genes in the popular imagination. Genes are not destiny. It is a stunningly common misconception that genetic influence on a trait implies that the trait is inflexible and incapable of modification, whereas a role for environmental risk factors means great flexibility and ease of modification. This idea is just plain wrong. Many traits that genes influence can be easily modified. The effects of the single-gene disorder of phenylketonuria can be effectively reversed by a simple modification of diet. Millions of people in the United States are taking cholesterol-lowering drugs that are quite effective at reducing their genetically influenced levels of cholesterol. Depression, although genetically influenced, can be effectively treated by both pharmacological and psychotherapeutic means. In contrast, many environmental effects are relatively irreversible. Severe social deprivation, head trauma, serious malnutrition, and severe physical or sexual abuse can produce long-lasting and sometimes irreversible changes in an individual's emotional and cognitive functioning. There is no close relationship between the degree to which a trait is influenced by genetic and environmental factors and the malleability of that trait.

Third, an even more sinister misconception held by some individuals is that researchers interested in genetic sources of individual differences in humans have dark, reactionary, and/or eugenic motives at heart. Genetic theories of human individual differences have been badly misused in the past. However, to tar an entire scientific field for the past misdeeds of racist or eugenic zealots is irrational. Were this logic to be applied widely in science, it would result in the cessation of many areas of research, to the detriment of mankind. We are both clinicians who have observed firsthand the suffering that psychiatric and substance use disorders inflict on our patients, friends, and family and those close to the sufferers. Our motive for conducting this effortful work over many years has been to use the best science we could to understand the etiology of psychiatric and substance use disorders so as to enable better prevention and treatment. There is no deeper political agenda at work here.

OUR PHILOSOPHY OF SCIENCE

A few words are also in order about the approach we have taken toward the science you will be reading about in this book. First, we believe there is an objective truth to be learned about the causes of human psychiatric and substance use disorders. We recognize that human beings are the most complex organisms we know about and that many factors make it difficult to obtain definitive results in human research. However, by conducting careful and thoughtful scientific research, we believe we can begin to untangle this complexity and contribute to the amelioration of these debilitating conditions.

Second, the VATSPSUD is an example of observational and not experimental science. That is, in important ways our study bears more resemblance to other observational sciences such as geology and astronomy than it does to laboratory genetics. In laboratory studies, for example with rodents or fruit flies, the scientist can have complete control over both the genetic composition and the environment of individual organisms. By contrast, in observational sciences, all the scientist can do is observe and interpret the world as presented to him or her. In our study, neither genetic nor environmental risk factors were in any way under our control. All we could hope to do was to record carefully the relevant observations and attempt, through thoughtful interpretation, to uncover etiological principles. Because we cannot do experiments, we can never be completely sure that we have ruled out the impact of hidden biases on our findings. We have tried to address the biases we are aware of, but our results are still vulnerable to those biases we do not know about.

Third, because of the nonexperimental nature of our area of research, it is important to recognize that *there is no such thing as a definitive study*. No study in human behavioral and psychiatric genetics, including this one, is without significant flaws or limitations.

Fourth, we are firm believers in an approach to scientific inquiry that has been called *inference to the best explanation* (Okasha, 2002). Scientists begin with the desire to test a particular hypothesis. They then attempt to collect as much information relevant to this question as possible, both in their own studies and in studies of others reported in the literature. Taking all these data, a scientist poses the following question: *Can this entire set of data be best explained by my hypothesis, or are there hypotheses that would better explain these observations?* Darwin's wonderful and epoch-making book *The Origin of Species* (1859) can be best understood as one long application of *inference to the best explanation* to arrive at the claim that natural selection provides the best available explanation for a wide variety of patterns observed in nature. This model, which suggests that science is a continuing, integrative, and cumulative process of refining explanatory models, is particularly appropriate for the subject matter of this book. It helps us emphasize that our goal is to provide the best possible explanation given current knowledge. We are not claiming to be in full possession of the truth.

One final comment is in order. In the writing of this book, we faced a dilemma. On the one hand, it is important to set the results of our research in the context of other relevant investigations in the fields of psychiatry and substance abuse. On the other hand, this book deals with such a wide set of disorders and research questions that to do careful literature reviews in each relevant area would require us to write a textbook of psychiatric epidemiology and genetics with thousands of references and long, dry chapters. A compromise was needed. We have provided brief reviews of the relevant literature, often citing a few representative studies or a good review article. Readers who are interested in more details may consult the works cited or the original journal articles in which much of this work has appeared. The reason for the brevity of our references to other literature is not that we are unaware of the valuable contributions of our colleagues. Instead, it is that we value the clarity of the presentation that we provide to you, our reader.

CHAPTER TWO

Methodology Used in the VATSPSUD

In this chapter we describe the methods used to identify and recruit study participants, select measures, and conduct our assessments. We also summarize the evidence for the validity of our measures and procedures.

ORGANIZATION AND TERMINOLOGY

The VATSPSUD consists of two parallel studies. The first is of women from female–female twin pairs and their parents. We refer to the twin portion as the FF study and the parent portion as the FFP study. The second study is of men and women from male–male and male–female twin pairs. We refer to this as the MM/MF study.

A few comments about terminology are in order. We use the terms *disorder*, *syndrome,* or *psychopathology* rather than *disease* to refer to clinical diagnoses. The term *disease* implies that the condition has a well-understood etiology, and this is not the case for the conditions we study.

We use the terms *twin* and *respondent* to refer to the member of the twin pair responding to a question. *Cotwin* refers to the respondent's twin. About 1% of the participants in our study are members of triplet and quadruplet births. We do not want to slight these individuals, who had to be particularly patient during the interviews because they were asked the cotwin questions multiple times. However, for simplicity, we use the terms *twins* and *pairs* to refer to all participants, including those from multiple sibships.

It is also worth considering what terms to use to describe differences between males and females. For the most part, our study is not able to distinguish whether the differences we find between men and women are due to biology or culture. Because some of the differences appear to be based on biological sex, we consider it inaccurate to refer to these as gender differences. We therefore opted to use the terms *sex* and *sex differences* to encompass both chromosomally defined sex (i.e., XX or XY) and culturally defined gender. In referring to study participants, we alternate between use of male and female pronouns. We are aware of the degree to which women have been slighted in biomedical research and are pleased that the VATSPSUD has helped to remedy this situation in the field of psychiatric genetics. Our clinical vignettes more often feature women than men, not because we consider women to be more pathological but because more of our research has derived from the FF sample.

SAMPLES

We describe the samples as they existed at the time of this writing (in late 2005). The analyses reported in the remainder of the book include descriptions of the results from previously published papers, as well as new analyses conducted for the book. Careful readers may note small discrepancies between sample sizes as reported in this book and in our papers. These differences reflect the changing nature of the databases. As anyone who has conducted large-scale field work can tell you, there is never a final data set. No matter how carefully we check the data prior to data entry, inconsistencies will be found at the analysis stage, requiring further data cleaning or dropping some participants from analyses. Even determining the numbers of participants can be difficult. Early published analyses include a handful of individuals who are no longer included because we subsequently found that they did not meet our inclusion criteria (e.g., they were not born in Virginia or they were born outside our birth cohort) or because twins no longer wished to participate and requested removal of their interviews from the database. Accumulation of more information, including DNA samples, has led us to change zygosity assignments of a handful of twin pairs.

In planning this book, we considered running all of our analyses again on a standard data set with our "final" sample. Ultimately we decided against this because we consider it extremely unlikely that any meaningful differences in results would be obtained. When you have sample sizes of thousands of twins, inclusion or exclusion of a handful of individuals makes no practical difference.

Selection and Recruitment

The twins in our study were identified through the Virginia Twin Registry (VTR). The registry was begun in 1980 by Walter Nance and Linda Corey, professors in the Department of Human Genetics at Virginia Commonwealth University. Multiple births were identified from birth records compiled by the Virginia Department of Health Statistics, which maintains a database containing the birth date, sex, race, and parent names of all individuals born in the Commonwealth of Virginia. Initially this work was done by hand (a research assistant went through all the birth certificates since 1918), but more recently VTR records have been updated by computer files.[1]

Contact information for the twins (or in the case of juvenile twins, their parents) is obtained by matching names and birth dates to state records, such as those of the Department of Motor Vehicles. This is quite successful for identifying individuals who have remained in Virginia and obtained driver's licenses, but less so for identifying individuals who have left the state or have changed their names (e.g., after marriage).

One limitation of our study is the absence of twins from ethnic minority backgrounds. At the time we were designing the first study, previous questionnaire studies with VTR participants had obtained much lower participation rates among nonwhite twins. Because only about 20% of native-born Virginians in this age range are nonwhite, we estimated that we would be able to interview fewer than 100 twin pairs—far too few to provide reliable estimates of heritability. On this basis, we judged that we could not expect to have adequate sample sizes of ethnic minority twins to enable us to analyze them as a separate group. For this reason, only pairs classified on birth certificates as white were eligible for study inclusion. We now regret the decision and look forward to the completion of several more representative twin studies now underway in the United States.

The Female–Female Twin Study

As we described in the Introduction, for scientific and practical reasons, the VATSPSUD began with female–female (FF) twin pairs. The design of the FF studies is summarized in Figure 2.1. We first targeted pairs who were born between 1934 and 1970. The registry identified 1,176 FF pairs in whom both had returned at least one questionnaire in the past several years, and these formed the wave 1 sample (FF1).

Of these 2,352 women, 2,164 (92.0%) were interviewed in FF1, including both members of 1,033 pairs. The complete pairs include 590 MZ pairs, 440 DZ pairs, and 3 pairs whose zygosity could not be determined. Of those twins who did not participate, 156 refused, 23 were lost to follow-up, and 9 did not refuse outright but could not be scheduled during the study time frame. Wave 1 interviews were conducted from January 1987 through July

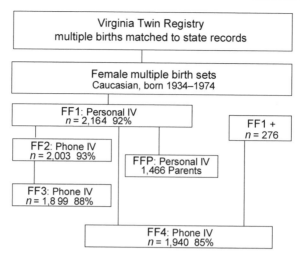

FIGURE 2.1. Design of the VATSPSUD female–female (FF) study. IV = interview; FF1–FF4 = waves 1–4 of FF twin study; FFP = FF parent study.

1989. The FF1 study also included several self-report measures. These are available for about 95% of participants.

After the FF1 sample was "complete," we continued to enroll women and to administer the FF1 interview through July 1994. Individuals who had been eligible for FF1 but had refused or had not been located were contacted again and asked to participate; 34 of these 188 were interviewed. Another 339 twins born from 1970 to 1974 were contacted for the study as they turned 18, and of these, 242 were interviewed. We refer to the 276 individuals in these two groups as FF1+. Combining FF1 and FF1+, 2,440 women were interviewed out of 2,691 eligible, representing 90.7% of all those we attempted to interview using the wave 1 protocol. (Cooperation rates were somewhat lower for the FF1+ group because it was an unfunded component of the study and we spent less effort attempting to recruit those who were initially uninterested). The FF1+ interviews were conducted simultaneously with collection of the second and third interview waves. Therefore, FF1+ participants were not studied again until the fourth interview, and their parents were not included in the parent study.

Our wave 2 (FF2) interviews began in March 1989 and were completed in July 1991. Twins were eligible to participate if they were part of the original FF1 sample (i.e., not in FF1+). Of these 2,164 women, 2,003 (92.6%) completed the wave 2 interview, including both members of 938 pairs. Of those who did not participate, 127 refused, 33 were lost to follow-up, and 1 was too ill to participate. The average interval between waves 1 and 2 was 17.3 months (SD = 3.8, range = 12–49).

The wave 3 interview (FF3) was begun in November 1992 and completed in April 1995. Twins were eligible to participate if they were included in FF1 (even if they did not complete FF2). Of the 2,164 eligible women, 1,899 (87.8%) were interviewed, including 854 complete pairs. Of those who did not participate, 222 refused, 5 were lost to follow-up, 10 were deceased, 4 were too ill to participate, and 24 did not refuse outright but could not be scheduled during the study time frame. Among women participating in the FF2 and FF3 studies, the average interval between these two interviews was 45.0 months (SD = 4.0, range = 30–53).

Wave 4 (FF4) began in June 1995 and was completed in April 1997. Twins were eligible to participate if they were part of the FF1 or FF1+ samples and had not died (n = 9) or refused further contact (n = 136) as of their last interview. Of the 2,295 eligible women, 1,940 (84.5%) were interviewed, including 827 complete pairs. Of those who did not participate, 253 refused, 31 were lost to follow-up, 3 were deceased, 1 was too ill to participate, 2 did not complete the interview, and 65 did not refuse but could not be scheduled during the study time frame. Among the original FF1 participants, the average interval between FF3 and FF4 was 31.5 months (SD = 6.8, range = 13–49). Among those participating in the FF1+ and FF4 studies, the average interval between these interviews was 36.1 months (SD = 8.8, range = 17–58).

For both the FF and MM/MF studies, waves were timed so that at least 1 year had elapsed between interviews. This was done so that "past year" events and symptoms from one interview would not overlap with those assessed at the next interview. Interview events were timed by the month of occurrence. In practice, the length of the "past year" and the minimum interval between interviews depended on the day in the month an interview occurred. For example, a twin who was interviewed in August 1989 would report about events occurring from August 1, 1988, until the day of the interview. She would be eligible for her next interview beginning in September 1990.

Details of the variables used in our analyses are presented in the context of the chapters describing our results. We present here some demographic information. At the time participants completed the FF1 (or FF1+) interview, they ranged in age from 18 to 54, with a mean of 29.3 years (SD = 7.7). Years of formal education ranged from 4 years to doctoral degrees (coded as 20 years), with a mean of 13.5 (SD = 2.1). Median annual income was in the $12,000–15,000 range for personal earnings and $35,000–40,000 range for household income. As of our last contact, about 67% of the sample were married, 5% were living with a partner, 10% were separated or divorced, < 1% were widowed, and 17% were single. The majority of the sample described their religious affiliation as Protestant (83%), with the remainder Roman Catholic (9%), Jewish (1%), other (5%), and none or no preference (2%). The majority of respondents were currently employed (82%). Among the remainder, 2% were looking for work, < 1% were retired, 1% were disabled, 13% were keeping house, and 2% were students. Occupational status was rated by interviewers using our adaptation of the 7-point Hollingshead scale

(Hollingshead, 1957). Among those who were currently working or had ever worked, 27% of participants fell in the upper two levels (professional and upper management), 21% were in level 3 (middle management, small business), 35% in level 4 (clerical), 3% in level 5 (skilled labor, small farms), and the remaining 14% in levels 6 and 7 (semiskilled and unskilled labor).

The Female–Female–Parent Study

As part of our original grant from the National Institute of Mental Health, we obtained funding to interview the biological parents of the FF sample. We attempted to interview all living parents of complete pairs from the original FF1 sample (i.e., 1,030 pairs with known zygosity), regardless of their role in rearing the twins. We identified 1,698 living parents and were able to interview 86.7%, including 855 mothers and 617 fathers. The rest refused to be interviewed or were too ill to participate. The sample includes 567 families in which both parents were interviewed.

The Male–Male/Male–Female Twin Study

The basis for entry into the MM/MF study differed somewhat from that for the FF study. We recognized that requiring FF pairs to be known to the VTR and to have returned questionnaires may have led to a sample selected for cooperativeness. For the MM/MF study, we therefore attempted to enroll eligible twin pairs even if they had not previously participated in research. This meant that we were starting with a sample that was more difficult to locate and might be less cooperative than the FF sample. Therefore, instead of relying on mailed questionnaires as our first contact, we chose to conduct a telephone interview. The design of the MM/MF study is summarized in Figure 2.2.

In 1992 we obtained from the VTR names and (last known) addresses of 9,415 individuals from white MM and MF pairs born from 1940 to 1974. We selected this age range to be comparable with the FF study.[2] Because at least one member of each pair had to be successfully "matched" to state records to obtain contact information, we were unlikely to include pairs of which both twins had left the state prior to obtaining driver's licenses.

The wave 1 interview (MF1) was conducted between March 1993 and October 1996 and complete interviews were obtained from 6,812 individuals (5,092 men and 1,720 women). Of those who did not participate, 1,163 refused, 862 could not be located, 127 were deceased, 31 were too ill to participate, and 388 did not refuse outright but could not be scheduled during the study time frame. There were also 32 individuals who completed part of an interview but ceased the interview prior to the psychopathology sections, so that their interviews are considered incomplete. This represents a 72.3% completion rate among those who were eligible (i.e., excluding twins deceased prior to the study).

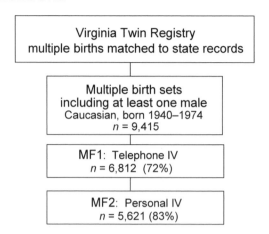

FIGURE 2.2. Design of the VATSPSUD male–male/male–female (MM/MF) study. IV = interview; MF1–MF2 = waves 1–2 of MM/MF twin study.

Individuals were eligible for the wave 2 interview (MF2) if they had completed wave 1. As with the FF study, interview waves of the MM/MF study were conducted at least 12 months after the prior interview. Wave 2 was conducted between April 1994 and October 1998. Complete interviews were obtained for 5,621 individuals, 82.5% of those who had completed MF1. Of those who did not participate, 851 refused, 51 were lost to follow-up, 24 were then deceased, 2 were too ill to participate, and 263 did not refuse outright but could not be scheduled during the study time frame. Among individuals completing both interviews, the interval between waves 1 and 2 ranged from 12 to 66 months, with a median of 15.3 and an average of 19.0 (SD = 8.7).

As of this writing, we have recently completed a third wave of data collection with twins from MM pairs. The goal of this study is to understand influences on substance use initiation and lifetime patterns of substance use. Analysis of the data from this study is now underway.

At the time they completed the MF1 interview, participants ranged in age from 19 to 57, with a mean age of 35.1 years (SD = 9.1). Years of formal education ranged from 1 year to doctoral degrees (coded as 20 years), with a mean of 13.4 (SD = 2.6). About 59% of the sample were married, 13% were separated or divorced, < 1% were widowed, and 28% were single. Of those not married at the time of interview, 20% were living with a partner.

Religious affiliation, employment, occupational status, and income were assessed as part of the MF2 interview. Religious affiliation was predominantly Protestant (75%), with the remainder divided among Roman Catholic (8%), Jewish (1%), other (2%), and no preference (14%). The majority of respondents were currently employed (88%). Among the remainder, 3% were looking for work, < 1% were retired, 3% were disabled, 4% were keeping house, and 2% were students. Employment varied by sex: 91% of males were currently employed and less than 1% of the remainder described themselves as keeping house, whereas the values for women were 78% and 15%, respectively. The median annual household income level was approximately $45,000 for both men and women. Median income from personal earnings was $18,000 for women and $30,000 for men. There was a good spread of occupational status: 22% of participants fell in the upper two levels (professional and upper management), 19% were in level 3 (middle management, small business), 21% in level 4 (clerical), 19% in level 5 (skilled labor, small farms), and the remaining 19% in levels 6 and 7 (semiskilled and unskilled labor).

Representativeness of Our Samples

Virginia is a diverse state, geographically and culturally. It ranges from the Washington, DC, suburbs of northern Virginia to the shipbuilding military hub of the Tidewater area in the southeast to the horse and tobacco farms of the central region to the coal-mining mountainous areas of the far west. The economic and educational characteristics of Virginia are near the national median, suggesting that the results from our study can be generalized to individuals from other regions.

As discussed earlier, one limitation of our sample is that it is restricted to individuals whose birth records identified them as white. We were interested to see whether we could identify other characteristics that were associated with study participation (or refusal) and that might give clues as to the representativeness of the study.

We selected a long list of demographic variables, including sex, age, educational level, occupation, religious affiliation, employment and marital status, and parenting status (defined as having children in the home or not), as well as some indicators of psychopathology, including ever having had a depressive period lasting at least 2 weeks, a period of drinking too much, and use of illicit substances. We then studied whether any of these variables were associated with study refusal or dropping out of later waves of the study.

As is found in most studies of twins, identical twins were somewhat more willing than fraternal twins to agree to participate in the study and to continue their participation in subsequent interview waves. Although we do not know for sure why this is the case, identical twins seem to be more invested in their identity as twins, and this may lead them to be more interested in involvement in twin research. Probably for similar reasons, DZ twins from same-sex pairs were more likely to agree than were those from opposite-sex pairs.

In addition to zygosity, the following variables predicted participation in subsequent interview waves: being female, higher educational level, older age, Protestant religious affiliation, and an absence of drinking problems. These findings are similar to those observed in other longitudinal studies. Overall, the magnitude of the effects was small. The largest effect was that the average educational level of participants in the FF studies increased by about one-half year between the FF1 and FF4 studies (from 13.5 to 14.2 years).

ASSESSMENT

In this section we describe the basis for our decisions on what constructs to assess. We finish the section by describing the selection and training of our interviewers and handling of the data.

Overview

A number of factors guided our selection of measures. These included: the overall goal of the particular wave of study, the need to balance breadth of coverage of many topics with adequate measurement, the use of the same measures that were used in prior waves, and the desire not to overburden the study participants. We often selected abbreviated versions of measures (or constructed short forms ourselves). The wording of some measures was adapted to fit an interview format (i.e., rather than a self-report question-naire). The major source for our measures of psychopathology and substance abuse/dependence was the Structured Clinical Interview for DSM-III-R, devel-oped by Robert Spitzer and colleagues at Columbia University (Spitzer, Williams, & Gibbon, 1987). As the study went on, we adapted a number of the sections to assess the revised criteria (DSM-IV), as well as the original ver-sion.[3] The constructs assessed across the entire study are summarized in Sidebar 2.1. Details and references to particular measures are provided in the chapters that follow.

The focus of each wave differed by study. FF1, FF2, and FFP interviews were funded by the National Institute of Mental Health and focused on occur-rence of and risk factors for major depression and anxiety disorders, although they also included eating disorders and alcoholism. FF3 was funded by a pri-vate donor (Rachel Brown Banks). It also assessed depression and anxiety but had a greater focus on smoking. FF4 was funded jointly by the National Insti-tute on Alcohol Abuse and Alcoholism and the National Institute on Drug Abuse and included a detailed assessment of alcohol and illicit drug use, abuse, and dependence.

FF1 and FFP were designed as in-person (face-to-face) interviews. This was done to establish greater rapport and because we believed assessment of some of the older parents might be difficult by telephone. About 10% of these interviews were conducted by telephone, primarily because the respondents were living outside Virginia. The remaining interviews (FF2, FF3, and FF4) were designed as telephone interviews, but about 5% of these were conducted in person. This occurred when respondents resided in an institutional setting (long-term nursing care, jail, or prison), when they had hearing impairments,

SIDEBAR 2.1. Content of the Twin Interviews

Demographics: age, marital status, household composition, children, education, occupational status, employment, income, religious affiliation

Twin variables: physical similarity, contact frequency (as children, adolescents, and adults), relationship quality

Childhood risk factors: loss of parent, neglect, physical abuse, sexual abuse[a]

Recent risk and protective factors: past-year stressful life events, social support, marital quality, role satisfaction

Psychological factors: personality traits, coping styles, optimism, altruism

Psychopathology: major depression, generalized anxiety, panic disorder, phobias, anorexia nervosa,[a] bulimia,[a] conduct disorder, antisocial personality, treatment history

Substances: use, abuse, and dependence on caffeine,[b] tobacco, alcohol, and illicit drugs (cannabis, sedatives, stimulants, cocaine, opiates, hallucinogens, and inhalants), parental attitudes toward alcohol use, alcohol expectancies

Family psychopathology:[c] major depression, generalized anxiety, smoking,[d] alcoholism

Interviewer ratings: respondent cooperativeness, interview quality, household characteristics

[a]Females only; [b]MM/MF study participants only; [c]asked about biological parents and cotwin; [d]cotwin only.

and when they expressed a preference for face-to-face interviews. Our use of phone interviews was largely the result of budgetary concerns. They were, on average, considerably less expensive than face-to-face interviews.

The content of the MM/MF interviews was parallel to that of the FF study. The information collected in MF1 was a combination of that collected in the questionnaires prior to FF1 and in the FF1 interview (excluding assessment of lifetime anxiety). As mentioned previously, our first contact with the MM/MF sample was by telephone. We decided that our detailed assessment of alcohol and drug use would be more acceptable during a second contact with the twins and better conducted as an in-person interview. Thus our MF2 interview is a combination of material from the FF2, FF3, and FF4 interviews but with less emphasis on eating disorders and childhood sexual abuse than in the FF interviews. About 20% of the MF2 interviews were conducted by telephone, usually because the respondents were living outside Virginia. A larger proportion of interviews in MF2 were done by telephone than for FF1 because the MM/MF sample included more individuals who had moved out of state; more males were in the military and stationed elsewhere temporarily; and more males wanted to be interviewed by telephone than in person. (Some stated that this was more private than being interviewed at home in proximity to their wives and children.)

Because of advice given to us by Ron Kessler early in the planning of the project, all of our interviews tried to establish an expectation of our twins that they would engage in what has been called "effortful responding." Prior survey research has shown that respondents react to the cues given by interviewers. If an interviewer seems to be in a hurry to get done and is impatient when the respondent stops to ponder a question, the respondent will tend to give short answers and not work hard to remember accurately. If, by contrast, the interviewer goes slowly and asks the respondent to think hard about the questions, he or she will typically try harder to provide accurate information.

For example, in each interview, we included a section that inquired about psychiatric and substance use problems during the respondent's entire life. After introducing the material to be covered in that section and explaining how it related to earlier parts of the interview, we always began by having the interviewer read the following statement to the twin:

> "Since these questions cover a long time period, please take your time to think back over your entire life before answering. Accurate responses are *very* important for this study."

Several interviews included self-report components. Material was formatted as self-report when it was believed, based on prior literature, that the information obtained would be more valid or reliable if not reported to an interviewer. This pertained to topics that were socially stigmatizing (childhood sexual abuse, conduct disorder, and antisocial personality symptoms) and items with response formats or reading levels that made them easier to administer in questionnaire form (e.g., personality scales, drinking motivations).

Assessment of Zygosity

Classification of same-sex pairs as identical (monozygotic, or MZ) and fraternal (dizygotic, or DZ) was conducted using a combination of questionnaire responses, photographs, and DNA testing. For female pairs, zygosity was initially determined on the basis of blind review by two experienced twin researchers using photographs in combination with standard questions about height, weight, physical similarity, and the frequency with which the twins had been mistaken for each other as children (Eaves et al., 1989). Blood samples were obtained from both members of 119 pairs of uncertain zygosity and analyzed using DNA markers (Spence et al., 1988).

By the mid-1990s DNA testing was easily conducted using samples of cheek cells (rather than blood samples, which are much more costly to collect and process). As part of the FF4 and MF2 studies, we collected DNA from all twins willing to contribute samples. Using these samples, we validated our earlier FF zygosity classifications by DNA testing from an additional 269 twin pairs, oversampling those for whom our prior zygosity assignment was questionable. On the basis of these tests, zygosity was changed for 12 pairs (4.5% of those tested), suggesting a correct original classification rate of at least 95% for the entire sample. Zygosity of MM pairs was initially determined by the algorithm developed on the FF sample and refined based on genotyping information from 227 MM pairs.

We interviewed as many members of triplet and quadruplet sets as were willing. Assignment of zygosity was done for each possible pair (i.e., three possible pairs for triplets, six possible pairs for quadruplets). It turned out to be a challenge to include all of the information from these individuals. In some analyses we handled this by including all possible pairings (i.e., some individuals contributed to more than one pair). In other cases, we randomly selected one pair per family and dropped others from the analyses.

Assessment Procedures

Although our interviews use a structured format, they still require clinical judgment and understanding. We required that our interviewers have an undergraduate degree in some form of behavioral science (usually psychology, social work, or psychiatric nursing), as well as a master's degree in a clinical area or 2 years of clinical experience.

Training for in-person interviews consisted of 2 full weeks of classroom training plus home practice sessions. Telephone interview training included a week of classroom training plus home practice. Whenever participants were willing, we audiotaped the interviews and used the tapes to monitor the interviewers' performance and adherence to the specified format. Each interview was reviewed for quality and consistency by two senior staff members prior to data entry. Some specialized ratings of life events (see Sidebar 8.4) were made by senior interviewers and editors based on audiotapes and reviews of interviewer notes.

For the FF1–FF2 interviews, Kendler reviewed each interview book and made a clinical diagnosis based on the psychopathology sections. After we (C.A.P. and K.S.K.) had reviewed and made diagnoses for about 1,500 MF1 interviews, we decided to compare our diagnoses with those obtained by a computer algorithm. We found that they agreed over 98% of the time. We therefore decided to eliminate the clinical diagnostic review, but required that two experienced clinician-interviewers review each protocol to ensure that the information put into the computer algorithm would be as accurate as possible.

Interview Validity and Reliability

We took a number of precautions to ensure that our interviews were as accurate and unbiased as possible. Members of a twin pair were interviewed separately by different interviewers. An interviewer sometimes conducted both the FF1 and FF2 interviews with the same twin, but in later assessments and in the MM/MF study, this was rarely done. Interviewers who were assigned members of a twin pair sometimes contacted each other with details of how to get in touch with a twin, but they were instructed never to discuss the content of interviews. The interview data were entered and verified (entered a second time) using menu-driven computer screens.

We conducted several substudies to assess the reliability of our interview and coding procedures. In FF1, we assessed interviewer reliability by having a second interviewer sit in during 53 interviews and code a second interview book. The results of this study supported the reliability of our interview procedures. (Details can be found in early publications based on the FF sample.) We also conducted repeat interviews (by an interviewer who had not previously interviewed the respondent or cotwin) within 2 to 8 weeks of the original interview with 194 respondents in the FF4 study and 191 respondents in the MF2 study. The similarity of the original and repeat interviews provides an index of *test–retest reliability*. These results are reported in Chapters 4 and 5.

We report two statistics to index the level of agreement across the two assessments. The first is the tetrachoric correlation, as defined in Chapter 3. The other is the kappa statistic (κ), which represents agreement corrected for chance. Correcting for chance is important for infrequent conditions. For example, imagine that we have an interview that classifies 10% of individuals as having a disorder and 90% of individuals as unaffected. Then we administer the interview to the sample again and again obtain the 10:90 split. We look at the frequencies and find that 84% of the time respondents are assigned to the same categories in both interviews. At first glance, 84% seems like excellent agreement, but in fact we should not claim that our procedures are reliable unless they result in consistent classifications at a higher rate than that expected by chance.

We would expect that by chance alone, 82% of the sample (i.e., 0.1*0.1 + 0.9*0.9) would obtain the same classification from both interviews. Thus the 84% value represents only a 2% improvement out of the 18% possible (i.e., 100%–82%). This represents a κ of 0.11 (0.02/0.18). Although there is some disagreement about the interpretation of the κ statistic, generally values higher than +0.80 are regarded as excellent, values from +0.60 to +0.80 as good to very good, values from +0.40 to +0.60 as fair to good, and values below +0.40 as poor to fair.

Confidentiality

In regard to the confidentiality of the interviews and data collection procedures, interview materials were all labeled by a study ID number, never by a participant's name. Of necessity, identifying information was mailed to field interviewers but was kept locked away when not in use. After our studies were complete, we destroyed the database containing name and address information. This means that we cannot link names of individuals to their interview records.[4]

NOTES

1. Subsequently, the registry was expanded to include twins born in North Carolina and South Carolina, and it is now known as the Mid-Atlantic Twin Registry (MATR).

2. Although birth years for the FF sample ranged from 1934 to 1974, very few pairs were born prior to 1940.

3. DSM-III-R and DSM-IV are the third revised and fourth editions of the *Diagnostic and Statistical Manual of Mental Disorders*, respectively (American Psychiatric Association, 1987, 1994). The DSM contains the criteria used in the United States for diagnosing psychiatric and substance use disorders.

4. A linking file is maintained by the MATR so that a twin wishing to withdraw from the study could do so. However, the MATR does not have access to our study materials, and we would need special permission to obtain the linking information from the MATR.

CHAPTER THREE

Twinning and Twin Models

In humans, there are two very different kinds of twins. By far the better understood, in terms of biological mechanism, is dizygotic (DZ) twinning. Normally in humans, the female reproductive cycle releases (or, more technically, ovulates) a single egg in each reproductive (or menstrual) cycle. Sometimes, however, the system "misfires" and, instead of releasing one egg, it releases two. If the woman who has just had such a misfiring has sexual intercourse during the 2–3 days after ovulation (during which time she is fertile) and no contraception is used, the two eggs may be fertilized by two different sperm. This will produce DZ twins who are, genetically, just like other full brothers and sisters: The twins come from two different eggs from the same mother and two different sperm from the same father.[1]

After being secreted from the ovaries, the eggs migrate down the Fallopian tubes (usually one from each side, but sometimes both from the same side). It is in these tubes that the eggs are typically fertilized by sperm. In the case of DZ twins, the two fertilized eggs then continue their migration down the tubes and into the uterus, where they implant in random locations in the lining. The embryos start to develop, each producing a fully separate placenta, a distinct inner membrane (the amnion), and a distinct outer membrane (the chorion). Sometimes, by chance, the two fertilized eggs implant close to one another in the womb. In this case, as the placentas grow, they meet and appear to merge, although actually remaining structurally separate. A microscopic examination of the fused placentas would reveal that they were indeed separate, but usually this cannot be seen just by looking at them in the delivery room. Same-sex DZ twins with fused placentas are sometimes a source of confusion, because some physicians, seeing what appears to be a single placenta, incorrectly conclude that the twins are monozygotic.

The most common natural cause of DZ twinning appears to be a subtle "overdrive" of the ovaries by the control hormones secreted by the "master" gland in the brain, the pituitary. Rates of DZ twinning are higher among older mothers (being highest from age 35 to 40), women who have already had several children, and women who are physically larger. DZ twinning differs widely by ethnic group. It is most common in Africans, of intermediate frequency in Europeans, and rarest in Asians (Cunningham, MacDonald, & Gant, 1989). DZ twinning also appears to run in families, apparently for genetic reasons, but only on the mother's side. Fathers do not appear to have much to do with twinning. Multiple births have become more common in recent years due to the increased use of fertility drugs, which increase the chance that multiple eggs will be ovulated. Like regular pairs of brothers and sisters, DZ pairs come in three kinds—male–male, male–female, and female–female—in what is close to a 1:2:1 ratio, as expected by chance.

By comparison, monozygotic (MZ) twinning remains something of a biological mystery. A single egg is fertilized by a single sperm. Then, for reasons that are poorly understood, the egg splits into two separate eggs, resulting in two individuals who, at least at the start of life, are genetically identical. The biggest factor affecting the biology of MZ twinning is the timing of the splitting. If the egg splits within the first 3 days after fertilization (typically before the egg implants in the uterine wall), each fetus will implant on its own and develop a separate placenta and its own separate amnion and chorion. Such early-splitting twins make up 20–30% of all MZ twins. From the perspective of the obstetrician, these early-splitting MZ twins cannot be distinguished from DZ twins.

More commonly, the split occurs between days 4 and 8 after fertilization, usually soon after the fertilized egg has implanted in the wall of the uterus. In this case, the twins share a single placenta, as well as the outer and earlier developing of the two membranes (the chorion) but have distinct inner membranes (amnions). This type accounts for 70–80% of MZ twins. If the split occurs between 8 and 12 days after fertilization, then the twins share both their inner and outer membranes and are therefore floating together in a single amniotic sac. This is risky because the umbilical cords sometimes get entangled. Fortunately, such late-splitting twins are rare—about 1% of MZ pairs. Finally, if the twins split after about 12 days, they are unable to separate completely and form as conjoined (or as they used to be termed, "Siamese") twins. Fortunately, such pairs are extremely rare. Being genetically identical, MZ twins are always of the same sex.

Unlike DZ twinning, MZ twinning is not related to maternal age, the number of prior offspring, maternal size, or ethnic background. MZ twinning also does not appear to run in families, although this is under some dispute. By and large, MZ twinning appears to be a rare but rather wonderful accident of nature that occurs at a modest but steady rate.

There is a huge literature on the epidemiology of twinning, but here we summarize only a few salient facts. Readers interested in more details may consult Keith, Papiernik, Keith, and Luke (1995). Before the widespread use of fertility drugs, twins constituted about 1 out of 80 pregnancies in women of European populations in Europe and North America (MacGillivray, 1986). In most of these countries, about one-third of the twins in the population are MZ; one-third, same-sex DZ; and one-third, opposite-sex DZ.[2]

REPRESENTATIVENESS OF TWINS

Twins and twinning are fascinating topics of study in their own right. As geneticists, however, we are interested in them primarily because they provide a way for us to understand the causes of variation in behavior among people in general. For the purpose of our studies, it is therefore important that twins be representative of the rest of the nontwin population. On a broad array of factors, twins do not appear to be any different from nontwins (termed *singletons*). There are two exceptions to this general rule. First, because the human womb was basically designed for one—and it is (pardon the pun) a stretch to have two—twins have a modest but significantly higher rate of prenatal and perinatal complications. Compared with singletons, twins are more often premature at birth and have a higher probability of low birthweight and several kinds of birth complications. Because of this, twins more often have disorders that arise from these complications. Second, twins are more prone to have delays in language development, at least in part because they have each other to communicate with. They may be less interested in learning to communicate with the outside world. However, they seem to catch up in their language skills by the early years of elementary school.

Surprisingly few studies have examined whether twins differ from singletons in their risk for psychiatric disorders. We are aware of four studies that have examined whether the rates of hospitalization for psychiatric disorders differ in adult twins versus singletons (Chitkara, MacDonald, & Reveley, 1988; Kendler, Pedersen, Farahmand, & Persson, 1996b; Kringlen, 1967; Rosenthal, 1960). All of these studies found no evidence that twins differed in this respect. In the most recent and thorough of these studies, we, along with colleagues from Sweden, studied admission rates using the excellent national data available in that country. We could find no evidence that admission rates for schizophrenia, bipolar illness, severe depression, or "neurotic" depression differed either between twins and singletons or in MZ versus DZ twins (Kendler et al., 1996b).

A number of studies, most of which used symptom rating scales rather than formal diagnostic procedures, have compared twins and singletons in childhood and adolescence. The eminent child psychiatrist Michael Rutter, reviewing this literature, concluded that twins and singletons appear to be broadly comparable in their levels of psychiatric problems (Rutter & Redshaw, 1991). In summary, although the evidence is not as extensive as we would like, the available results suggest that twins are representative of the general population with respect to prevalences of psychopathology.

ANALYSIS BASICS

In this section we describe some basic principles governing the way in which we conduct analyses in this book and present the results. We confine our discussion to model fitting and aspects of analyses that are specific to twin research. We assume that the reader has a basic familiarity with the concepts of means, variances, and correlations. Other statistical concepts are described later in the book in the context of particular analyses. Readers can obtain more details of twin modeling principles in a book by Neale and Cardon (1992).

Twin-Pair Similarity

Many of our analyses rely on estimates of twin-pair similarity—how closely the members of a twin pair resemble each other for a measure or disorder. The type of statistical estimate of similarity employed depends on the type of variable being studied. When we study continuously scaled or multiple-category variables (such as scores on personality scales or symptom counts), we use Pearson (product–moment) correlations. We use tetrachoric correlations for two-category (i.e., binary or dichotomous) variables and polychoric correlations for variables with just a few (but more than two) categories. In this book, we use r to represent a correlation, regardless of the type.

Estimation of tetrachoric and polychoric correlations relies on the assumption that the categories represent values that would be obtained if cutoffs were applied to a normally distributed variable (see Sidebar 3.1). When studying an illness or disorder, we assume that there is a normal distribution of liability to develop the disorder. Individuals who have the disorder are assumed to lie above a *threshold* of liability and individuals without the disorder to have a below-threshold level of liability. This concept is illustrated in Figure 3.1. The scatterplot shows the scores of 50 twin pairs on a liability dimension to which we have applied the (arbitrary) scores of 0 to 7. Now assume that individuals with a liability score of 4 or higher are "affected" with a disorder and that those below 4 are unaffected. These thresholds are illustrated in the figure by the dashed lines. Applying the thresholds to the scores for twin 1 and twin 2 results in four categories: both twins affected, twin 1 affected but twin 2 unaffected, twin 2 affected but twin 1 unaffected, and both twins unaffected. The number of pairs in each of these categories is shown in the upper table in the right portion of Figure 3.1. The tetrachoric correlation estimated

SIDEBAR 3.1. Tetrachoric Correlations

The concept of a tetrachoric correlation can most easily be explained by a story. Imagine you were given a research assignment to determine the correlation in height between 100 pairs of fathers and their sons. You explained the project to your research assistant and gave him a high-quality tape measure, telling him to measure everyone to the nearest inch. However, he was rather lazy and disregarded your instructions. All he did was to record whether the 100 fathers and their 100 sons were taller or shorter than 5'10". When you see the results, at first you are in despair—instead of 100 pairs of measurements of height, all you have is a 2 × 2 table that tells you the number of father–son pairs in which both were short, the father was tall and the son was short, the father was short and the son was tall, and both were tall. But then a statistically minded friend tells you about the tetrachoric correlation. She tells you that if you are willing to assume that height is approximately normally distributed in the general population—a safe assumption—then calculating the tetrachoric correlation from that 2 × 2 table will exactly reproduce what you would have gotten with a true correlation (if your research assistant had done what he was told to do). In essence, you are calculating the father–son correlation in "liability" to being tall. The accuracy of your estimate will be poorer because you have thrown away information, but it is (approximately) equal to the correlation for height that you would have obtained if you had the precise measurements. You are greatly relieved, and very thankful to Karl Pearson for developing this statistic back in 1901.

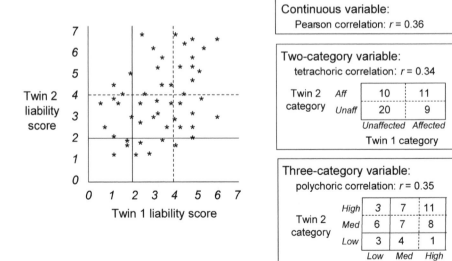

FIGURE 3.1. Correlations based on scores of 50 twin pairs.

from the data in this table is 0.34 and represents the correlation in the twin pairs for the liability for the disorder. This is the reason that, in the literature, tetrachoric correlations are sometimes called *correlations of liability*.

Next we consider a three-category example. In Figure 3.1, this is illustrated by dividing the twins into Low, Medium, and High categories based on cutoffs of 2 and 4, resulting in nine categories for the pairwise data. The number of pairs in each of these cells is shown in the 3×3 table. The polychoric correlation estimated from these data is 0.35. For comparison, the Pearson correlation coefficient based on the "true" liability scores is 0.36.

The values from different correlation estimates are not always this close. In this example, we know the tetrachoric is close to the true value, but in practice we would not be very confident about tetrachoric correlations estimated from 50 pairs of twins. The 95% confidence interval (CI) for the tetrachoric estimate of 0.34 is quite broad, ranging from –0.01 to 0.68. There is slightly more precision for the three-category polychoric correlation ($r = 0.35$, 95% CI = 0.10, 0.62). (See section on statistical significance and precision later in this chapter for a description of CI.)

When the disorder is very infrequent (i.e., has a high threshold), there is lower statistical power to estimate the tetrachoric correlation, and it may differ markedly from the correlation based on the "true" scores. For example, applying a cutoff score of 5 to the data in Figure 3.1 results in an estimated tetrachoric correlation of 0.50, with a 95% CI of –0.08 to 0.85. The major reason the sample sizes in VATSPSUD are so large is that we wanted to obtain estimates that are as accurate as possible, even for uncommon disorders.

Multiple-Threshold Test for Continuum of Measurement

For some analyses, we use multiple-category variables to represent a theoretical gradation of liability. For example, in analyses of phobic disorders, we assign twins to three categories: no fear, fear without phobia, and phobia. By using data from twins (or other pairs of relatives), we are able to test whether the data are consistent with this ordering of categories.[3] That is, we can test whether these three categories represent differing levels of severity on a single continuum of liability. For example, assuming that twins are correlated for liability, we would predict that, relative to the probabilities in the whole sample, if twin 1 has a low score, then twin 2 is more likely to have a low score than a medium or high score.

Comparison of the observed pattern of scores with those expected based on ordered categories can be used to calculate a chi-square statistic. For the three-category variable shown in Figure 3.1, the chi-square for the multiple-threshold test is 2.2, well below the value of 3.84 required for a 1-degree-of-freedom test based on a significance level of $p < 0.05$. This means that these data are consistent with (but not proven to be) a single dimension of liability.

Basics of Twin Models

The goal of twin analysis is to estimate the sources of individual differences in liability to develop a disorder. We assume that a person's liability arises from genetic and environmental factors, which combine over development. In a basic twin design, we can identify the relative contributions of three components. *Additive genetic factors* (often abbreviated *A*) are so called because they are assumed to arise from multiple genetic loci whose effects combine additively.[4] *Shared environmental factors* (traditionally abbreviated *C* for "common") are factors that are shared by family members and make them more similar, such as parental rearing styles, social class, familial attitudes, and, for twins, the intrauterine environment. Finally, *individual-specific environmental factors* (abbreviated *E*) are those that are not shared by family members. For example, this might represent experiences in childhood that one twin does not share with his cotwin and environments to which the twins are exposed upon leaving home. It is important to note that when the study is based on a single variable (rather than multiple measures of liability or assessments on multiple occasions), the specific environmental component also includes measurement error. We consider this issue more fully in Chapter 12.

To avoid possible confusion, we need to discuss the meaning of what we call shared, common, or family environment. (All three of these terms are used interchangeably by twin researchers. We generally use the term *shared environment* because elsewhere in this book we use the term *common* to refer to common factors in models based on factor analysis). The best way to approach this is by contrasting the two concepts of *objective* and *effective* shared environment. Let's say that a pair of female twins, Martha and Megan, grew up in a home with an abusive alcoholic stepfather, who is equally abusive to both of them. *Objectively*, their stepfather was surely part of their shared environment. However, since early childhood Megan was more self-assured than her sister and developed a particularly strong bond with her mother. Martha was more irritable and hard to get along with and was not as close with her mother. Whereas Megan was able to cope pretty well with the harsh treatment from her stepfather—through both her temperament and support from the mother—Martha was much more vulnerable. *Effectively*, the stepfather's behavior had a quite different impact on the twin sisters, contributing to a higher risk for future mental health problems in Martha than in Megan.

Twin modeling estimates only *effective* environment. Shared environment is measured indirectly as the resemblance in twin pairs above and beyond that accounted for by genes. So the behavior of Megan and Martha's stepfather—which *objectively* affected them equally—would not contribute much to shared environment as seen in twin modeling because it *effectively* contributed to differences between them rather than to similarities.

The distinction between these two kinds of shared or family environment is important to keep in mind, because failure to appreciate this creates confusion in interpreting the results from twin studies. In many areas of the social sciences, when investigators study families, they are examining *objective* effects. (Indeed, because they typically study one child per family, they could not study effective environment even if they wanted to). When such investigators come to look at twin studies, they assume that our measure of shared environment reflects objective effects—but it does not. Thus, if a twin study finds little evidence of shared environmental effects, this does not mean that family environment has no effect, only that the effect is not to make twins more similar.

The relative contributions of the three components are estimated by comparing the similarity of MZ and DZ twin pairs. MZ twins within a pair resemble one another because they share all of their genetic and shared environmental factors, whereas DZ pairs share (on average) half of their genetic variation plus the shared environmental component. To the degree that pair resemblance among MZ pairs exceeds that of DZ pairs, this implies that genetic factors are contributing to liability. If MZ and DZ pairs are equally similar, this indicates that shared environmental, but not genetic, factors are contributing to pair resemblance. To the extent that members of MZ pairs are dissimilar, this implicates the role of individual-specific environmental sources. See Sidebar 3.2 for details on how genetic and environmental estimates are calculated.

The results from twin studies are typically reported in terms of proportions of variance. The proportion of variation due to genetic factors is referred to as *heritability.*[5] This is a frequently used concept that is not always well understood. Because heritability coefficients are proportions, the heritability estimate from one study can be larger than that from a different study either because the genetic variance is larger or because the environmental variance is smaller. This means that heritabilities estimated in markedly different cultures may not be comparable. See Sidebar 3.3 for more details on interpretation of heritability coefficients.

Structural Models and Model Fitting

Many of our analyses employ model fitting implemented using structural equation modeling (SEM) software programs. The term *model* is used because the proposed structure usually represents a simplification of the true process underlying the relations among the observed variables. Furthermore, the model represents just one hypothesized portrayal; there may be several possible explanations of the process.

The model structure produces a set of mathematical equations that summarize the expected variable characteristics (thresholds or means, variances, and correlations). The SEM program tests the model by calculating the discrepancy between the observed data characteristics and those implied by the model. This discrepancy is summarized by one or more indices of model fit.

SIDEBAR 3.2. Calculating Twin-Model Estimates

The logic of our approach to twin data can be easily illustrated. Let's begin with two key equations:

1. $r_{MZ} = a^2 + c^2$
2. $r_{DZ} = \frac{1}{2}a^2 + c^2$

The first equation means that the correlation in liability between MZ twins is the result of all the additive effects of genes (because MZ pairs share all their genes) and their shared environment. By contrast, in the second equation, the correlation in liability between DZ twins is the result of half of the effect of the additive genes (because DZ pairs share, on average, half of their genes) and their shared environment.

If we have estimates of the values of r_{MZ} and r_{DZ}, we can rearrange the terms in these formulas to calculate a^2, c^2, and e^2 as shown in equations 3–5. Anyone who remembers the basics of high school algebra should be able to derive these equations from 1 and 2, so we will leave that to the interested reader.

3. $a^2 = 2(r_{MZ} - r_{DZ})$
4. $c^2 = 2r_{DZ} - r_{MZ}$
5. $e^2 = 1 - r_{MZ}$

Equation 3 says that if you want to estimate the proportion of genetic variance (a^2) of a disorder, take the difference between the MZ and the DZ correlation and double it. Equation 4 says that if you want to estimate the proportion of shared environment (c^2), double the DZ correlation and subtract from that the MZ correlation. Finally, equation 5 indicates that the proportion of individual-specific environment (e^2) can be calculated as the remainder after subtracting the MZ correlation from 1. All of these calculations assume that the MZ and DZ correlations are known with equal accuracy. Because this is never precisely true, estimates obtained algebraically will differ somewhat from those obtained using statistical software.

The following table shows examples of results from four hypothetical twin studies, including rough estimates of a^2 and c^2.

	Pair correlations		Proportions of variance		
	r_{MZ}	r_{DZ}	a^2	c^2	e^2
Trait 1	0.60	0.60	0%	60%	40%
Trait 2	0.60	0.30	60%	0%	40%
Trait 3	0.80	0.40	80%	0%	20%
Trait 4	0.60	0.40	40%	20%	40%

The results for trait 1 are what you might observe for a measure such as religious affiliation. Twin resemblance is high and equal in MZ and DZ twins. Twin similarity, our analysis would suggest, is due entirely to the effects of shared environment. For traits 2 and 3, twin resemblance is due entirely to genetic effects, with trait 2 having

(continued)

SIDEBAR 3.2. *continued*

moderately high and trait 3 high heritability. Trait 4 is the most complex, in that the twin results provide evidence that familial resemblance is due both to genetic and to shared environmental factors.

The formulas and the table suggest three rough rules of thumb for interpreting twin data that examines one trait at a time. First, if the MZ correlations are approximately twice as large as the DZ correlations (as seen for traits 2 and 3), twin resemblance is probably due entirely to genetic factors. Second, if MZ and DZ correlations are approximately the same magnitude (as seen for trait 1), twin resemblance is probably due entirely to shared environmental effects. Third, if the size of the DZ correlation is between 50 and 100% of that seen in MZ pairs (as seen for trait 4), then it is likely that both genetic and shared environmental effects are operative.

In practice, the ability of twin studies to resolve sources of individual differences depends on three factors. First is the nature of the variable being studied. Twin studies have much more power with a continuous than with a dichotomous variable. If the variable is dichotomous, there is more power with a common than with a rare trait. A second factor is the sample size, and a third is the subtlety of the question. VATSPSUD was designed to give us moderate power to distinguish, for a common disorder, between models that attribute all of the familial aggregation to genes and those that attribute it to shared environment. We have limited power to answer more subtle questions, such as whether familial resemblance for these disorders is due entirely to genetic effects (e.g., heritability of 40%) or mostly to genetic effects with a small contribution from the shared environment (e.g., heritability of 30%, shared environment of 10%).

SEM is useful when estimates are based on several sources of information (in the parlance of simultaneous equations, when there are more equations than unknowns). For example, to estimate liability thresholds, we "average" across the prevalences observed for twins 1 and 2 from both MZ and DZ pairs.[6] SEM is also useful for comparing or combining estimates from different groups (e.g., males and females).

The model-fit statistics provide an absolute measure of model fit and can also be used to compare the fits of alternative models. As is common in twin studies, we tested alternative models by dropping components (i.e., the genetic and/or shared environmental effects) and seeing if the simpler model fit our data. In general, simpler models (those with fewer parameters) are preferred if they do not result in substantially worse fit. For example, we can estimate a model separately for males and females, then obtain a numerical index of the change in fit when the parameters are required to be equal across males and females. Based on this index, we can make a judgment about whether males and females differ significantly in the sources of liability.

Statistical Significance and Precision

In research reports, statistical estimates are accompanied by a numerical index of their precision, such as standard errors or probability levels. In this

SIDEBAR 3.3. Interpretation of Heritability Coefficients

When first confronted with a heritability statistic, a typical reaction is "so what does this mean?" It is like learning about a new scale for height or temperature but being given no guidelines with which to orient oneself. The table that follows lists a few benchmarks for estimates of heritability in human populations.

Heritability	Human traits/diseases
0%	• Language • Religion
20–40%	• Myocardial infarction • Lung cancer • Breast cancer • Personality • Asthma
40–60%	• Plasma cholesterol • Adult-onset diabetes • Blood pressure
60–80%	• Weight • Intelligence
80–100%	• Height

These estimates are not precise results from meta-analysis but broad estimates based on having read and reviewed the relevant literature (Kendler, 1983; King, Rotter, & Motulsky, 2002; Lichtenstein et al., 2000). We suggest that, for purposes of interpretation, heritability levels in humans can be usefully divided into five groups.

The first group of traits effectively has *zero heritability*. Here we pick as paradigmatic two traits that run very strongly in families: religious affiliation and language. That is, Baptists tend to beget Baptists, Jews beget Jews, and Buddhists beget Buddhists. Similarly, the language children speak is always that of their caregivers (at least until they enter school). We have good evidence that genes do not contribute to individual differences for either of these traits. Instead, these characteristics "run in families" because of a process called social learning or cultural transmission.

For the second group of traits, with *moderate heritability*, genetic factors account for 20–40% of population individual differences. The risk for heart attack (more technically, myocardial infarction) fits in this category. Genes that influence lipid and cholesterol metabolism make significant contributions to risk, but other factors, including diet, level of stress, and smoking, are also important. Most twin and adoption studies of the major dimensions of personality also suggest heritability in this range (Loehlin, 1992). Nearly all cancers also have moderate levels of heritability (Lichtenstein et al., 2000), as does asthma.

The third group of traits, which have *moderately high heritability*, include two well-studied biomedical traits: plasma cholesterol and blood pressure. For these traits, heritability ranges from 40 to 60%: Genes and environment make approximately equal contributions to the trait. Plasma cholesterol has been quite well studied. Indi-

(continued)

SIDEBAR 3.3. *continued*

vidual differences are about equally due to a variety of genes that influence cholesterol absorption, transport, synthesis, and degradation and to environmental influences, the most important being the amount of cholesterol consumed in the diet. Another common medical disorder—adult-onset diabetes—also has moderately high heritability.

The fourth group of traits, which have *high heritability* in the range of 60–80%, includes two well-studied traits: weight and intelligence. As might be expected, weight is a bit less heritable than height because it is more influenced by environmental factors such as diet and levels of exercise. Intelligence has been extensively studied in family, twin, and adoption studies, with nearly all heritability estimates in the range of 50 to 70%. Very few biomedical conditions have values this high, but heritabilities in this range have been found for two severe psychiatric disorders—schizophrenia and bipolar illness—that were not studied in VATSPSUD because of their relative rarity.

The fifth group, with *very high heritability*, contains only one very well-studied trait: human height. A large number of studies going back to the early days of the 20th century suggest that the heritability of height in human populations is close to 90%. Estimates nearly as high are found for the size of other body parts (including the brain). Having studied many adult MZ pairs, we can attest to the fact that such twins rarely differ in height by more than half an inch. Aside from cases with substantial malnutrition or trauma, differences among people in height are almost completely determined by the genes they inherited from their parents.

---

book, we report the 95% CIs around our estimates. These represent the range of values within which we would expect the estimate to fall 95% of the time if the hypothesized model represents the "true" model for the data.

The reader should keep in mind that for some types of estimates there are theoretical lower or upper boundaries and the 95% CI will not be symmetrical. For example, the 95% CI for a proportion of variance estimated at 0.75 might range from 0.30 to 1.00; it is asymmetrical because the upper limit cannot exceed 1.0. The 95% CI is thus a better portrayal of the range of possible values than assuming a symmetrical estimate (e.g., ±2 * standard error). See Sidebar 4.2 for more details about CIs for the estimates from twin models.

Path Diagrams

SEM analyses are often portrayed as path diagrams. Figure 3.2 shows a precise representation of a SEM for a basic twin analysis. We describe this diagram in some detail because we use path models throughout the book to portray our analyses and display the numerical results. The boxes represent observed variables (the measures we obtain from our interviews and questionnaires). In Figure 3.2, the observed variables are binary and represent the presence or absence of disorder X for twins 1 and 2. Ovals are used to represent unobserved, or latent, variables—those that are inferred from the characteristics of the observed variables. One-headed arrows represent direct effects of

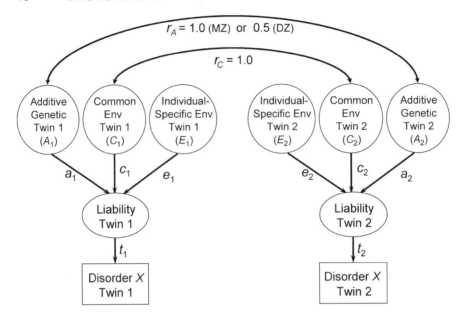

FIGURE 3.2. Basic twin model to estimate genetic and environmental sources of liability to a disorder. Env = environment.

one variable on another (e.g., regression weights or factor loadings), whereas two-headed arrows represent indirect effects (correlations), without any sense of one variable affecting the other.

Figure 3.2 includes a latent variable for each twin, representing the liability to develop disorder X. As described earlier, the pair correlations of liability are inferred based on the frequencies of X in twin 1 and twin 2. Variation in liability arises from the three components, which are all unmeasured variables. Based on the principles of genetic segregation and twinning, the correlation between the genetic components (r_A) is fixed to be 1.0 for MZ pairs and 0.50 for DZ pairs. Based on the assumptions of the twin model, the correlation between the shared environmental components (r_C) is fixed at 1.0 for both types of twins. By definition, the specific environmental components (E) are not correlated across members of a twin pair (i.e., $r_E = 0$ and is not shown). We use lower-case letters to indicate the quantities that are estimated in the analysis (technically, *parameters*). In Figure 3.2, these include additive genetic variance (a), shared environment (c), individual-specific environment (e), and the location of the threshold (t) on the liability dimension. The subscripts on these variables ($_1$ and $_2$) correspond to twin 1 and twin 2. For most models, these estimates are equated across twins 1 and 2. The variance in liability associated with each component is calculated as the square of each of these quantities (i.e., a^2, c^2, e^2), and the total variance in liability is the sum of the three variances ($a^2 + c^2 + e^2$).

Figure 3.3 shows a reduced version of our path diagram that is similar to the diagrams we use throughout this book. This diagram represents the same model as Figure 3.2, but it has been simplified for clarity of presentation. We omit the latent variable representing liability from the diagram, but it is implied whenever we analyze a categorical outcome. Rather than showing the raw estimates of a, c, and e (which need to be squared and sometimes standardized for interpretation), we display the variance proportions, shown in white boxes.

Throughout this book, we have attempted to emphasize the big picture and substantive results and interpretations, rather than dwelling on the details of the analyses. For readers who, like us, share a penchant for methodological minutiae, technical details can be found in footnotes, appendices, and the original publications describing these studies.

NOTES

1. If a woman has intercourse with two different men in the 2–3 days after ovulating two eggs, it is possible that the eggs will be fertilized by the sperm of two different fathers, producing "dizygotic half-siblings." However, such cases are very rare and, for the purposes of this book, can safely be ignored.

2. We do not discuss here "higher order" births in any detail. As described in Chapter 2, our study did include a small number of triplets and one set of quadruplets. Triplets can come in all varieties; they can arise from one, two, or three separate eggs. Some are "trizygotic" in that all three triplets are related to each other genetically as regular brothers and sisters. They can be monozygotic, with all three being genetically identical. Or two of the triplets can be identical and the third dizygotic to his or her two identical triplets. Quadruplets can also come in all varieties, but we leave it to our readers to work these out!

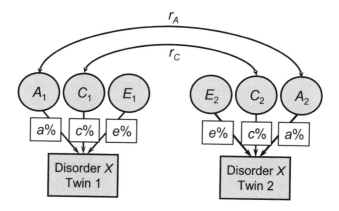

FIGURE 3.3. Simplified portrayal of basic twin model.

3. In fact, similar tests could be conducted for any pair of variables that one would expect to be moderately correlated.

4. There are other genetic mechanisms, including dominance (when alleles at a locus do not combine additively) and epistasis (when the alleles from different loci interact), which we do not consider here. Twin models are not at all powerful in their ability to detect such effects, especially in the presence of additive genetic effects. In this book, we focus solely on additive genetic effects because, even in the VATSPSUD, our ability to detect dominance or epistasis is low.

5. Several definitions of heritability can be estimated in other behavior genetic designs. The definition employed here is the proportion of variance attributable to additive genetic effects, known in the literature as narrow-sense heritability.

6. It is not precisely an average because the estimates are weighted by the number of observations, which may differ for MZ and DZ pairs.

PART II

GENETIC RISK

CHAPTER FOUR

Internalizing Disorders

In Part II of this book we take the perspective of genetic epidemiologists and examine the results from our studies of twin resemblance. This chapter describes our studies of the common *internalizing disorders*. In the next chapter, we present similar analyses of the *externalizing disorders*. These terms arose from child and adolescent psychiatry. *Internalizing* disorders are characterized by *internal* suffering, usually manifested in anxiety or depression. *Externalizing* disorders are characterized by acting out in the external environment either by antisocial behavior or by taking psychoactive substances. As clinicians commonly say, individuals with internalizing disorders make themselves miserable, whereas individuals with externalizing disorders make people around them miserable.

The internalizing disorders studied in VATSPSUD include major depression, panic disorder, generalized anxiety, and phobias. We begin each section with a description of the clinical features of the disorder and summarize briefly what is known about its prevalence in adults in the general population. We then describe how we assessed the disorder in our sample, present the results from our twin analyses, and discuss how the results fit into the larger literature on genetic influences on risk for developing these disorders.

MAJOR DEPRESSION

Major depression (MD) is a particularly complex psychiatric disorder that includes alterations in mood and emotion, in capacity to experience pleasure and be interested and involved in the activities of the world, in neurovegetative functions (e.g., appetite, body weight, and sleep), in cognition (e.g., inappropriate guilt), and in psychomotor activity (e.g., agitation or retardation). MD is one of the oldest well-recognized syndromes within medicine, having been described in medical texts since ancient times (Jackson, 1986). MD is also a public health problem of substantial magnitude because it is both relatively common and associated with considerable impairment in occupational and psychosocial functioning. A recent World Health Organization review predicts that by the year 2020, MD will be second only to cardiovascular illness in the total disease burden imposed on humankind worldwide (Murray & Lopez, 1996).

Epidemiological studies have produced a wide range of estimates of population prevalence for MD (Boyd & Weissman, 1981). The most widely quoted values for the lifetime prevalence (the percentage of individuals who at some time in their lives would meet criteria for a disorder) of MD in the United States is from the National Comorbidity Survey (NCS) and is based on interviews conducted between 1990 and 1992 (Kessler et al., 1994b). Using DSM-III-R criteria, this study reports lifetime prevalences for MD to be 12.7% for men and 21.3% for women. A second NCS study, completed in 2003, reported lifetime prevalences for MD slightly lower than those found in the original NCS (Kessler et al., 2003).

Figure 4.1 shows the prevalences of lifetime MD and the other internalizing disorders among male and female twins from same-sex pairs participating in the VATSPSUD. As defined by DSM-III-R, MD is a very common disorder in our study, experienced by 34.4% of women and 28.5% of men sometime in their lifetimes. We also included a more narrow definition of MD (see Sidebar

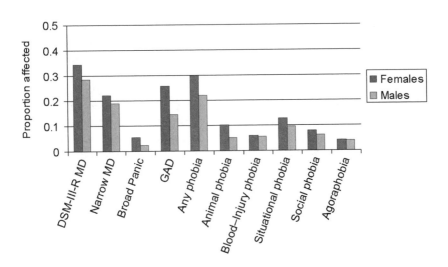

FIGURE 4.1. Lifetime prevalences of internalizing disorders in twins from same-sex pairs. MD = major depression; GAD = generalized anxiety disorder.

4.1). Prevalences based on this definition were substantially lower: 22.2% in women and 18.9% in men.

The VATSPUD prevalences for MD are considerably higher than those found in the NCS. Two possible reasons for this are (1) that our methods detected episodes that would have been missed in other studies, and (2) that our methods exaggerated symptoms and identified episodes that did not actually meet criteria. We believe the evidence is consistent with the first explanation. In contrast to the NCS, the VATSPSUD used several procedures that increase the detection of MD, including employing clinically trained interviewers who used an interview that relied on clinical judgment and repeated assessments of MD.[1] Other evidence comes from an important recent study of MD among adolescents who were followed with repeated assessments up to the age of 21 (Wells & Horwood, 2004). The results of this study suggest that MD is very common (37% met criteria for MD based on at least one interview), that the forgetting of prior episodes occurs frequently, and that people rarely "make up" depressive episodes.[2] We interpret these results to indicate that the high prevalences of MD found in our study are likely to be valid.

Genetic and Environmental Influences

A large number of family studies conducted since the early decades of this century have consistently shown that MD runs (or more technically "aggregates") in families (Tsuang & Faraone, 1990). A meta-analysis of five modern studies that met rigorous methodological criteria found that first-degree relatives of individuals with MD have a nearly threefold increased risk of developing MD compared with control samples (Sullivan, Neale, & Kendler, 2000). There have been three adoption studies of MD, and two of these found significant genetic effects on risk for MD. However, none of the adoption studies met modern methodological criteria. Earlier twin studies that did not use modern methods and that were based on hospitalized cases (e.g., Bertelsen, Harvald, & Hauge, 1977) suggested that MD has a genetic component. However, when we began our study, the relative role of genes and environment in contributing to the familial aggregation of mild to moderate MD (the kind most common in the general population) had not yet been investigated using modern research methods.

Our estimates of twin-pair resemblance for lifetime DSM-III-R and narrowly defined MD are summarized in Figure 4.2. Consistent with prior family studies, we found strong evidence of resemblance for MD within twin pairs. We highlight four aspects of these estimates: First, for male and female twins, resemblance was consistently greater among MZ than among DZ pairs. Second, for both MZ and DZ pairs, resemblance among female pairs was higher than among males. Third, the patterns of twin resemblance for the narrow and DSM-III-R definitions of MD are quite similar. Fourth, as will often be seen in this book, despite our large sample size, the degree of resemblance for MD in these twin pairs is known with only modest accuracy. For example, for

SIDEBAR 4.1. Assessment of Major Depression (MD)

The DSM-III-R definition of MD (American Psychiatric Association, 1987)—which is the version used most commonly in this volume—includes three major requirements: (1) an episode of at least 2 weeks' duration, (2) the presence of at least five of nine so-called "A" criteria (of which at least one must be either depressed mood or loss of interest/pleasure), and (3) that the disorder cannot be better understood as resulting from medical illness, the effects of medication, or grief.

In the VATSPSUD, we assessed, in separate sections of our interviews, MD in the year prior to interview and lifetime MD prior to the past year. When we considered "lifetime" MD in this and other chapters, we combined these two separate assessments so that an individual was regarded as having a positive lifetime history of MD if he or she reported an episode that met criteria in the past year and/or prior to the past year.

Our assessment methods differed for these two time periods.

In our "lifetime minus the past year" assessment, we used a slightly adapted version of the SCID interview for DSM-III-R diagnoses (Spitzer & Williams, 1985). Two probe questions were used:

1. "Looking back over your life (except the last year), have you ever had a time when you were feeling depressed or down for at least 7 days in a row?"
2. "What about a time lasting at least 7 days when you were uninterested in things or unable to enjoy the things you used to?"

Individuals who responded positively to one or both of these probes were then asked about the remaining symptomatic criteria for MD for the episode in their lives that they identified as the worst. Those positive for three or more symptoms were then asked for further details, including number and length of lifetime episodes, age at onset, and whether they had received treatment.

For assessing episodes of MD occurring during the previous year, our approach was different. Everyone was asked about 16 symptoms of depression, which included all the DSM-III-R criteria. Several of the individual criteria, however, were "disaggregated" into several different questions. For example, we asked separate questions about weight gain and weight loss and about insomnia and hypersomnia. Individuals who indicated that they experienced two or more symptoms were then asked which symptoms co-occurred, and we reconstructed the syndromes that they had experienced. In the analyses presented in this chapter, we also employ a narrower definition of MD, which requires a minimum duration of illness of 4 weeks (instead of the 2 required by DSM-III-R) and the presence of significant episode-related impairment.

For many of our diagnostic categories, we assessed test–retest reliability, having the same twins interviewed twice by different interviewers with the same interview protocol. For MD, 375 individuals were reinterviewed, with an average interval of 30 days between interviews. For lifetime DSM-III-R MD, the test–retest reliability was reasonably good ($r = 0.88$, $\kappa = 0.66$ [95% CI = 0.58, 0.74]). For narrowly defined MD, it was a bit lower but still in the good range ($r = 0.79$, $\kappa = 0.54$ [95% CI = 0.45, 0.63]).

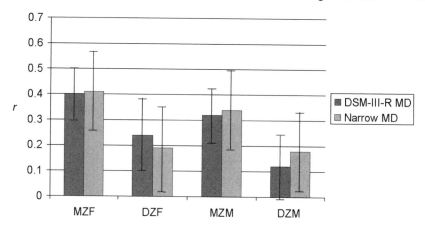

FIGURE 4.2. Similarity of same-sex twin pairs for lifetime history of major depression (MD). MZF = monozygotic female; DZF dizygotic female; MZM = monozygotic male; DZM = dizygotic male; r = correlation coefficient.

DSM-III-R MD, the correlation in MZ female twin pairs is 0.40 with a 95% CI of 0.29–0.51. (See Appendix 4.1 for sample sizes, pair correlations, and 95% CI for all the disorders described in this chapter.)

The next step was to analyze the pair-resemblance information using statistical models for twin data. We concentrate here on the substantive results. (Chapter 3 contains a description of our model-fitting approach and numerical details can be found in Appendix 4.2.)

The estimated genetic contributions to risk for lifetime MD are shown in Figure 4.3 and details can be found in Appendix 4.3. Four aspects of these

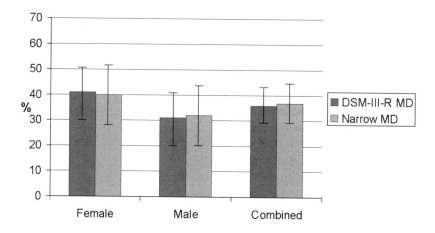

FIGURE 4.3. Estimated genetic proportions of variance in risk for major depression (MD). Bars indicate 95% confidence intervals based on AE models.

results are noteworthy: First, for both men and women, twin-pair resemblance for liability to (or risk for) lifetime DSM-III-R MD could be explained largely or entirely by genetic factors. For both men and women, genetic factors account for 30–40% of the variation in liability to lifetime MD. The estimated genetic effects were similar for MD defined according to DSM-III-R and based on our narrow definition. The estimates of heritability based on males and females combined were 36% for DSM-III-R MD and 37% for narrowly defined depression.

Second, we were unable to find evidence of shared environmental contributions to the etiology of MD. Contrary to expectations of some major segments of the mental health community, twin studies have found that for mood and anxiety disorders, the effects of shared environment are quite modest. We return to this issue in later chapters.

Third, in the full models, the confidence intervals around our estimates of the genetic and shared environmental effects are quite large and, except for the genetic estimate in males, include zero (see Sidebar 4.2 and Appendix 4.3).

Fourth, estimates for individual-specific effects are substantially higher than for either genetic or shared environmental effects. In analyses that include only one assessment of MD, we cannot distinguish how much of the individual component is due to errors of measurement versus "true" individual-specific environmental effects. We know that some of these individual-specific effects are due to error from not having measured MD with perfect reliability. We return to this issue in Chapter 12, in which, by using two time points of measurement, we can begin to distinguish measurement error from true environmental effects.

SIDEBAR 4.2. Confidence Intervals

When attempting to estimate sources of liability to a dichotomous trait such as MD (that is, individuals are categorized as either affected or unaffected), the twin method is a blunt tool. The CIs are larger for the genetic and shared environmental estimates compared with the specific environment because the genetic and shared environmental estimates are correlated with each other (they are both indices of familial resemblance), whereas specific environment is independent of the other estimates.

As described in Chapter 3, one way to evaluate the importance of genetic and environmental estimates is to drop them from the model (i.e., set them equal to zero) and see what effect this has on the statistical fit of the model. For nearly all the disorders presented in this chapter, dropping the shared environmental effects did not worsen the model fit. Consequently, a "reduced" model that includes only genetic and individual-specific environmental effects can be considered preferable to the full model because it is consistent with the data and is simpler. In Appendices 4.3 and 5.3 we report the CIs for the full models and for reduced models that had significantly improved fit relative to the full model for that disorder.

Discussion and Implications

Our findings in the VATSPSUD are similar to those obtained subsequently by other investigators in other populations. MD has been studied in five other community and clinical samples of twins in which the evaluations were based on diagnostic criteria assessed by structured interviews. Our study is most comparable methodologically to two large population-based twin studies: one of twins of both sexes in Australia (Bierut et al., 1999) and the other of male pairs from the U.S. Vietnam Era Twin Study (VETS, Lyons et al., 1998). Like ours, these studies found no evidence for the influence of shared environmental factors. Heritability estimates for MD were similar: 24% in men and 44% in women in the Australian study and 36% in the men from the Vietnam Era Twin Registry. Our findings can also be usefully compared to the largest clinically ascertained twin study of MD completed to date (McGuffin, Katz, Watkins, & Rutherford, 1996). Heritability estimates based on this sample were somewhat higher than those we obtained for males (58%) but very similar to our results for females (38%).

In collaboration with Patrick Sullivan and Michael Neale, Kendler conducted a meta-analysis of all these studies (Sullivan et al., 2000). We formally tested the similarity of the results and found that the heritability estimates did not differ statistically. Heritability for lifetime MD across all these samples was estimated to be 37% (95% CI = 33%, 42%).

These results have a number of implications for how we define and think about major depression. First, they suggest that genetic factors are just as important in mild forms of depression as in more severe forms. Although there is a tendency in the field to think that disorders defined more narrowly are more severe and likely to be "more genetic," we found that the role of genetic and environmental factors in the etiology of more narrowly defined MD closely resembles that found for depression diagnosed using the rather broad DSM-III-R criteria. That is, there was no evidence from a genetic perspective that narrowly defined MD is a better definition for genetic or biological studies. Indeed, in a paper based on our female sample in which we compared twin resemblance for a number of other definitions of MD, we found a modest trend for the narrowest definitions of MD to be the least heritable (Kendler, Neale, Kessler, Heath, & Eaves, 1992b). These results undercut a common conception of psychiatric disorders—that the severe disorders are medical conditions with strong biological components, whereas milder syndromes are just "problems of living" best understood from a social-psychological perspective. Furthermore, these findings support the validity of our diagnostic approach to MD. If our relatively high rates of depression arose because we detected many "false positive" cases, the heritability of MD should have increased when we used the narrower definition. This did not happen.

Another implication of our results is that they provide a hint that the importance of genetic risk factors in MD may differ in men and women. When we analyzed the sexes together, the difference was not statistically significant.

In Chapter 9, we reconsider this question of differing levels of heritability of MD in men and women and address another question about sex differences that is subtler and more interesting: Do men and women differ *qualitatively* in their genetic and environmental risk factors? For example, do the genetic risk factors for MD in women overlap completely with those in men, or are there some genetic factors that predispose to MD in only one sex?

PANIC DISORDER

Panic disorder is one of the most dramatic of psychiatric conditions. Its defining feature is the "panic attack." Panic attacks are rapid-onset and relatively short-lasting periods of intense anxiety that are usually accompanied by a number of physical and psychological symptoms. The most typical physical symptoms are cardiovascular, especially rapid heart rate and chest pain; respiratory, particularly the feeling of being short of breath or choking; and gastrointestinal, most frequently nausea. The most common psychological symptom, in addition to the feeling of intense anxiety, is the fear of dying or "losing control."

Panic attacks probably represent the misfiring of a neural system built into us to respond to situations of extreme danger. Almost all of us have had one or more times of extreme fright—perhaps just avoiding a car collision or right before opening night of a high school play—when we have experienced symptoms that closely resembled those of a panic attack. A panic attack is the occurrence of a fright response when there is no actual danger. It is as if the body is generating a dramatic false alarm.

In full-blown panic disorder, panic attacks occur frequently and often unpredictably. Prior to the publication of the DSM-III in 1980, no distinction was made between panic disorder and other forms of what was then known as anxiety neurosis. Based largely on the pioneering work of the psychiatrist Donald Klein—who showed that individuals with panic disorder had relatively specific and often dramatic responses to low doses of antidepressants—the crafters of DSM-III subdivided the old category of anxiety neurosis into panic disorder and generalized anxiety disorder (GAD), which is distinguished by sustained periods of high levels of free-floating anxiety. Since that time, panic disorder has been rapidly accepted as a valid psychiatric disorder in the United States and many other areas of the world. Many individuals who suffer from panic disorder are substantially disabled by their attacks, often developing phobic avoidance of places or situations in which these attacks are likely to occur.

One important practical problem in analyses of panic disorder is its relative rarity. When we applied full DSM-III-R criteria for panic disorder, we found lifetime prevalence rates in VATSPSUD of 1.1% in males and 3.2% in females. These rates lie between those found in the Epidemiologic Catchment Area Study (1.0% in males and 2.1% in females; Eaton, Dryman, & Weissman, 1991) and those reported in the first National Comorbidity Survey (2.0% in males and 5.0% in females; Kessler et al., 1994) and are therefore likely to be broadly representative of U.S. adults.

However, even with the large numbers of individuals studied in VATSPSUD, the low prevalences of panic disorder meant that our sample contained rather few cases, and this made it difficult for us to get stable estimates from standard twin models. As we noted in Chapter 3, the ability of twin studies to partition resemblance between relatives into genetic and environmental sources when studying a dichotomous trait is critically dependent on the frequency of the disorder (Neale, Eaves, & Kendler, 1994a). We therefore investigated several broader definitions of panic.

Our most stable and (we believe) valid results for this disorder were obtained using a multiple-threshold definition model (but, as we discuss later, even here we had some difficulty). This definition included three categories based on lifetime history of panic symptoms: broad panic disorder, panic attacks that did not meet criteria for broad panic disorder, and no panic symptoms (see Sidebar 4.3). Broad panic disorder had a lifetime prevalence of 5.5% and 2.4% in female and male twins, respectively. Another 7.0% of female and 3.4% of male twins had panic attacks but did not meet criteria for broad panic disorder.

Genetic and Environmental Influences

When we began our study, relatively little was known about genetic influences on panic disorder. The single twin study that had then been conducted suggested that genetic factors played only a modest role in the development of this disorder (Torgersen, 1983). However, that study was based on a small sample, containing only 29 pairs of twins in which one or both had panic disorder. Despite the absence of strong evidence, there was a widespread belief that panic disorder was a distinct and highly heritable condition. Several studies had shown that panic disorder or panic-like syndromes strongly aggregated in families (Crowe, Noyes, Persico, Wilson, & Elston, 1988; Crowe, 1990). Feeding the excitement were results of an analysis of the inheritance pattern of panic disorder in pedigrees that suggested that the disorder might be the result of a single autosomal dominant gene (Pauls, Bucher, Crowe, & Noyes, 1980).

The left portion of Figure 4.4 displays twin-pair correlations for the broad definition of panic disorder in male and female twins from VATSPSUD. For the sake of simplicity, we have not included the CI in this figure (or subsequent figures) showing pair correlations, but these estimates are available in Appendices 4.1 and 5.1. As we saw with MD, in both sexes the MZ pair correlations exceed those for DZ pairs. However, even using our broad

SIDEBAR 4.3. Assessment of Panic

The DSM-III-R criteria for panic disorder include the occurrence of an attack without an external stimulus, repeated attacks within a month or recurring worry about having another attack, development of a full-blown attack within 10 minutes, and at least 4 of 13 possible symptoms.

We based our assessment of a lifetime history of panic disorder on the SCID interview for DSM-III-R. A single probe question was used to evaluate the criterion of the fear being unexpected:

> "Thinking back over your entire life, have you ever had a spell or attack when you suddenly felt frightened or extremely uncomfortable in a situation in which you didn't expect to feel that way?"

Our interviewers were explicitly trained to discount incidents in which the panic attacks occurred in response to real danger or to a clear phobic stimulus (e.g., someone with a snake phobia who had barely avoided stepping on a snake).[a] If the response to the probe question was still positive, we then assessed the remaining criteria, including questions about the maximum number of attacks in any 4-week period, the longest duration of worry about another attack, and the time required for the attack to develop (from the first symptom to a full attack). We asked the twin to identify the worst attack she or he remembered clearly and asked which of the 13 individual symptoms occurred.

We developed a definition of "broad panic disorder" that required at least two panic attacks per month, the emergence of a full attack within 30 minutes, and at least 4 of the 13 symptoms. We tested the validity of our definition in two ways: First, the multiple-threshold model provides a statistical test to determine whether the categories examined—here, broad panic disorder and panic attacks without meeting criteria for broad panic—really represent different measures of severity of the same underlying condition. These models passed this test easily. Second, we examined several external variables to validate our definition of panic-like syndromes, including panic-associated avoidance and panic-associated treatment seeking. We found surprisingly little difference on these variables between those who endorsed our broad panic and those who met full DSM-III-R criteria for panic disorder (Kendler, Gardner, & Prescott, 2001b). These results led us to feel reasonably comfortable with using this broad definition. For our twin analyses we employed a three-category definition of panic: no symptoms, panic attacks without broad panic, and broad panic.

The test–retest reliability of our panic definitions among 194 MF2 participants was in the good range: for any panic attacks, $\kappa = 0.53$ (95% CI = 0.23, 0.83) and for the three-category definition, $\kappa = 0.44$ (95% CI = 0.17, 0.71).

---

[a]Discriminating between what did and did not represent a real danger proved to be more challenging than we had expected. This problem is illustrated by the following case, which caused much debate among the senior staff of the VATSPSUD:

> Janet (not her real name) was a 54-year-old married twin who lived, along with her husband, in a remote area of western Virginia. She had always felt mildly uncomfortable when

(cont.)

SIDEBAR 4.3. *(continued)*

her husband traveled for his job. This concern became greater when a break-in and robbery was reported in a nearby town. Janet reported that her "attacks" started during the first business trip her husband had taken after she heard about the robbery. Each time, her attacks began with her "hearing" some unusual noise, such as the sound of footsteps outside. She would rush out, in a full-blown panic, convinced that someone was trying to break into the home, but always find no one there.

Did Janet have true panic attacks? Was she really in danger, living on her own in a remote area? We eventually decided to be conservative and not rate these as panic attacks. We were confronted with a number of such uncertain cases. If Janet's interview had been conducted on a different day or by a different interviewer, the information obtained might have led us to make a different decision. This story illustrates the impossibility of obtaining perfect measurement of psychiatric disorders.

definition, we observed only one pair of DZ male twins who both had panic disorder. This led to some difficulty estimating the correlation in this group.

The right portion of Figure 4.4 presents the genetic estimates based on our full model. As would be expected from the twin correlations, the results suggest that the heritability of panic-like syndromes is higher in males than in females (36% vs. 23%). However, not surprisingly given the imprecision of the correlations, these estimates are not significantly different in males and females. The estimated genetic proportion based on the model combining the sexes is 32%, with no evidence for shared environmental effects (see Appendix 4.3 for details).

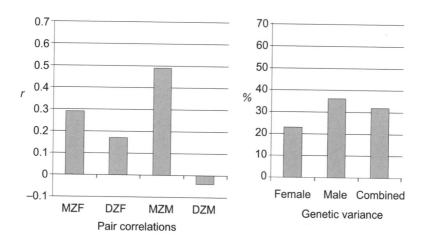

FIGURE 4.4. Pair similarity and estimated genetic variance for lifetime history of broadly defined panic disorder in same-sex twin pairs.

Discussion and Implications

The most interesting aspect of our results for panic disorder is how similar they are to the results obtained for the other mood and anxiety disorders we studied. Our expectation that panic disorder would stand out as having an especially high heritability was not realized. Since the first publications based on the VATSPSUD, panic disorder has also been examined in the VETS study (Scherrer et al., 2000). This study reported a heritability estimate for panic disorder of 43%, a bit higher than ours but within the confidence interval of our estimates.

In an earlier study of panic disorder with just our female–female sample (Kendler, Neale, Kessler, Heath, & Eaves, 1993d), we had used the twin method to ask a simple but clinically relevant question. Some individuals with panic disorder start to avoid going places—such as crowded shopping malls or even church—where their panic attacks might occur. We wondered whether panic disorder with such symptoms of avoidance and panic without any such avoidance behavior are qualitatively different from one another or whether they represent different levels of severity of the same underlying condition. Using the multiple-threshold model, our answer was clearly the latter. Our results suggest that individuals who experience panic disorder with avoidance—which in the extreme leads to agoraphobia (see the description later in this chapter)—have a more severe form of the same underlying condition as individuals who have panic disorder without avoidance.

We remained somewhat puzzled by the inconsistency between our findings of modest twin resemblance for panic disorder and the results of several early family studies that found the risk for panic disorder to be more than 10 times greater in relatives of individuals with panic disorder than in controls (e.g., Crowe, Noyes, Pauls, & Slymen, 1983; Mendlewicz, Papadimitriou, & Wilmotte, 1993). However, more recent studies have reported much lower familial aggregation for panic disorder, findings more consistent with our own results (e.g., Fyer et al., 1996; Maier, Lichtermann, Minges, Oehrlein, & Franke, 1993). One explanation is that all major family studies of panic disorder to date have been carried out using clinically ascertained probands who may be a quite selected and more severe sample than individuals in the community with panic disorder (Eaton et al., 1991). This is relevant because the etiological importance of familial/genetic factors might differ in treated and untreated cases of panic disorder. Alternatively, it is possible that studies of panic disorder in the general population may include a large proportion of people who do not have "true" panic disorder. As reflected in the case history of "Janet" (see Sidebar 4.3) and prior definitions of anxiety disorders, distinguishing between panic and nonpanic forms of anxiety is problematic, in part because panic attacks may occur as part of other anxiety disorders (Argyle & Roth, 1989; Marks, 1987).

GENERALIZED ANXIETY DISORDER

As noted in our discussion of panic disorder, prior to the development of DSM-III, what we now call generalized anxiety disorder (GAD) was part of the broad syndrome of anxiety neurosis. For good reason, the architects of DSM-III believed that panic disorder was sufficiently distinctive to become its own category. Phobias and obsessive–compulsive disorder also became separate categories. This left the question of what to do with the remaining patients who presented with anxiety as a prominent clinical feature but who did not manifest the paroxysmal severe attacks characteristic of panic disorder. The decision was to create a new category with the somewhat awkward name of "generalized anxiety disorder." The underlying logic was this: Whereas panic disorder was defined by brief attacks of severe anxiety, GAD would be characterized by relatively persistent, generalized, and "free-floating" anxiety. DSM-III-R listed 18 individual symptoms covering a broad range of physical, cognitive, and emotional aspects of anxiety.

Whereas panic disorder took off as a diagnostic category, GAD has remained something of a "poor stepchild" among the anxiety disorders. Some researchers and clinicians consider it to be a wastebasket category, not representing a true syndrome but used for individuals who do not fit neatly into the definitions of other anxiety disorders. Nowhere is the confusion about this syndrome more clearly demonstrated than in the wide shifts that have occurred in the required minimum duration of illness. In its first incarnation in the Research Diagnostic Criteria (Spitzer, Endicott, & Robins, 1975), GAD, like MD, required a minimum of 2 weeks' duration of symptoms. In DSM-III, without any empirical basis, the minimum duration was set at 1 month. Then DSM-III-R, on the basis of what some (ourselves included) regard as rather slender evidence, expanded the minimum duration to 6 months!

The criteria used to define GAD in the VATSPSUD are described in Sidebar 4.4. In nearly all of our analyses, we have used a 1-month duration of illness. Based on this definition, GAD was a relatively common lifetime disorder, diagnosed in 25.9% of women and 14.7% of men in our sample. These values are much higher than those reported in the NCS (6.6% in females and 3.6% in males), but these results are not comparable because the NCS used much more restrictive criteria.[3] When we applied to the VATSPSUD criteria similar to those used in the NCS, we obtained rates close to those found in the NCS: 3.5% in males and 5.8% in females (Hettema, Prescott, & Kendler, 2001b).

The results of our twin study of GAD are summarized in Figure 4.5. For both males and females, pair resemblance is higher for MZ than for DZ pairs. As with MD, resemblance for GAD is higher in MZ female than in MZ male pairs. Heritability of GAD is modest in both sexes, and no evidence was found for any role of shared environment in the etiology of GAD.

SIDEBAR 4.4. Assessment of Generalized Anxiety Disorder (GAD)

The DSM-III-R definition of GAD—the version used most commonly in this volume—includes 18 individual symptoms of anxiety divided into three broad categories of motor tension, autonomic hyperactivity, and vigilance and scanning. A minimum of 6 such symptoms are required to meet diagnostic criteria.

As in our assessment of MD (see Sidebar 4.1), we assessed GAD in two sections of our interviews: in the year prior to interview and lifetime GAD prior to the past year. Individuals were regarded as having a positive lifetime history of GAD if they reported an episode that met criteria in the past year and/or prior to the past year.

Our assessment methods differed for the two time periods.

In our "lifetime minus the past year" assessment, we used a slightly adapted version of the SCID interview for DSM-III-R diagnoses (Spitzer & Williams, 1985). A single probe question was used:

> "Thinking back over your entire life, except the last year, have you ever had a time when for at least 1 month you were anxious, nervous, or worried more days than not?"

For assessing GAD during the previous year, however, we used two probes, a variant of the preceding one and a second probe reflecting the somatic features of anxiety:

1. "During the last year, have you had a time lasting at least 5 days when you felt anxious, nervous, or worried most of the time?"
2. "During the last year, have you had a time lasting at least 5 days when most of the time your muscles felt tense or you felt jumpy or shaky inside?"

If one or both of the probe questions was answered positively, individuals were then asked whether, during their worst episode of anxiety, they had experienced the 18 specific "D" criteria for DSM-III-R GAD. If the answers to at least three of these questions were positive, we then asked several follow-up questions about the focus of the anxiety, the number and longest duration of prior episodes, age at onset, and treatment history.

In forming diagnoses, we did not use DSM-III-R criterion "C," which requires that GAD not be diagnosed if it occurs only during an episode of MD. For the analyses reported in this chapter, we use a 1-month minimum duration rather than the 6 months specified by DSM-III-R.[a]

The test–retest reliability of GAD was calculated for 194 individuals reinterviewed with an average interval of 30 days between interviews. For 1-month GAD, the test–retest reliability was fair: $\kappa = 0.33$ (95% CI = 0.14, 0.51).

[a]A contentious issue in the conceptualization of GAD is its relationship with MD. Not infrequently, these disorders co-occur in the same individual at the same time. We chose to ignore this criterion because we did not want to prejudge the nature of the relationship between GAD and MD. We examined the impact of applying this diagnostic rule on results of our twin modeling

(continued)

SIDEBAR 4.4. *(continued)*

and found it was modest (Kendler, Neale, Kessler, Heath, & Eaves, 1992b), a result we took as further justification for our approach.

We also took an empirical approach to defining a minimum duration of illness (Kendler et al., 1992b). Requiring 6 months of illness resulted in lifetime prevalence rates about one-fourth those needed for a definition requiring a 1-month duration. Based on the multiple-threshold model (see Chapter 3), we found that individuals with shorter or longer durations of GAD could be seen as having differing levels of severity of the same underlying condition. Because we had much more statistical power with the more common 1-month definition of GAD, we have used this definition in nearly all subsequent analyses in the VATSPSUD.

As with most of the other disorders studied in this chapter, the model that required equal estimates for men and women did not fit significantly worse than the model allowing sex differences. The estimated genetic proportion based on combining the sexes was 28% (95% CI = 2%, 38%).

Discussion and Implications

Only two other meaningful twin studies of GAD have been conducted. Among 49 twin pairs in which one twin was seen in a clinical treatment setting and had an anxiety disorder, the risk for GAD was higher among the MZ (40%) than among the DZ (10%) cotwins (Skre, Onstad, Torgersen, Lygren, & Kringlen, 1993), a result consistent with a strong genetic effect. In the study using methods most similar to ours, Scherrer et al. (2000) examined GAD

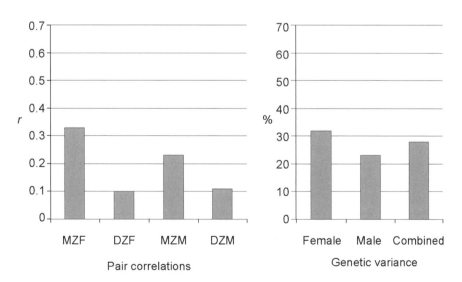

FIGURE 4.5. Pair similarity and estimated genetic variance for lifetime history of generalized anxiety disorder in same-sex twin pairs.

with a minimum 1-month duration in 3,362 male twin pairs from the VETS. The lifetime prevalence in this sample was a bit lower than in ours (12.3%). The estimated heritability of GAD was 38%, somewhat higher than that obtained in the VATSPSUD but within the confidence intervals of our estimates. As in our study, there was no evidence for an effect of shared environment on risk for GAD.

Our findings lead to two observations that have particularly interesting implications for the definition and etiology of GAD. First, the heritability of GAD is only slightly lower than that of panic disorder. This argues against the hypothesis that when anxiety neurosis was divided by the architects of DSM-III into panic disorder and GAD, all the biological cases of anxiety neurosis were classified as panic disorder and those classified as GAD constitute a "ragbag" set of cases arising from psychosocial dysfunction. It appears that the contribution of genetic factors is of similar magnitude for both the paroxysmal severe anxiety attacks in panic disorder and the chronic free-floating anxiety of GAD.

A second observation is that the heritability of GAD is similar to that obtained for MD. Both conditions are characterized by chronic dysphoria (unpleasant mood). This raises the interesting question of the relationship between the genetic risk factors for MD and GAD. We will examine this in some detail in Chapter 11.

PHOBIAS

Phobias are a common type of anxiety disorder characterized by a relatively persistent, irrational, and dysfunctional fear of specific objects or situations. The assessment of what is irrational and dysfunctional requires some judgment. For example, fear of being attacked when walking alone at night may be reasonable in some areas of our cities and should not form the basis for a psychiatric diagnosis.

We spare the reader the typical table seen in many textbooks of abnormal psychology containing literally dozens of Greek terms for specific kinds of phobias. From a research perspective, the more pragmatic issue is finding the optimal way to group the wide diversity of individual phobias. As is common with such diagnostic questions, among mental health researchers, there are "lumpers" and "splitters." The most influential lumpers in recent times have been the authors of the recent DSM editions (American Psychiatric Association, 1980, 1987, 1994), which reduce the richness of phobias to three classes: agoraphobia, social phobia, and simple (or specific) phobia. The extreme splitters would argue that every feared object deserves its own phobia subtype.

In the VATSPSUD, we decided to take a middle ground. We assessed a lifetime history of phobias using an adaptation of the Phobic Disorders section of the Diagnostic Interview Schedule (DIS), Version III-A (Robins & Helzer, 1985), which in turn was based on the DSM-III criteria. We assessed 22 specific unreasonable fears grouped into five categories: animal phobia, blood–injury phobia, situational phobia, social phobia, and agoraphobia (literally "fear of open places" but now defining a broader syndrome).

Our approach differed from that adopted in the DSMs by dividing the category of simple or specific phobia into three distinct groups: animal, situational, and blood–injury. We were concerned that irrational fears of animals and specific situations—especially closed-in places and high places—might be partly etiologically distinct. Phobias of physical injury or seeing blood differ in one important way from the more typical phobias (Marks, 1988). In individuals with typical phobias, exposure to the phobic stimulus (such as snakes, heights, or public speaking) reliably produces increased activity in the *sympathetic* nervous system as manifested by increases in pulse rate and blood pressure, as well as sweating and flushing. By contrast, when individuals with blood–injury phobias are exposed to phobic stimuli (such as needles or blood), they typically experience increased *parasympathetic* activity, manifested by a slowing of the heart rate and a reduction in blood pressure, leading to pallor and sometimes fainting.

In addition to classification of phobia types, another important diagnostic issue is how one determines whether a fear is associated with dysfunction. Three criteria that have been used to judge dysfunction are level of distress, degree of functional impairment, and treatment seeking. In the VATSPSUD, we employed a definition of significant objective impact on behavior (see Sidebar 4.5).

Theories of Etiology

Phobias are of particular interest to genetic epidemiologists because there are several well-developed competing etiological theories that can be tested with data from twins. We focus here on three of them, each of which suggests that phobias arise mainly from one of the three domains of risk factors included in our twin models: individual-specific environment, family environment, or genes.

One school of thought theorizes that phobias arise as a result of classical conditioning from the accidental pairing of benign stimuli with fear-inducing objects or situations (Eysenck, 1979; Marks, 1987; Rachman, 1977; Watson & Rayner, 1920). For example, you could develop a lifelong fear of dogs because, as a 3-year-old child, you had the terrifying experience of being knocked down and bitten by a large dog. This theory postulates that phobias should be entirely environmental in origin. Furthermore, it would predict that any twin resemblance for phobias should result only from the correlated exposure among family members to such a coincidental pairing of stimuli. For example, twins might share a phobia of dogs because they were both attacked by the vicious dog owned by the next-door neighbor. Given that exposure to phobic stimuli is expected to be mostly random, this etiological theory would predict that most of the risk for phobias is due to individual-specific environ-

SIDEBAR 4.5. Assessment of Phobias

Diagnostic criteria for phobias require a persistent irrational fear, accompanied by dysfunction or impairment. We assessed lifetime history of specific fears of 22 objects or situations by asking:

"Have you ever had an unreasonable fear of . . . ?"

If the respondent answered yes, we asked additional questions to address whether the fear was unreasonable and whether avoidance of the feared object or situation had ever had a significant objective behavioral impact on his or her life. For example, behavioral impairment would be indicated if a respondent with fear of flying turned down a desired job promotion and a needed pay increase because the new job required extensive airplane travel, or if a respondent with fear of snakes repeatedly refused to go on family camping trips despite resulting marital strife. The behavioral impairment also could be as simple as an individual with a fear of elevators always taking the stairs, even if that meant climbing many flights in hot weather. Respondents who suffered substantial distress from their irrational fears but never changed their behavior to avoid the feared objects were not rated as having a phobia.

The fears were grouped into five classes:

1. *Animal phobia*—bugs, spiders, mice, snakes, bats, other animals
2. *Blood–injury phobia*—sight of blood, needles or injections, dentists or hospitals, certain diseases (such as cancer or AIDS)
3. *Situational phobia*—tunnels, other closed places, bridges, airplanes, other high places
4. *Social phobia*—meeting new people, giving a speech, using public bathrooms, eating in public
5. *Agoraphobia*—going out of the house alone, being in crowds, being in open spaces

We also formed a category of "any phobia," which included the preceding categories plus responses to the item: "Is there anything else you've been unreasonably terrified to do or be near?" and which did not fit in one of the other categories (e.g., fear of water or darkness).

The test–retest reliability for our assessment of phobia was calculated based on 383 individuals reinterviewed with an average interval of 30 days between interviews. The test–retest reliability estimates were fair to good: any phobia, $\kappa = 0.45$ (95% CI = 0.34, 0.55); animal, $\kappa = 0.40$ (95% CI = 0.23, 0.56); blood–injury, $\kappa = 0.30$ (95% CI = 0.10, 0.51); situational, $\kappa = 0.43$ (95% CI = 0.29, 0.57); social, $\kappa = 0.44$ (95% CI = 0.25, 0.63); and agoraphobia, $\kappa = 0.50$ (95% CI = 0.27, 0.74).

ment (i.e., experienced by one twin in a pair but not the other), with a bit due to shared environmental factors such as the dog next door.

Social learning theory provides the basis of another etiological theory of phobias. Among human and nonhuman primates, the fear of objects or situations can be learned from observing the fear responses of others (Bandura, 1986). Many phobias begin in childhood (Burke, Burke, Regier, & Rae, 1990), when other family members, particularly parents, are potential sources for their "vicarious" acquisition. For example, if you repeatedly see your mother scream and jump up on a chair when she sees a mouse in the kitchen, it is not unreasonable that you may acquire the same reaction without ever having been, yourself, directly traumatized by a mouse (and despite the substantial exposure to benign views of mice, such as Mickey and Minnie). If the social learning theory of phobia acquisition is correct, this would predict that phobias are entirely environmental in origin but that many of the environmental factors would be shared among members of a twin pair (who would both be exposed to their parents as possible phobic role models).

As first observed by Darwin (1877), the choice of feared objects and situations in phobias is not random (Marks, 1987; Ohman, 1986). This has been explained by two related theories of inherited phobia-proneness: (1) a preparedness to develop conditioned fears of certain stimuli (Seligman, 1971) or (2) innate fears that require no learning (Gray, 1982). Both theories suggest that through natural selection man has evolved an inherited predisposition to form phobic reactions to certain stimuli. (The theories differ as to whether exposure plus subsequent conditioning is required to manifest this predisposition.) Both theories provide an explanation as to why individuals are more prone to form fears of snakes, spiders, rats, and high places than of objects that are considerably more dangerous in the modern world, such as handguns, electric outlets, and knives. This would occur, the theories predict, because only objects or situations that reflected true danger over the tens of thousands of years of human evolution would produce phobia-proneness. Guns, knives, and electric outlets are too new in evolutionary time to have yet produced enough selection for fears of them.

If there is an inherited form of phobia-proneness, it is likely that it would have evolved through a process called *stabilizing selection* (Hartl, 1980). Stabilizing selection arises when having a moderate level of a trait is more "fit" from an evolutionary perspective than having a high or low level. In the case of phobias, it was probably best for our ancestors to be moderately afraid of what the world threw at them. If phobia-proneness was too low, they would get into danger too easily. If phobia-proneness was too high, they would spend too much time and energy on their fears and avoid many situations that could lead to good things such as food, safety, and sexual relations. Stabilizing selection results in substantial additive genetic variation in populations (Hartl, 1980; Lande, 1976; Mather, 1966). Thus the inherited-phobia-proneness theory predicts that there should be significant genetic influences on the predisposition to phobias.

Phobias were quite common in the VATSPSUD. The lifetime diagnosis of any phobia was met by 30.0% of the females and 21.9% of males in our sample. Figure 4.1 shows the prevalences for each of the phobia subtypes. They range from a low of about 4% for agoraphobia to a high for situational phobias of 13% in females and 10% in males. These values are similar to those found in national epidemiological studies. Based on DSM-III-R definitions, the NCS examined three types of phobias, for which they found the following lifetime prevalences (combined across males and females): agoraphobia, 6.7%; simple phobia, 11.3%; and social phobia, 13.3% (Magee, Eaton, Wittchen, McGonagle, & Kessler, 1996). In the Epidemiologic Catchment Area Study, the lifetime prevalences of any phobia varied widely between sites, ranging from 7.8% in New Haven to 23.3% in Baltimore (Robins et al., 1984).

Genetic and Environmental Influences

We describe the results separately for our twin analyses of any phobia and each phobia subtype, as the pattern of results differed for some subtypes. As shown in Figure 4.6, twin resemblance for the lifetime diagnosis of any phobia was substantially greater in MZ than in DZ pairs for both FF and MM twin pairs. The results from our model fitting are summarized in Figure 4.7 (and details are in Appendices 4.2 and 4.3). For females, the full model estimates the heritability of liability to any phobia to be 31%, and the effect of the shared environment is zero. The pattern of results in males is very similar except that the heritability estimates are somewhat smaller. Examining the two sexes together, we found (as we did for all the phobia subtypes) that heritability estimates in females and males were not significantly different. The estimated genetic variance based on the combined sample is 27%.

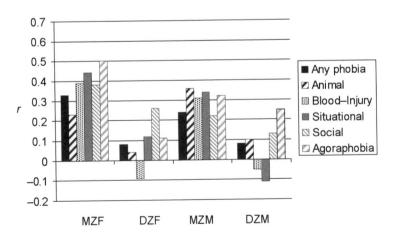

FIGURE 4.6. Similarity of same-sex twin pairs for lifetime history of phobias.

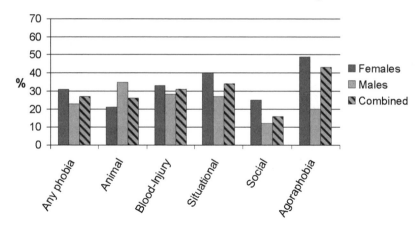

FIGURE 4.7. Estimated genetic proportions of variance in risk for phobias.

Animal Phobia

In the course of our work with the VATSPSUD, we came to regard animal phobia as the "archetypal" phobia. The definition was simple and the phobic stimulus easily and clearly delineated—an irrational fear of any living creature that significantly influenced behavior. We found a large sex difference in prevalence of animal phobias, with lifetime prevalence estimates of 10.4% in females and 5.2% in males. The pattern of twin resemblance in Figure 4.6 shows modest twin similarity that is greater in MZ than in DZ pairs and is a bit larger in males than in females. When examining the two sexes separately, we found no evidence for shared environmental effects. The estimated heritability of animal phobias was rather higher in males than in females, but this was not a significant difference. The estimated heritability of animal phobias based on combining the male and female data is 26%.

Blood–Injury Phobia

Blood–injury phobias were, along with agoraphobia, the rarest in the VATSPSUD, with lifetime prevalence rates of 6.0% and 5.8% in females and males, respectively. This lack of a sex difference in prevalences is noteworthy—something rarely seen in anxiety disorders, in which female preponderance is the rule.

As noted earlier, blood–injury phobia stands out from all the other phobias. We hypothesized that the pattern of twin resemblance for blood–injury phobia might differ substantially from that of other, more "typical" phobias. As shown in Figure 4.6, the twin-pair correlations for MZ pairs are similar to those seen for the other phobia subtypes. The DZ correlations are a bit unusual in that they are actually negative in both males and females. However, the confidence intervals around these correlations are very broad and not really different (from a statistical perspective) from those seen for most of the other subtypes (see Appendix 4.1).

The results of twin modeling are shown in Figure 4.7. Heritability for blood–injury phobia was estimated to be about 30% in both males and females, with no evidence for shared environmental factors. When we combined the data across the sexes, heritability was estimated at 31%.

Situational Phobia

Second perhaps to animal phobias, our category of situational phobias includes the most typical kinds of phobic fears—closed-in places, high places, and airplanes. It was the most common class of phobias, with lifetime prevalences of 13.0% in females and 9.5% in males. The pattern of resemblance, shown in Figure 4.6, is similar to that seen for the other phobias (except perhaps for the negative DZ correlation in male pairs).

Our results suggest no evidence for shared environmental effects on liability to develop situational phobias. All the pair resemblance was estimated to be due to genetic factors. When the sexes were examined together, the estimated heritability was estimated to be 34%. The remaining liability was due to individual-specific environmental effects.

Social Phobia

Along with agoraphobia, social phobia includes a set of phobic stimuli that are somewhat less circumscribed than those seen with the more typical animal and situational phobias. In the VATSPSUD, our assessment asked explicitly about four fears: meeting new people, giving a speech, using public bathrooms, and eating in public. The prevalence for lifetime social phobia in our sample was 8.0% in females and 6.3% in males.

Pair resemblance for social phobia was similar to that seen for other phobias among MZ twins but somewhat different for DZ pairs (Figure 4.6). The correlation in DZ pairs was higher than half that seen in MZ twins, and this trend is particularly marked in females. This means that for both males and females, there was evidence for both genetic and shared environmental effects. When we combined the data for males and females, the sources of risk for social phobia were estimated as 17% genetic and 15% shared environmental, with the remaining 68% due to individual-specific environmental effects.

Agoraphobia

Although the literal meaning of agoraphobia is "fear of the marketplace" (*agora* in Greek), the term has come to have a rather different meaning. We operationalized it as an irrational fear of going out of the house alone, being in crowds, or being in open spaces. Of all the phobias, agoraphobia has perhaps the most diffuse, nonlocalized kind of phobic stimuli. In this way, it is an atypical phobia.

As shown in Figure 4.6, twin resemblance for agoraphobia was particularly strong in female MZ pairs, and the difference in resemblance in MZ and DZ pairs was more pronounced in females than in males. As would be expected from this pattern, when the sexes were examined separately (Figure 4.7), heritability of liability to agoraphobia was considerably higher in females than in males, and there was a modest shared environmental effect for males.

Despite the large differences in parameter estimates between males and females, these were not significantly different. We do not know whether this result means that the sources of individual differences in agoraphobia are the same in the two sexes or that they are different but that we lack the power to detect the difference because agoraphobia is a relatively infrequent disorder. Our analysis combining male and female twins suggested that individual differences in liability to agoraphobia were due only to genes and individual-specific environment. The level of heritability, 43%, was higher than that seen with most other phobias.

Discussion and Implications

In a recent review and meta-analysis of family and twin studies on anxiety disorders with our colleague Jack Hettema (Hettema, Neale, & Kendler, 2001a), we identified four family studies of phobias that met our inclusion criteria for methodological quality. The results of these studies agreed well with one another in suggesting that phobias clearly ran in families, with close relatives of an individual with phobias having a substantially increased risk of having a phobia themselves. Nearly all of the twin studies of "phobia" have in fact relied on self-report questionnaires that assessed fears rather than on interviews that diagnosed clinical phobias (Neale & Fulker, 1984; Phillips, Fulker, & Rose, 1987; Rose, Miller, Pogue-Geile, & Cardwell, 1981; Rose & Ditto, 1983; Stevenson, Batten, & Cherner, 1992; Torgersen, 1979). These studies have consistently suggested that genetic factors contribute to these phobia-like fears. Twin studies of clinically defined phobias, aside from those coming from the VATSPSUD (Kendler, Neale, Kessler, Heath, & Eaves, 1992c; Kendler, Karkowski, & Prescott, 1999b; Kendler, Myers, Prescott, & Neale, 2001c; Neale et al., 1994b), have been few and far between. Two earlier studies had sample sizes too small for useful analysis, although both found concordance rates to be higher in MZ than in DZ pairs (Carey & Gottesman, 1981; Torgersen, 1983). Recently, one study of social phobia in adolescent female twins reported heritability estimates of 28% and, in contrast to our findings, no evidence for shared environmental effects (Nelson et al., 2000).

What can we conclude from our twin study of phobias? First, we would argue that the results support the inherited phobia-proneness model. Genetic effects were detected for any phobia and for each of the five phobia subtypes. The magnitude of such effects ranged from quite modest (for social phobia) to moderately robust (for agoraphobia in females).

Second, with the possible exception of social phobia, we found no consistent evidence for shared environmental effects on phobias. These results are inconsistent with the predictions of social learning theory for phobias if, as seems plausible, parents or other household members are prime models from whom phobic fears are learned. Our results do suggest that if social learning plays any role in the etiology of phobias, it is most likely to have its effects on social phobia.

Third, the largest proportion of risk for phobias was the result of individual-specific environment. What is unclear is what proportion of these effects reflects true environmental factors—such as those predicted by the conditioning theory of phobia formation—and what reflects unreliability of measurement. We do know that the reliability of our definitions of phobias was far from perfect, so there is surely some error in our measurement. (We consider the effects of measurement error on heritability estimates for phobias in Chapter 12.) However, these results are at least partly consistent with the conditioning theory of phobia formation.

Fourth, when we began these analyses, we wondered, given the dramatic differences in its clinical presentation, whether blood–injury phobia would prove to be very different from the other phobias. At least with respect to the broad breakdown of risk factors into their genetic and environmental constituents, it does not look different from the other, more typical phobias.

Fifth, these results do not address what are perhaps the most interesting questions about the role of genetic and environmental risk factors in phobias. For example, how closely related are these risk factors for the individual phobia subtypes? Would we find one large set of genetic risk factors that predisposes to all phobia subtypes—so that the type of phobia that an individual develops is solely the result of particular environmental experiences? Or would we find distinct genetic risk factors for the individual phobias? Are there environmental risk factors that predispose to more than one phobia subtype? We address these and other complex questions in Chapter 11.

SUMMARY

What are the "take-home messages" from this chapter—our first look at common psychiatric disorders through the eyes of the psychiatric geneticist? We would emphasize two. First, genetic factors make significant but not overwhelming contributions to individual differences in risk for the common mood and anxiety disorders. This was true for all the disorders we examined. Second, with the possible exception of social phobia, we found no convincing evidence that shared environment contributes substantially to risk for these conditions.

These results are just a start. Think of them, perhaps, as the opening themes of a symphony. We have not asked how valid the assumptions of the twin method are when applied to these disorders. We have not examined how the genetic and environmental estimates might change when we correct for the effects of measurement error (recalling that our estimates of individual environment are confounded with measurement error). We have not explored the specificity of the genetic and environmental risks for these individual disorders, nor whether genetic effects in males and females are the same or different. Finally, we have not asked how genetic risk factors might relate to or interact with environmental risk factors. These important issues will be examined closely in Parts IV and V of this book.

NOTES

1. Some evidence suggests that the more detailed the questioning about MD, the higher the observed prevalence. In the Lundby study, which used repeated personal interviews over 25 years of all inhabitants of a delimited area in Sweden (Hagnell, Lanke, Rorsman, & Ojesjo, 1982), lifetime risks for MD in a birth cohort somewhat younger than our sample (born 1957–1972) were even higher than in the VATSPSUD: 30% for men and 49% for women.

2. Participants were interviewed at ages 15, 16, 18, and 21. At age 21, 18% of the sample reported a lifetime history of MD. However, if all four interviews were examined together, 37% of the sample reported meeting lifetime criteria for MD at least once. Furthermore, very few individuals at age 21 described depressive symptoms occurring earlier in their lives that they had not reported when they were younger.

3. The NCS required 6 months' minimal duration and eliminated cases in which the GAD episodes occurred only when the individual also had MD.

APPENDIX 4.1. Sample Sizes, Prevalences, and Pair Resemblance for Internalizing Disorders

Disorder	Sex	n	Prevalence (%)	Zygosity	No. of pairs	Tetrachoric correlation	95% CI	Odds ratio*	95% CI
Major depression (MD)	F	2,154	34.4	MZ	673	0.40	0.29, 0.51	3.02	2.15, 4.23
				DZ	469	0.24	0.10, 0.38	1.90	1.29, 2.80
	M	2,929	28.5	MZ	857	0.32	0.21, 0.43	2.45	1.78, 3.39
				DZ	644	0.12	-0.02, 0.25	1.38	0.96, 1.99
Panic disorder (three-level)	F	1,996	Attacks = 13.6 Broad = 5.5	MZ	555	0.29	0.11, 0.47	a	
				DZ	381	0.17	-0.04, 0.39	a	
	M	2,921	Attacks = 5.2 Broad = 2.0	MZ	701	0.40	0.17, 0.62	a	
				DZ	484	-0.04	-0.44, 0.36	a	
Generalized anxiety disorder (GAD)	F	2,154	25.9	MZ	596	0.33	0.20, 0.47	2.61	1.73, 3.93
				DZ	434	0.10	-0.06, 0.27	1.33	0.85, 2.09
	M	2,929	14.7	MZ	701	0.23	0.07, 0.40	2.15	1.26, 3.68
				DZ	485	0.11	-0.09, 0.31	1.43	0.76, 2.68
Any phobia	F	1,925	30.0	MZ	501	0.33	0.19, 0.47	2.51	1.66, 3.80
				DZ	326	0.08	-0.10, 0.26	1.24	0.76, 2.02
	M	2,922	21.9	MZ	701	0.24	0.10, 0.37	2.00	1.34, 2.99
				DZ	484	0.08	-0.09, 0.26	1.29	0.77, 2.16
Animal phobia	F	1,925	10.4	MZ	501	0.23	0.00, 0.46	2.28	1.03, 5.04
				DZ	326	0.04	-0.25, 0.33	1.15	0.42, 3.16

	N	%		Pairs	r	95% CI	OR*	95% CI
M	2,922	5.2	MZ	701	0.36	0.10, 0.62	4.59	1.64, 12.89
			DZ	484	0.10	-0.26, 0.46	1.55	0.34, 6.97
Blood–injury phobia F	1,925	6.0	MZ	501	0.39	0.13, 0.65	4.66	1.74, 12.49
			DZ	326	-0.09	-0.52, 0.35	0.68	0.09, 5.32
M	2,921	5.8	MZ	701	0.31	0.07, 0.56	3.59	1.40, 9.18
			DZ	484	-0.05	-0.46, 0.36	0.80	0.10, 6.17
Situational phobia F	1,925	13.0	MZ	501	0.44	0.26, 0.62	4.51	2.38, 8.53
			DZ	326	0.12	-0.13, 0.37	1.48	0.66, 3.30
M	2,921	9.5	MZ	701	0.34	0.15, 0.52	3.37	1.74, 6.54
			DZ	484	-0.11	-0.39, 0.17	0.64	0.19, 2.16
Agoraphobia F	1,925	6.1	MZ	501	0.50	0.26, 0.74	7.55	2.87, 19.83
			DZ	326	0.11	-0.27, 0.50	1.59	0.34, 7.33
M	2,922	4.0	MZ	701	0.32	0.01, 0.63	4.25	1.18, 15.33
			DZ	484	0.25	-0.08, 0.58	2.88	0.80, 10.42
Social phobia F	1,925	9.1	MZ	501	0.38	0.16, 0.60	4.06	1.83, 8.98
			DZ	326	0.26	-0.02, 0.55	2.59	0.97, 6.91
M	2,922	6.3	MZ	701	0.22	-0.03, 0.46	2.38	0.95, 5.97
			DZ	484	0.13	-0.19, 0.44	1.70	0.49, 5.97

aNot calculated because definition had more than two categories.
*Odds ratio is odds of a twin being affected if the cotwin has the disorder versus if the cotwin does not have the disorder.

APPENDIX 4.2. Model-Fitting Information: Change in Fit Relative to Full Model for Male and Female Twin Pairs Analyzed Separately

Disorder	Model	df	LRT Females	LRT Males
Major depression	AE	1	0.3*	0.0*
(MD)	CE	1	3.1	5.0
	E	2	52.2	31.8
Panic disorder	AE	1	< 0.1	0.0*
	CE	1	< 0.1	2.4
	E	2	11.8	8.9
Generalized anxiety	AE	1	0.0*	0.0
disorder (GAD)	CE	1	4.1	0.9
	E	2	21.8	8.3
Any phobia	AE	1	0.0*	0.0*
	CE	1	3.9	1.5
	E	2	18.9	11.7
Animal phobia	AE	1	0.0	0.0*
	CE	1	0.8	1.3
	E	2	3.3	6.5
Blood–injury phobia	AE	1	0.0*	0.0*
	CE	1	2.0	1.3
	E	2	6.0	4.9
Situational phobia	AE	1	0.0*	0.0*
	CE	1	3.6	3.2
	E	2	18.1	7.9
Agoraphobia	AE	1	0.0*	0.2
	CE	1	2.8	0.2
	E	2	13.0	5.8
Social phobia	AE	1	0.3	0.0
	CE	1	0.5	0.1
	E	2	13.1	3.2

Note. LRT is likelihood ratio test, representing the fit of this model compared to the full (ACE) model.
*Best-fitting model by Akaike's Information Criterion (AIC; Akaike, 1987); if no *, full model is best (or the fits of AE and CE cannot be distinguished).

APPENDIX 4.3. Parameter Estimates from Full and Best-Fitting Models, for Females, Males, and Sexes Combined

Disorder	Group	Model	Test of sex differences[a]	a^2 (%)	95% CI	c^2 (%)	95% CI	e^2 (%)	95% CI
Major depression (MD)	Females	Full		32	0, 51	8	0, 37	60	49, 72
		AE		41	30, 51	—		59	48, 70
	Males	Full		31	4, 41	0	0, 21	69	59, 79
		AE		31	20, 41	—		69	59, 80
	Combined	Full	1.1*	36	12, 43	2	0, 30	62	52, 72
Panic disorder	Females	Full		23	0, 45	6	0, 36	71	55, 89
	Males	Full		36	0, 56	0	0, 39	64	44, 88
		AE		36	12, 56	—		64	44, 88
	Combined	Full	0.2*	32	0, 44	0	0, 35	68	56, 82
Generalized anxiety disorder (GAD)	Females	Full		32	1, 44	0	0, 24	68	56, 81
		AE		32	19, 44	—		68	56, 81
	Males	Full		23	0, 38	0	0, 29	77	62, 93
		AE		23	8, 38	—		77	62, 92
	Combined	Full	1.3*	28	2, 38	0	0, 21	72	62, 82
Any phobia	Females	Full		31	0, 44	0	0, 24	69	56, 83
		AE*		31	17, 44	—		69	56, 83
	Males	Full		23	0, 35	0	0, 26	77	65, 91
		AE		23	10, 35	—		77	65, 90
	Combined	Full	0.6*	27	5, 36	0	0, 18	73	64, 83
Animal phobia	Females	Full		21	0, 41	0	0, 30	79	59, 100
	Males	Full		35	0, 58	0	0, 42	65	42, 92
		AE		35	8, 58	—		65	42, 92

(continued)

APPENDIX 4.3. (continued)

Disorder	Group	Model	Test of sex differences[a]	a^2 (%)	95% CI	c^2 (%)	95% CI	e^2 (%)	95% CI
Animal phobia (cont.)	Combined	Full	0.7*	26	0, 42	0	0, 28	74	58, 91
Blood–injury phobia	Females	Full		33	0, 57	0	0, 38	67	43, 93
		AE		33	7, 57	—		67	43, 93
	Males	Full		28	0, 51	0	0, 38	72	50, 97
		AE		28	3, 51	—		72	49, 96
	Combined	Full	< 0.1*	31	0, 47	0	0, 28	69	53, 88
Situational phobia	Females	Full		40	0, 57	0	0, 34	60	43, 78
		AE		40	22, 57	—		60	43, 78
	Males	Full		27	0, 45	0	0, 25	73	55, 92
		AE		27	8, 45	—		73	55, 92
	Combined	Full	1.0*	34	12, 46	0	0, 30	66	54, 79
Agoraphobia	Females	Full		49	0, 69	0	0, 48	51	31, 77
		AE		49	23, 69	—		51	31, 77
	Males	Full		20	0, 61	14	0, 49	66	39, 94
	Combined	Full	0.6*	43	0, 60	0	0, 48	57	41, 77
Social phobia	Females	Full		25	0, 59	14	0, 49	61	41, 83
	Males	Full		12	0, 42	8	0, 35	80	58, 99
	Combined	Full	1.7*	16	0, 45	13	0, 38	71	55, 87

[a]Change in LRT comparing MF equality and MF different models; all tests $df = 2$.
*Consistent with male–female equality (based on AIC).

CHAPTER FIVE

Externalizing and Substance Use Disorders

In this chapter we describe the results from VATSPSUD for twin analyses of externalizing, eating, and substance use disorders. There is often resistance to the notion of genetic influences on conditions that are typically viewed as arising from poor self-control and/or deprived environments. These disorders obviously have a volitional component different from that seen for the mood and anxiety disorders. That is, whereas anxiety and depressive conditions are things that people "have," these disorders relate to things that people "do." However, in our study and in others, the genetic influences on liability are as large (or larger) for substance use disorders as for mood and anxiety disorders. In this age of widespread acceptance of biological psychiatry and the pharmacological treatment of mood states, we should not forget that until recently there was great skepticism about the existence of genetic influences for any psychiatric condition (e.g., Szasz, 1984).

We first consider antisocial behavior in childhood and adulthood and then disorders associated with misuse of licit and illicit substances, and we conclude by examining bulimia. As in Chapter 4, we describe the clinical features of each disorder and summarize what is known about its prevalence in the general population. We include sidebars describing how we assessed the disorder in the VATSPSUD, present the results from our twin analyses, and discuss how these results fit into the larger literature on genetic influences. Details of our analyses of externalizing disorders can be found in Appendices 5.1–5.3. The chapter concludes with a discussion of how genetic and environmental factors might contribute to risk for liability to develop these disorders.

81

ANTISOCIAL BEHAVIOR

Antisocial behavior is typically grouped into two clinical disorders based on the age of the person affected. Conduct disorder (CD) refers to antisocial behaviors occurring in childhood and early adolescence (usually defined as before age 15, but sometimes before 18). CD encompasses several types of deviant behavior, including delinquency (skipping school, running away from home, lying), property crime (theft, vandalism, setting fires), cruelty (torturing animals), and violent or aggressive behavior (starting fights, assault, robbery, rape).

Antisocial personality disorder (ASP) refers to behaviors displayed in late adolescence and adulthood. The DSM-III-R defines ASP as a "pervasive pattern of disregard for and violation of the rights of others" (American Psychiatric Association, 1987, p. 649) as evidenced by three or more of the following behaviors: illegal activities, deceitfulness, impulsivity, aggressiveness, recklessness, consistent irresponsibility, and lack of remorse. The DSM also requires a history of CD for the diagnosis of ASP. However, so that we could view these two syndromes as distinct entities, we did not use this criterion in the VATSPSUD. We therefore employ the term *adult antisocial behavior* (AASB) to refer to our definition (see Sidebar 5.1).

These disorders are characterized by a habitual pattern of behavior, not just isolated incidents. Individuals with CD and ASP engage in these behaviors intentionally. A boy who gets into fights because he cannot control his anger when taunted by the neighborhood bully has poor impulse control but probably does not have CD. A woman who is a heavy drug user may be neglectful of her children and unable to hold a job, but she may not have ASP. Another important feature of CD and ASP is that individuals with these disorders commonly experience little remorse for their actions. This is the classic feature of sociopaths: They are not constrained by society's rules and may even enjoy flouting them.

Clinical studies suggest that the rates of CD are much higher among boys than girls. However, epidemiological studies suggest that the sex difference is less marked. One cohort study of 15-year-olds found that CD occurred among 8.6–12.1% of males (depending on the definition employed) compared with 7.5–9.5% of females (Fergusson, Horwood, & Lynskey, 1993). Some researchers argue that these sex differences exist because the definition of CD reflects disruptive behaviors that are more often shown by males and that are likely to lead to treatment or incarceration. Girls may engage in other sorts of behavior that are equally antisocial but are less noticeable and not illegal, including lying, manipulative behavior, and acting out sexually. Some evidence suggests that CD problems in females tend to be limited to adolescence, whereas males are more likely to have enduring patterns of antisocial behavior (Fergusson & Horwood, 2002; Moffitt, Caspi, Rutter, & Silva, 2001). Most individuals with CD appear to grow out of their behaviors as they become more mature. The prevalence of antisocial behavior among adults is much lower.

SIDEBAR 5.1. Assessment of Antisocial Behavior

In the VATSPSUD we used items based on DSM-III-R criteria to assess conduct disorder (CD) and adult antisocial behavior (AASB). CD was assessed in the MF1, MF2, and FF4 interviews; AASB was assessed at MF2 and FF4. The interviews used the same criteria but somewhat different response formats, which are described here.

CONDUCT DISORDER

We assessed CD using 11 items inquiring about the frequency of playing hooky from school, running away overnight, telling lies, stealing, starting fires, engaging in vandalism, being cruel to animals, starting fights, using a weapon in a fight, hurting others, and committing robbery.[a] Individuals were considered to meet criteria for CD if they were positive for three or more items. We formed two sets of diagnoses: CD-15, which indicates whether or not individuals met criteria for CD prior to age 15, and CD-18, which indicates whether or not they met criteria for CD prior to age 18.[b]

In our MF1 interview, we asked the CD items in a yes/no format: for example, "Before the age of 18, did you play hooky a lot from school?" Individuals were considered positive for a criterion if they answered "yes." We then asked, "How old were you when this began?"

Based on feedback from the interviewers in our MF1 study, we were concerned that the items were being underendorsed, perhaps because respondents were reluctant to admit to these behaviors to an interviewer. Evidence from other studies had suggested that behaviors seen as socially unacceptable are more frequently disclosed when more anonymous data collection methods are used. When it came time to design our FF4 and MF2 interviews, we therefore placed the items in a self-report questionnaire, which asked, "Please indicate how often you did these things during two periods: (a) when you were age 14 and younger, and (b) when you were age 15 to 17." The response choices were: 6+, 3–5, 1–2, and 0. For each item we chose a cutoff (1–2 or 3–5) that most closely matched the wording of the DSM criterion. Responses were used to code the CD-15 and CD-18 variables, as previously detailed. The analyses described in this chapter are based on the CD-18 definition as assessed in the FF4 and MF2 interviews.

ADULT ANTISOCIAL BEHAVIOR

We use the term AASB to distinguish our definition from the DSM definition of antisocial personality disorder (ASP), which requires a history of CD. Although it is common for antisocial behavior in adulthood to be preceded by CD, we decided not to make this a requirement, so that we could study how the two disorders co-occurred.

AASB was assessed in the MF2 and FF4 interviews as part of a self-report questionnaire. We used 17 items based on DSM-III-R ASP criteria. These asked the frequency with which respondents, since the age of 18, had: quit a job without having another lined up, borrowed money without plans to repay it, run up bills they couldn't afford to pay, drifted without a regular place to live, conned someone, took advantage of someone, neglected their children, were irresponsible at work, got fired, stole or

(continued)

destroyed property, were arrested, were convicted of a crime, caused an accident because of driving under the influence, put themselves or others in danger through reckless behavior, got into physical fights, intentionally injured someone, and/or hit a spouse or romantic partner.

The response choices for these items were: never, 1–2 times, 3–5 times, and more than 5 times. Responses to the 17 items were combined to reflect the seven DSM criteria, using what we judged to be the most appropriate cutoff score for each item. Individuals who were positive for three or more criteria were counted as having AASB.[c]

The test–retest reliability of our assessment of antisocial behavior was calculated for 295 individuals who were reinterviewed with an average interval of 30 days between interviews. The test–retest reliability for CD-18 was $\kappa = 0.65$ (95% CI = 0.51, 0.80) and for AASB was $\kappa = 0.42$ (95% CI = 0.09, 0.74), representing good to fair reliability.

---

[a]We did not ask an item corresponding to the rape criterion. In other data sets that we examined, the few people admitting to this behavior all endorsed a sufficient number of other symptoms to meet CD criteria. We decided the additional information that might be obtained from a few respondents was not worth the risk of offending many others.

[b]We are grateful to two of our colleagues, who conducted the original analyses of antisocial behavior in the VATSPSUD and created the algorithms for forming these diagnoses. Rise Goldstein studied CD among the FF pairs. Kristen Jacobson studied CD among male pairs and AASB among male and female twins.

[c]We did not fully assess the DSM criterion that the individual feel no remorse for his or her behavior. It was our judgment that the reliability with which this could be rated using self-report or interviewer judgment was too low to be useful.

Results from Twin-Pair Models

In the VATSPSUD we used modifications of the DSM-III-R criteria for antisocial behavior (see Sidebar 5.1). The analyses presented here are for cases of CD that began before age 18. Figure 5.1 shows the lifetime prevalences in our sample of the disorders described in this chapter. Based on our definitions, 4.4% of females and 19.1% of males from same-sex VATSPSUD pairs met criteria for CD. These values are somewhat higher than those found in some epidemiological studies, particularly among males. For CD, this may be because we used retrospective assessments among adults of behaviors before age 18, whereas other studies are based on interviews of adolescents about recent antisocial behavior. It is also possible that our use of a self-report method (rather than an interview) encouraged greater endorsement of antisocial behaviors. A study in Australia based on telephone interviews of adult twins found prevalences of CD similar to ours: 3% in women and 18% in men (Slutske et al., 1997).

In the VATSPSUD, 2.4% of females and 8.3% of males met criteria for AASB. These values are also difficult to compare with epidemiological studies that have used DSM-defined ASP (which requires a history of CD, as well as

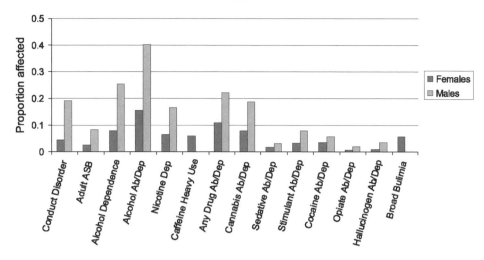

FIGURE 5.1. Lifetime prevalences of externalizing and substance use disorders among twins from same-sex pairs. ASB = antisocial behavior; Ab/Dep = abuse/dependence.

adult symptoms). However, our results do show the usual pattern of sex differences and decline of rates between adolescence and adulthood.

The twin-pair correlations and genetic variance proportions for CD and AASB are shown in Figure 5.2. (See Chapter 3 for discussion of pair correlations and twin-pair models.) These are among the few disorders for which we found evidence of sex differences. Among females, pair resemblance for CD and AASB was much stronger among MZ than among DZ pairs, leading to

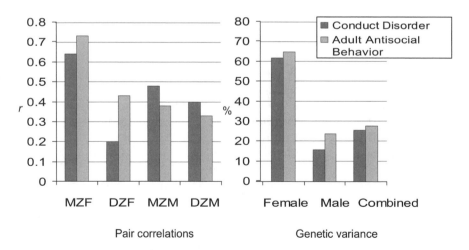

FIGURE 5.2. Pair similarity and estimated genetic variance for adolescent and adult antisocial behavior in same-sex twin pairs. MZF = monozygotic female; DZF = dizygotic female; MZM = monozygotic male; DZM = dizygotic male.

genetic estimates of over 60%, with little evidence of shared environmental effects. In contrast, male MZ and DZ pairs were more similar, leading to modest estimates of genetic and shared environmental effects. Among males, the estimated proportions of variance for CD were 16% genetic, 32% shared environment, and 52% specific environment. For AASB, the estimates were 24% genetic, 19% shared environment, and 57% individual-specific factors.

As noted in Chapter 4, we have limited ability to detect sex differences when the prevalence of the disorder is low in one or both sexes. Because of this, we could not reject the hypothesis that males and females have equal estimates. The estimated proportions of variance based on combining the sexes for CD were 26% genetic, 25% shared environment, and 49% individual-specific environment. For AASB, the estimates combined over sex were similar: 28% genetic, 22% shared environment, and 50% specific environment. (See Appendix 5.3 for CIs for these estimates.)

Genetic Influences: Evidence and Implications

Twin studies of antisocial behavior have covered a range of outcomes and methods, from questionnaire studies of aggression to interview studies of antisocial personality. Overall, the results support the existence of both genetic and shared environmental influences on liability to CD (Thapar & Scourfield, 2002). Two studies using methodology similar to our own (retrospective reports of CD using structured interviews of adult twins from population-based registries) were conducted with males in the VETS and adult twins from an Australian volunteer registry. The estimates for CD from the VETS were 10% genetic, 30% shared environmental influences, and 60% specific environment (Lyons et al., 1995). The Australian study reported a heritability for DSM-III-R CD of 43%, with 25% shared environment and 32% specific environment, among females, and 65% heritability, 4% shared environment, and 31% specific environment among males (Slutske et al., 1997). However, these values were not significantly different between males and females, perhaps because of the low prevalences among females.

Most studies of adult antisocial behavior have reported heritabilities in the range of 30–60% and have found little evidence for influence of the shared environment (McGuffin, Moffitt, & Thapar, 2002). For example, the estimates from the VETS study were 43% genetic, 5% shared environment, and 52% individual-specific environment (Lyons et al., 1995).

What might it mean that there are genetic influences on antisocial behavior? Some research suggests that what is inherited is a predisposition to *behavioral disinhibition*. This cluster of behaviors includes poor impulse control, reduced ability to anticipate the consequences of one's behavior, and excessive emotionality (Iacono, Malone, & McGue, 2003; Slutske et al., 2002b). This hypothesis is consistent with the observation that most (but not all) individuals with CD grow out of their behavior. Children's behavior is motivated more by immediate rewards than by long-term outcomes. Maturity brings the ability to recognize consequences, inhibit behavior, and accept delayed gratification.

Another theory is that genetic factors influence liability for antisocial behavior by influencing physiological reactivity (Brennan et al., 1997). Some evidence suggests that people with antisocial behavior are less responsive in their physiological measurements (such as those obtained during a polygraph test). The idea is that these individuals may be less amenable to social control because they are constitutionally insensitive to punishment or the threat of punishment. If you have ice water in your veins, this will not necessarily cause you to become antisocial, but it might make it much harder for outside influences to modify your behavior.

Shared Environmental Influences

It is not surprising that there might be shared environmental influences on antisocial behavior among juveniles. Twins are often part of each others' peer groups, and it is likely that younger twins may be engaging in antisocial behaviors together. Shared environmental effects might also represent neighborhood and community effects. One might predict that, as the twins get older and their social networks diverge, the influences of the shared environment will decrease.

Critics of the twin method have sometimes claimed that all results from twin studies look basically the same: moderate heritability and no shared environment. The results for CD—in which shared environment has been reliably detected across multiple studies—belie this criticism. Although the twin method is often a blunt research tool, it has been shown to be sensitive enough to detect the shared environmental influences on CD.

The differing results from adolescent and adult twin studies have led to the proposal that there may be different forms of antisocial behavior with distinct causes (DiLalla & Gottesman, 1989; Moffitt, 1993). One form is thought to have strong environmental influences and to be limited to adolescence. Another form that is more genetically influenced persists into adulthood and is hypothesized to be less amenable to environmental intervention. We return to this issue in Chapter 10, where we describe some longitudinal twin analyses of antisocial behavior.

SUBSTANCE ABUSE AND DEPENDENCE

In this section we consider the results from the VATSPSUD for twin analyses of three licit (or legal) substances: alcohol, nicotine, and caffeine; and six illicit substances: cannabis, sedatives, stimulants, cocaine, opiates, and hallucinogens. We selected these substances because they were among those most commonly used and abused. However, misuse of several of the illicit substances was too infrequent (especially among women) to permit us to obtain precise estimates of genetic and environmental influence.

We defined illicit drug use as use of illicit substances or improper use of a prescription medication. Improper use was defined as using more than a doctor prescribed or for other purposes than a doctor prescribed. The classification of substances into the categories of licit and illicit is based more on historical events than on clinical criteria or pharmacological action. Many illicit substances are less addictive than those available legally or by prescription. The addictive potential of substances can be studied in animals by examining how hard they will work to obtain the substance after just a few exposures. In humans, a frequently used index of addictiveness is the proportion of regular users who become physically dependent. Based on these criteria, nicotine is one of the most addictive drugs.

In the VATSPSUD, we studied substance dependence and abuse. In broad terms, dependence refers to physiological (or sometimes psychological) dependence, whereas abuse refers to the adverse consequences of substance use that may occur with or without dependence. Sidebar 5.2 describes the criteria we used to define substance abuse and substance dependence.

The DSM applies the same criteria to most classes of substances, including alcohol, nicotine, and illicit drugs. However, not all criteria pertain equally well to all substances. Therefore we used alternative criteria for nicotine dependence and problem use of caffeine (see Sidebars 5.4 and 5.5).

We now turn to the twin-model results for each substance and how these compare with other studies in the literature. We end this section by discussing the implications of these results for understanding the etiology of substance use disorders.

Alcohol

In the VATSPSUD, over 92% of women and 97% of men reported that they had consumed a full drink at least once in their lives. Alcohol use disorders were common; 7.7% of women and 25.4% of men met DSM-IV criteria for alcohol dependence. (See Sidebar 5.3 for a description of our assessment of alcohol use disorders.) Another 7.8% of women and 14.8% of men met criteria for alcohol abuse without dependence (Kendler, Heath, Neale, Kessler, & Eaves, 1992a; Prescott, Aggen, & Kendler, 1999). These values are somewhat higher than those reported in some U.S. epidemiological studies (Kessler et al., 1994). However, this may be in part because of study differences in rates of abstinence. The prevalences of alcohol use disorders among drinkers in our sample are comparable to those observed among drinkers in other studies. For example, prevalences of DSM-IV alcohol dependence among female and male drinkers participating in a recent epidemiological study of alcohol disorders were 11.8% and 27.6%, respectively (Grant, 1997).

SIDEBAR 5.2. Substance Abuse and Dependence in the DSM

The distinction between substance abuse and substance dependence is sometimes murky, and the criteria for these disorders have been revised across editions of the DSM. For example, several criteria grouped under dependence in DSM-III-R are listed under abuse in DSM-IV.

In the VATSPSUD, the FF1–FF3 interviews were constructed based on DSM-III-R. The FF4, MF1, and MF2 interviews were created after DSM-IV was adopted (in 1994), and we constructed the interviews so that we could form diagnoses based on both DSM-III-R (to be comparable to our past research) and DSM-IV (to be comparable to other studies using the newer criteria). Like most of our work on substances, the analyses reported in this chapter were based on DSM-IV criteria.

Under DSM-IV, the abuse criteria include:

Use that is hazardous to oneself or others (e.g., using a car, machinery, guns, or knives while one is under the influence).
Legal problems or traffic accidents.
Use that interferes with responsibilities (such as work or school).
Use that interferes with relationships.

In the VATSPSUD, we defined an episode of abuse as a period lasting at least 4 weeks during which at least one of these four criteria was experienced.

Under DSM-IV, dependence is defined as having at least three of seven criteria:

Tolerance: needing to use more of the substance to get the same effect or getting less of an effect from using the same amount.
Withdrawal: experiencing physical symptoms associated with cessation of use, or using the substance (or a substance from a related class) to avoid withdrawal symptoms.
Inability to keep oneself from using, or using more than intended.
Persistent desire to quit or multiple failed attempts to quit or cut down on use.
Spending excessive amounts of time obtaining, using, or recovering from use of the substance.
Giving up important occupational or social activities in favor of substance use.
Continuing to use despite serious medical or psychological consequences.

In the VATSPSUD, an episode of dependence was defined as a period lasting at least 4 weeks, during which three or more of these criteria were experienced.

In the DSM, the same criteria are applied to all substance classes, including nicotine, caffeine, alcohol, prescribed medications, and illicit drugs. However, it is readily apparent that some criteria are not equally applicable to all substances. Except for underage users, obtaining alcohol and nicotine does not present much of a problem, whereas access may be a major preoccupation for users of illicit substances. Except in extreme amounts, it is not hazardous to use caffeine. Similarly, not all substances have

(continued)

SIDEBAR 5.2. *(continued)*

a clear withdrawal syndrome. Cannabis is eliminated very slowly from the body, and even heavy users who stop abruptly will not typically experience physical symptoms of withdrawal (although they may have psychological symptoms). These considerations led us to alter the criteria used to define problem use of nicotine and caffeine (see Sidebars 5.4 and 5.5).

In the DSM, abuse and dependence are rated hierarchically, so that one cannot be classified as having abuse if one also meets criteria for dependence. In the VATSPSUD, we did not use this hierarchical rule but rated the presence or absence of both disorders. It was thus possible to meet criteria for abuse and dependence, abuse only, dependence only, or neither.

For alcoholism, we had sufficient cases to consider both abuse and dependence. For caffeine and nicotine, the abuse criteria are not very meaningful. For illicit substances and misuse of prescribed substances, we often had too few cases to consider both disorders. In the analyses reported in this book, we have usually combined the cases into a category of abuse and/or dependence, abbreviated as abuse/dependence.

SIDEBAR 5.3. Assessment of Alcohol Use, Abuse, and Dependence

Alcohol disorders were assessed in the FF1, FF3 (for past-year only), FF4, MF1, and MF2 interviews. There were minor differences between interviews in the structure and detail of the items. The FF4 and MF2 interviews had the same format, and they form the basis for most of the analyses we report in this book. We describe the assessment procedure used in these interviews. Compared with the other interviews, they contained additional consumption questions and assessed more detailed follow-up questions about the particular criteria. We first asked a series of questions about frequency and quantity of alcohol consumption for the past year and for the year in which the twin drank most (if this was other than the past year). We then asked three probe questions:

1. "Think back about your use of alcohol over your entire life. Has there ever been a *period* in your life when you drank too much?"
2. "Has there ever been a *period* in your life when someone else objected to your drinking?"
3. "Has there ever been a *period* in your life when you would drink instead of working or spending time with hobbies, family, or friends?"

Interviewers were trained not to code single events but to require that periods lasted at least 7 days.

If the twin was rated positive for any of the probe questions or exceeded a drinking threshold, he or she was then asked a series of items to assess the abuse and dependence criteria. We used consumption information, as well as endorsement of

(continued)

SIDEBAR 5.3. *(continued)*

problems, because of the concern that not everyone who had experienced alcohol-related difficulties would identify them as a problem. The consumption thresholds were intended to identify approximately the top 25% of drinkers within each sex. Men were rated as above threshold if they reported a single-day consumption of at least 13 drinks or had consumed 7 or more drinks at least once a week for at least 4 consecutive weeks. The values for women were 7 drinks and 4 drinks, respectively.

We next asked a series of items to assess lifetime presence of the abuse and dependence criteria. When items were answered positively, follow-up items were used to assess their severity or duration. If one or more symptoms were endorsed, we asked the person his or her age at the onset of the first symptom, the number of episodes, and the duration of the longest episode. We formed syndromes by identifying those symptoms that clustered together (similar to the syndromes for MD; see Sidebar 4.1). We then asked the person's age at onset of the syndrome and the duration of the longest episode.

We did not score abuse and dependence hierarchically but rated the presence or absence of both. It was therefore possible to meet criteria for both abuse and dependence, abuse only, dependence only, or neither. We used the multiple-threshold model (see Chapter 3) to explore the scaling among the different categories. Relatively few individuals met criteria for dependence without abuse, and they were not distinguishable from individuals who met criteria for both dependence and abuse. The results of our analyses are consistent with abuse and dependence being on the same continuum of severity. Consequently, we have conducted analyses using alcohol dependence (AD), alcohol abuse and/or dependence (AAD), and a multiple-threshold (MT) definition consisting of three categories: unaffected, abuse only, and dependence with or without abuse. For some analyses we have used a definition of problem drinking that includes individuals who endorsed one of the probe criteria but did not meet diagnostic criteria for alcohol abuse or dependence.

The analyses described in this chapter are based on the DSM-IV AD and AAD definitions as assessed in the FF4 and MF2 interviews. The test–retest reliability for these definitions was calculated for 382 individuals reinterviewed with an average interval of 30 days between interviews. The value for AD was $\kappa = 0.72$ (95% CI = 0.61, 0.82) and for AAD was $\kappa = 0.74$ (95% CI = 0.66, 0.82).

Genetic and Environmental Influences

The left side of Figure 5.3 displays the twin-pair correlations for liability to alcohol disorders. For both dependence and abuse/dependence, MZ twin pairs are more similar than DZ pairs. The correlation for dependence among DZ female pairs appears unusually low, but it does not differ significantly from the other DZ correlations; the relatively small number of pairs in this group and the relatively low prevalence of dependence among women means that this correlation has a particularly wide confidence interval ($r = 0.07$, 95% CI = –0.26, 0.41).

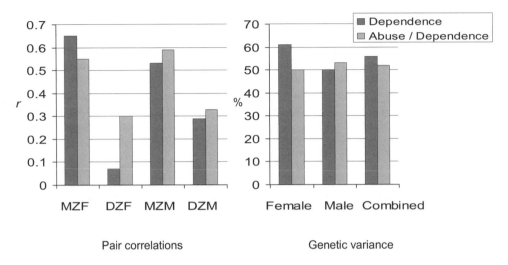

FIGURE 5.3. Pair similarity and estimated genetic variance for lifetime history of alcoholism in same-sex twin pairs.

The heritability estimates, shown in the right side of Figure 5.3, are similar for both disorders in both sexes, ranging from 50 to 61%. The estimates did not differ significantly across males and females. The estimates combined across sex for alcohol dependence were 56% genetic, 0% shared environment, and 44% specific environment; for alcohol abuse/dependence, they were 52% genetic, 6% shared environment, and 42% specific environment. The shared environmental estimate for abuse was not significantly different from zero.

The results of twin studies of males have consistently demonstrated a significant role for genetic factors in contributing to vulnerability to alcoholism. The heritability estimates in most studies are 50–60%. In contrast, the results from studies of female twins are less consistent. The earliest studies found low heritability for females, and this led to a widespread belief that alcoholism is "not genetic" in women. More recent studies have found heritability estimates more similar to those seen among males. Our results are close to those obtained in the study most similar to ours; analyses of interview data from the Australian twin registry found heritability estimates of about 60% for both males and females (Heath et al., 1997). We believe that the variability among studies of female twins is probably due to methodological differences in how the samples were found and measured and that the heritabilities from population-based studies provide the best estimates (see Prescott & Kendler, 2000).

Nicotine

Nicotine is the psychoactive substance found in tobacco products. Among VATSPSUD twins from same-sex pairs, 40% of females and 73% of males reported smoking regularly (defined as seven or more cigarettes a week) for a month or more at some point in their lives. As shown in Figure 5.1, 6.5% of females and 16.7% of males met criteria for our rigorous definition of nicotine dependence based on the Fagerstrom Test for Nicotine Dependence (FTND; see Sidebar 5.4). These rates are quite a bit lower than those reported by studies that used the broader DSM criteria. For example, in a subset of the National Comorbidity Survey, 24% of the sample met DSM-III-R criteria for lifetime nicotine dependence (Breslau, Johnson, Hiripi, & Kessler, 2001).

SIDEBAR 5.4. Assessment of Tobacco Use and Nicotine Dependence

We assessed tobacco use and nicotine dependence in our FF3 and MF2 interviews. In the MF2 interview we assessed all forms of tobacco use, including cigarettes, cigars, pipe smoking, snuff, and chewing tobacco. With the FF sample we asked about tobacco use only in the form of cigarettes, because very few women use other forms of tobacco.

We first asked a series of questions assessing the use of tobacco during the age when use was heaviest. Individuals who reported ever smoking regularly in their lifetimes (which we defined as seven or more cigarettes a week for at least 1 month) were asked items from the Fagerstrom Tolerance Questionnaire (FTQ; Fagerstrom & Schneider, 1989), a widely used scale among tobacco researchers. For the analyses reported here, we employed a modified version of the FTQ called the Fagerstrom Test for Nicotine Dependence (FTND; Heatherton, Kozlowski, Frecker, & Fagerstrom, 1991), which has been found to be a better index of dependence. The FTND is most applicable to cigarette smokers, but we also administered it (using modified wording) to individuals whose tobacco use was in forms other than cigarettes. Example items include: how soon after waking one smokes the first cigarette, whether one smokes while sick in bed, and whether it is difficult to refrain when smoking is forbidden. We administered several other items constructed to assess the DSM-III-R dependence criteria of withdrawal symptoms and failed attempts to quit.

For the analyses reported in this chapter, we used a cutoff on the FTND so that individuals with a score of 7 or higher were considered dependent and those with a lower score were considered unaffected. This is a strict cutoff, the same as that used to select participants for studies of nicotine withdrawal. Nonsmokers and individuals who experimented with tobacco but never became regular smokers were also classified as unaffected.

The test–retest reliability of the FTND was calculated for 193 individuals who were administered the MF2 interview twice. For classification as dependent or not dependent, the test–retest reliability was $\kappa = 0.75$ (95% CI = 0.62, 0.88).

Genetic and Environmental Influences

Figure 5.4 shows the pair correlations and genetic estimates for nicotine dependence. Among both females and males, MZ pairs are more similar than DZ pairs. The estimated proportions of variance for nicotine dependence were 52% genetic, 6% shared environment, and 42% individual-specific factors for females and 57% genetic, 11% shared environment, and 32% individual-specific factors for males. Not surprisingly, these values did not differ significantly between sexes; the combined estimates are 55% genetic, 11% shared environment, and 34% individual-specific factors. The shared environmental estimates were not significantly different from zero.

Most twin studies of nicotine dependence have used proxy measures, such as persistent smoking. These studies typically find moderate heritabilities (30–40%) and some evidence for shared environmental influences (see Li, Cheng, Ma, & Swan, 2003; Sullivan & Kendler, 1998). The VETS and Australian twin registry study also directly assessed nicotine dependence (using items developed from DSM-III-R criteria). In the VETS, the best-fitting twin model estimated heritability to be 60% and found that shared environmental effects did not contribute to liability to nicotine dependence (True et al., 1999). The Australian study found a heritability of 56% and little evidence of shared environmental effects for DSM-IV nicotine dependence (Lessov et al., 2004). Thus the available evidence suggests the importance of genetic factors and perhaps a small role for shared environmental factors in creating familial resemblance for nicotine dependence.

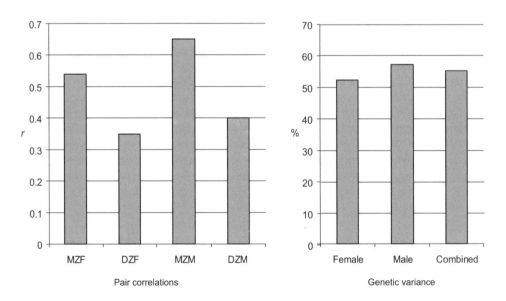

FIGURE 5.4. Pair similarity and estimated genetic variance for lifetime history of nicotine dependence in same-sex twin pairs.

Caffeine

Caffeine is the most commonly used psychoactive substance in the world. It is consumed primarily in the form of tea, coffee, and caffeinated sodas, but it is also found in chocolate. Caffeine is used daily by about 80% of the world's population (James, 1997).

The usual abuse and dependence criteria do not apply very well to caffeine. We assessed withdrawal and intoxication as defined by DSM-IV criteria, as well as heavy use and toxicity (see Sidebar 5.5). Although we assessed caffeine use in both male and female twins, the questions about other sequelae of caffeine use were administered only to female twins participating in the FF4

SIDEBAR 5.5. Assessment of Caffeine Use and Use-Related Problems

Caffeine use was assessed in our MF2 and FF4 interviews, but only the FF4 interview included questions about caffeine-related effects. Use was assessed for the year prior to interview and for the year of greatest use. Frequency of caffeine consumption was assessed by asking the typical number of days per month caffeine was consumed. Quantity was assessed separately for coffee, tea, and caffeinated soda in terms of average daily consumption (on days when caffeine was used). We converted use into approximate number of milligrams (mg) of caffeine using the following estimates: brewed coffee, 125 mg/cup; instant coffee, 90 mg/cup; tea, 60 mg/cup; and caffeinated soft drinks, 40 mg/can.[a] We calculated a *monthly use* variable by multiplying the average mg/day on days caffeine was used by the number of days per month caffeine was consumed. We defined a *heavy use* variable as daily or near-daily consumption of 625 mg of caffeine (i.e., the equivalent of five cups of brewed coffee).

We used seven items to assess problematic caffeine use.[b] Two items based on the DSM criteria assessed tolerance. Four items assessed caffeine withdrawal symptoms, including headaches, marked fatigue or drowsiness, marked anxiety or depression, and nausea or vomiting. These were taken directly from Appendix B of DSM-IV, in which criteria for caffeine withdrawal were listed as a syndrome "provided for further study." Another item asked about toxicity using a shortened list of the DSM-IV criteria for caffeine intoxication, including feeling ill, shaky, or jittery after caffeine use.

The test–retest reliability for these measures, based on 189 women interviewed twice, was good to excellent. The correlation for monthly use was $r = 0.77$ (95% CI = 0.70, 0.82). The test–retest reliability estimates for the categorical items were: heavy use, $\kappa = 0.76$ (95% CI = 0.62, 0.91), $r = .95$ (95% CI = 0.89, 1.00); withdrawal, $\kappa = 0.63$ (95% CI = 0.44, 0.81), $r = .86$ (95% CI = 0.73, 1.00); tolerance, $\kappa = 0.41$ (95% CI = 0.24, 0.58), $r = .68$ (95% CI = 0.49, 0.87); and toxicity, $\kappa = 0.60$ (95% CI = 0.47, 0.72), $r = .84$ (95% CI = 0.74, 0.95).

---

[a]These values are approximations; the actual amounts will depend on portion sizes and amount of coffee and tea used for brewing. The FF4 study was conducted before the widespread use of high-caffeine sodas. We did not measure caffeine consumption in food products, as these make very small contributions to overall caffeine consumption.
[b]Our colleague Debra Foley aided in the development of these items.

study. We therefore focus on them here. The prevalences among female twins were: heavy use in the past year, 6.1%; tolerance, 15.5%; withdrawal, 24.0%; and toxicity, 12.8%.

Genetic and Environmental Influences

The left side of Figure 5.5 shows pair correlations for our indices of caffeine use and use-related problems among female twins.[1] The values vary, but for all the indices the MZ pair correlations are significantly greater than the DZ pair correlations. The genetic estimates, shown in the right side of Figure 5.5, were: monthly use, 43%; heavy use, 77%; tolerance, 40%; withdrawal, 35%; and toxicity, 45%. There was no evidence for shared environmental influences on liability to caffeine use-related problems. In aggregate, these results suggest that genetic factors contribute to liability to levels of caffeine use, as well as to an array of caffeine-related problems.

To our knowledge, there have been no similar twin studies of caffeine use and use-related problems. Studies of caffeine consumption have been conducted using twins from national registries of male and female twins in Finland and Sweden and male twins participating in the World War II Veteran Twin Study (Carmelli, Swan, Robinette, & Fabsitz, 1990; Kaprio, Sarna, Koskenvuo, & Rantasalo, 1978; Pedersen, 1981). Heritability estimates from these studies ranged from 36 to 51%. The studies from the Scandinavian samples found some evidence for small shared environmental effects, but the other

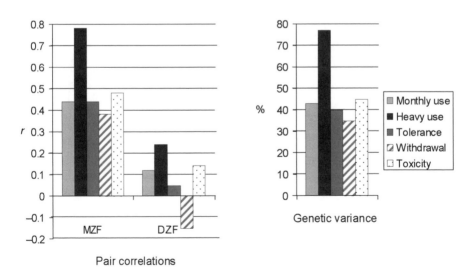

FIGURE 5.5. Pair similarity and estimated genetic variance for lifetime history of caffeine use and problem use among female twin pairs. Data from Kendler and Prescott (1999b, Table 1).

U.S. sample, like our own, did not. In sum, the available evidence supports the existence of moderate genetic influences on liability to use caffeine and to develop a range of problems associated with caffeine use.

Illicit Substances

Use of illicit substances (or misuse of prescription drugs) was quite common among VATSPSUD participants (Kendler, Karkowski, Neale, & Prescott, 2000a; Kendler, Karkowski, & Prescott, 1999d; Kendler & Prescott, 1998). More than 56% of males and 50% of females from same-sex twin pairs reported having tried such drugs at least once (see Sidebar 5.6). By far the most commonly used drug was cannabis (usually in the form of marijuana), which was used by 52% of males and 48% of females. Prevalences of other drug use among males were: sedatives, 11%; stimulants, 19%; cocaine, 17%; opiates, 6%; and hallucinogens, 14%. Among females, they were: sedatives, 8%; stimulants, 10%; cocaine, 14%; opiates, 3%; and hallucinogens, 10%.

Figure 5.1 shows the prevalences of drug abuse/dependence among males and females for six classes of illicit drugs and for the combined category of "any drug." Eleven percent of females and 22.3% of males met criteria for abuse/dependence for one or more substances. Males had significantly higher prevalences for all drug classes. By far the most common substance disorder was cannabis abuse/dependence (7.8% female, 18.6% male), followed by stimulants (3.3% female, 7.8% male), cocaine (3.6% female, 5.7% male), sedatives (1.8% female, 3.2% male), hallucinogens (0.9% female, 3.5% male), and opiates (0.6% female, 2.0% male).

The prevalences of use and abuse/dependence observed in our study are broadly similar to those obtained in recent U.S. epidemiological studies (Anthony, Warner, & Kessler, 1994; Substance Abuse and Mental Health Services Administration [SAMHSA], 1997). For example, the lifetime prevalence of cannabis use among adult participants in the NCS (Anthony et al., 1994) was 41% for females and 52% for males, very similar to the values we observed. These findings suggest that the VATSPSUD can be considered broadly representative of the U.S. adult population in terms of substance use and misuse.

Genetic and Environmental Influences

Figure 5.6 shows the twin-pair correlations for abuse/dependence for any substance and the individual drug classes. For all the categories but one (opiates in males), MZ pairs were significantly more similar than DZ pairs. Overall, the MZ pair correlations are the highest of all the disorders studied in the VATSPSUD, with most ranging from 0.60 to 0.80. The estimated genetic proportions of variance in liability to abuse/dependence are shown in Figure 5.7. There was no evidence for contributions of shared environmental effects ex-

SIDEBAR 5.6. Assessment of Illicit Drug Use, Abuse, and Dependence

Illicit drug use was assessed in our FF4 and MF2 interviews. We defined illicit drug use as use of an illicit substance or improper use of a prescription medication. *Improper use* was defined as using more than a doctor prescribed or use for other purposes than a doctor prescribed. Respondents who reported improper use were asked a series of questions about their age at first use and frequency and quantity of use over their lifetimes. These questions were organized by pharmacological class into cannabis, sedatives, stimulants, cocaine, opiates, hallucinogens, and "other" (most commonly inhalants and steroids). Preparations that included two or more substance classes were coded under both. Respondents were given or mailed (if interviewed by telephone) a page listing various classes of drugs and their common forms (including prescription and street names).

Based on their responses to the "use" items, individuals were routed one of three ways for each class of drugs:

1. Individuals who reported using drugs from a particular class 11 or more times in a month were asked all the DSM-IV abuse and dependence criteria for that substance (see Sidebar 5.2).
2. Those who reported using a class of substance at least 6 times in their lives but fewer than 11 times in a month were asked the DSM-IV abuse items for that substance. If they responded positively to any of the abuse items, they were asked the dependence items. If they responded negatively to all the abuse items, they skipped the dependence questions.
3. Individuals who had used drugs from a class fewer than 6 times in their lives were not asked any of the abuse or dependence items.

The abuse and dependence items were asked "for the time when you used the most." For those who were positive for one or more criteria, we also asked about their age at first symptom, the duration of their longest episode, whether they had sought treatment, and whether drug episodes overlapped with episodes of depression and alcohol-related symptoms (if such episodes were reported in prior sections of the interview).

The test–retest reliability for abuse/dependence was calculated for 383 individuals who received the MF2 or FF4 interview twice. The kappa coefficients and tetrachoric correlations for abuse/dependence were: any substance, $\kappa = 0.70$ (95% CI =0.60, 0.80), $r = 0.93$ (95% CI = 0.88, 0.98); cannabis, $\kappa = 0.65$ (95% CI = 0.53, 0.77), $r = 0.91$ (95% CI = 0.85, 0.98); sedatives, $\kappa = 0.63$ (95% CI = 0.39, 0.87), $r = 0.92$ (95% CI = 0.81, 1.00); stimulants, $\kappa = 0.70$ (95% CI = 0.51, 0.90), $r = 0.95$ (95% CI = 0.88, 1.00); cocaine, $\kappa = 0.67$ (95% CI = 0.48, 0.86), $r = 0.94$ (95% CI = 0.86, 1.00); opiates, $\kappa = 0.77$ (95% CI = 0.51, 1.00), $r = 0.97$ (95% CI = 0.92, 1.00); and hallucinogens, $\kappa = 0.66$ (95% CI = 0.35, 0.97), $r = 0.95$ (95% CI = 0.85, 1.00).

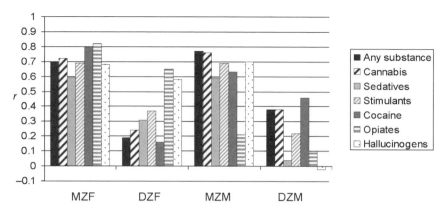

FIGURE 5.6. Similarity of same-sex twin pairs for lifetime history of abuse or dependence of illicit substances.

cept for cocaine abuse/dependence in males, for which the estimates were: genetic, 39%; shared environment, 26%; and individual specific, 35%. Except for cocaine and opiates, the estimates were very similar for males and females. Even for these drugs, the estimates were not significantly different across the sexes, again because of the low prevalences of these disorders.

There have been few twin studies of illicit substance use and abuse. Several studies have been conducted using twins identified in clinical settings, but the results are difficult to interpret because the samples were identified not because of their drug use disorders but because they were being treated for other disorders (e.g., alcoholism, psychosis, or affective disorders). A study of

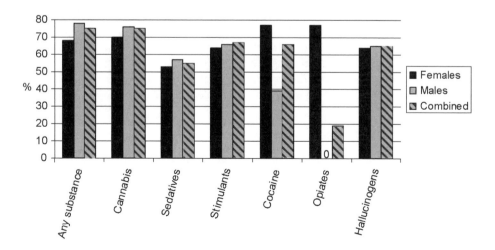

FIGURE 5.7. Estimated genetic variance in risk for substance abuse/dependence.

188 twin pairs identified through drug treatment centers reported heritability estimates for abuse/dependence on five of the same drug classes that were included in our study (all but hallucinogens). Heritability estimates among males were 57–78%, similar to those observed in our study. The results among females were more variable (0–73%) but with large confidence intervals due to the relatively small sample size of 66 female twin pairs (van den Bree, Johnson, Neale, & Pickens, 1998). The only twin study using a methodology similar to our own is the VETS (Tsuang et al., 1996). Among these male twins, genetic estimates were lower than those observed in our study for any drug (34%), for hallucinogens (25%), for cannabis (33%), and for sedatives (38%), but they were similar for stimulants (51%). The value for opiates (69%) was higher than that found among VATSPSUD males but similar to that found among females. The VETS also found evidence for shared environmental influences on any drug abuse/dependence (28%), cannabis (29%), hallucinogens (19%), and sedatives (6%).

In summary, the available evidence from twin studies of abuse/dependence on illicit drugs is consistent with our findings of at least moderate but possibly strong genetic influences and also of some evidence for shared environmental factors.

Genetic Mechanisms

As we noted at the beginning of this chapter, the idea that there are genetic influences on substance use disorders is often met with resistance. It is important to emphasize that what is inherited is a *predisposition* toward a pattern of behavior. There are no genes that code directly for developing a substance use disorder. Genetic influences are not destiny. There is still room for individual choice and environmental intervention.

Assuming we accept the evidence that genetic influences affect the development of substance use disorders, how might this occur? The details are not yet clear, but it probably involves a combination of three factors: specific drug mechanisms, general effects through the brain's reward pathways (regions and connections responsible for the experience of pleasure and reward), and indirect mechanisms via other genetically influenced behaviors.[2]

Specific Drug Effects

Specific drug mechanisms include genes that code for aspects of brain function that are likely to be specific to a particular class of substance. For example, genes are known to code for receptors in the brain that interact specifically with nicotine, opiates, and benzodiazepines (a group of prescription antianxiety drugs that includes Valium and Xanax). Some psychoactive substances such as alcohol probably act through several different discrete receptor systems, whereas others, such as cocaine and amphetamines, act largely by inducing release of specific kinds of neurotransmitters in the brain and/or by blocking their reuptake back into nerve terminals. Animal studies have shown that alterations of these genes can have dramatic effects on the responses to these drugs.

General Liability

The rewarding effects of most, and perhaps all, drugs of abuse appear to depend on common brain pathways that utilize the neurotransmitter dopamine (Koob & Le Moal, 1997). Genetic variation in the functioning of this "hedonic" (or pleasure-related) brain system is another way in which genes might influence risk for substance use disorders. For example, genetic differences may be associated with the degree of pleasure that is experienced on first using a drug, which in turn would relate to risk for further use and potential addiction.

Genetic variation may also influence an individual's experience of different aspects of drug effects on mood, anxiety, and mental alertness and unpleasant side effects such as drowsiness, nausea, or headaches. Different individuals may experience these effects to a greater or lesser degree or as more or less pleasurable or aversive. An active area of alcohol research is identifying motivations for drinking and studying how these relate to individual differences in risk to develop alcoholism. We describe some of this work in Chapter 15.

Other evidence relevant to general genetic mechanisms comes from studies of pharmacological treatments for addiction. Naltrexone, a drug that blocks opiate receptors, reduces craving not only for opiates but also for alcohol and possibly other drugs (Srisurapanont & Jarusuraisin, 2005). Furthermore, the effectiveness of this treatment varies with genetic differences among people (Oslin et al., 2003). We also know that genes can influence how drugs are absorbed in the body and then metabolized and excreted. Variation in any of these systems could have an impact on the liability to develop drug-related problems.

Indirect Effects

The third mechanism for genetic influence on substance disorder liability is through other genetically influenced characteristics. For example, some individuals may be more prone to abuse substances because of personality traits, such as risk taking or sensation seeking. Problems of impulse control increase the risk for the development of substance abuse, as well as for antisocial behavior. Such *mediating* variables (traits that lie in the pathway between genes and disorders) have been widely studied, and there is evidence that they may have a strong genetic basis (Hicks, Krueger, Iacono, McGue, & Patrick, 2004). Chapter 11 describes some of our research on this issue.

Individuals may also develop substance disorders because they are medicating themselves for symptoms of other psychiatric disorders, such as anxiety or depression. To the degree that these disorders are genetically influenced, this could lead to the patterns of familial resemblance for substance use disorders observed in the VATSPSUD and other genetically informative studies. We return to this issue in Chapter 11, in which we discuss studies that address general versus specific genetic risk for substance use disorders.

The Role of Environmental Factors in Liability to Substance Use Disorders

Studies of substance abuse may be difficult to compare across cultures or historical periods. Cultural acceptance of smoking (especially in women) has fluctuated greatly in the past several generations. Societal interventions, such as prohibition in the United States in the early 20th century or the opening of borders in Eastern Europe, rapidly affected the availability of substances. Such factors may lead to differences among studies of the relative importance of genetic and shared environmental factors in producing familial resemblance for substance use and abuse. As we saw for caffeine consumption, two studies conducted in Scandinavia found evidence for shared environmental factors, whereas this was not the case for the studies of U.S. twin samples.

As we described in Chapter 3, most psychiatric disorders are assumed to be multifactorial in origin, arising from a combination of genetic and environmental risk factors. For the other disorders studied in VATSPSUD, environmental risk is ubiquitous; no one has a stress-free life. But with substance abuse, a necessary risk factor is the availability and consumption of the substance.

Individuals must expose themselves to the substance before a genetic predisposition to develop dependence can be expressed. Exposure to this risk factor is incomplete, self-selected, and likely to be nonrandom with respect to genetic risk. Among individuals who have a family history of substance abuse (and are at above-average genetic risk), some will have increased environmental risk (the substance is in their environment) and others will have decreased environmental risk (associated with a repugnance for substance use that arises from witnessing its effects).

Exposure differs for different types of substances. Unlike alcohol, which nearly everyone tries, a substantial minority of the population does not use sufficient nicotine to become dependent, and many never even try illicit substances. It is possible that many individuals who have a genetic predisposition to become dependent never have the opportunity to express their liability.

The processes that determine exposure to a substance are likely to differ from those that affect development of addiction once drug exposure has occurred. Some evidence suggests that environmental factors shared by family members are important for exposure but less important for development of dependence contingent upon exposure. This may explain why the evidence for shared environmental factors is greater for illicit drugs than for more commonly used substances (alcohol, nicotine, and caffeine). We return to this issue in Chapter 12, in which we describe analyses that address the stage aspects of substance involvement.

BULIMIA

Bulimia nervosa is one of the newest of psychiatric disorders; it was first described as a clinical syndrome in 1979. The core symptom of bulimia is binge eating, wherein individuals consume unusually large amounts of food in relatively short time periods. During these binges—which might, for example, consist of a large-sized pizza followed by a box of cookies and a dozen donuts—individuals feel "out of control." Individuals with bulimia attempt to counteract the effect of this excess food consumption to reduce their chances of gaining weight. These compensatory behaviors can range from relatively normative activities such as excessive exercise to laxative abuse and, in the most extreme form, self-induced vomiting (or "purging"). Individuals with bulimia are typically quite preoccupied with their weight and body shape.

Of the major psychiatric disorders, bulimia has one of the largest differences in rates between the sexes. Although it does occur in males, it is so rare that even in our large sample we would not have found enough affected males to reach any useful conclusions. We therefore assessed this disorder only in women.

Bulimia is also unusual in one other way. In one sense, it is an internalizing disorder in that affected individuals tend to suffer, often feeling anxiety and guilt about their binge episodes. However, like the externalizing disorders, bulimia is characterized both by deviant behavior (that is, something people *do* rather than something they *have*) and problems with impulse control. We decided to include bulimia in this chapter, but it could have been placed in Chapter 4.

Bulimia is one of the psychiatric disorders in which empirical research supports an important etiological role for cultural factors. The prevalence of bulimia has significantly increased in Western countries in recent years, and in non-Western countries the prevalence is strongly related to the degree of contact with Western culture (Keel & Klump, 2003). For example, in the Pacific islands of Fiji, a substantial rise in eating disorder pathology in adolescent girls occurred after the introduction of television and the associated exposure to Western ideals about body image (Becker, Burwell, Gilman, Herzog, & Hamburg, 2002). These results suggest that the risk for bulimia is related to cultural models of ideal body size.

When we first examined bulimia in 1991, etiological models for the condition overwhelmingly emphasized intrapsychic and sociocultural mechanisms. Only two twin and no adoption studies of bulimia had been published, and the two twin studies included very small sample sizes (11 and 27 pairs, respectively).

In our sample of 2,163 women participating in the FF1 interview, 60, or 2.8%, met DSM-III-R criteria for bulimia. This is within the range of prevalences found in prior studies of bulimia among young female populations of 1.7–4.2% (Kendler et al., 1991a). Another 63 women had broadly defined bulimia (see Sidebar 5.7). Consistent with other epidemiological studies, we found that exercise was the most common compensatory behavior among those meeting criteria for bulimia, followed by strict dieting, self-induced vomiting, and fasting.

In our twin modeling, we examined both the narrow definition of bulimia (only those meeting DSM-III-R criteria) and our broad definition. The twin-pair correlations and genetic estimates are shown in Figure 5.8. The correlations were: MZ, 0.55 and DZ, 0.29 for the narrow definition; and MZ, 0.51 and DZ, 0.25 for the broad definition. For both narrowly and broadly defined bulimia, our best-fitting model included only genetic factors and individual-specific environment, with heritability estimates of 55% and 50%, respectively.

Since our initial report in 1991, results of studies examining bulimia or bulimic symptoms have been reported from two other population-based female twin samples. In the Australian Twin Registry, Wade, Neale, Lake, and Martin (1999) found that their best-fit model for bulimia estimated herit-

---

SIDEBAR 5.7. Assessment of Bulimia

The DSM-III-R criteria for bulimia nervosa include recurrent episodes of binge eating, a feeling of a loss of control during these episodes, compensatory behaviors designed to avoid weight gain, and overconcern with body weight and shape. We based our assessment of a lifetime history of bulimia on the SCID interview for DSM-III-R (Spitzer & Williams, 1985). A single probe question was used to evaluate the criterion of eating binges:

> "Have you ever in your life had eating binges during which you ate a lot of food in a short period of time?"

Our interviewers were explicitly trained to discount episodes in which the amount and kind of food consumed was within the normal range. If the response to this question was positive, we then assessed the remaining criteria, including recording the specific form of compensatory behavior (e.g. self-induced vomiting, laxative abuse, fasting).

Individuals who probably or definitely met all the DSM-III-R criteria were considered to be positive for narrowly defined bulimia. Those who met most but not all criteria but who were judged on review of the interview to have clinically significant bulimic symptoms were considered to have broadly defined bulimia.

Although we assessed bulimia in both the FF1 and FF3 interviews, we report results largely from the FF1 interview, for which we did not obtain a measure of test–retest reliability.

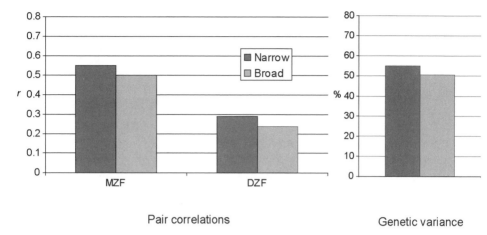

FIGURE 5.8. Pair similarity and estimated genetic variance for lifetime history of bulimia nervosa among female twin pairs. Data from Kendler et al. (1991, Tables 3 and 4).

ability at 62% and, like our study, found no evidence for shared environment. In postpubescent adolescents from the Minnesota Twin Registry, the best-fit model for eating disorder symptoms estimated heritability at 54% (Klump, McGue, & Iacono, 2003). These results, along with our original findings, suggest strongly that, as with all the other disorders that we have examined in VATSPSUD, a woman's vulnerability to bulimia is significantly influenced by her genetic makeup.

NOTES

1. The caffeine analyses were originally published in Kendler and Prescott (1999b).
2. Much of the evidence for these mechanisms comes from research on animals, particularly rodents, but also primates. Although animal analogues have their limitations (e.g., it is difficult to create animal equivalents for hazardous use or occupational interference), many aspects of drug dependence have parallels in animal behavior. It is relatively easy to measure how hard an animal will work to obtain a drug, whereas ascribing mental states (depression, anxiety) is much more problematic.

APPENDIX 5.1. Sample Sizes, Prevalences, and Pair Resemblance for Externalizing Disorders

Disorder	Sex	N	Prevalence (%)	Zygosity	No. of pairs	Tetrachoric correlation	95% CI	Odds ratio	95% CI
Conduct disorder	F	1,457	4.4	MZ	331	0.64	0.35, 0.92	16.05	4.09, 63.03
				DZ	203	0.20	−0.34, 0.74	2.39	0.27, 21.28
	M	2,756	19.1	MZ	633	0.48	0.35, 0.61	4.51	2.88, 7.05
				DZ	425	0.40	0.23, 0.57	3.44	1.99, 5.94
Adult antisocial behavior	F	1,486	2.4	MZ	345	0.73	0.44, 1.00	33.10	6.40, 171.2
				DZ	210	0.43	−0.12, 0.97	7.07	0.70, 71.76
	M	2,751	8.3	MZ	634	0.38	0.15, 0.61	4.43	1.89, 10.40
				DZ	422	0.33	0.10, 0.57	3.30	1.44, 7.56
Alcohol dependence	F	1,925	7.7	MZ	501	0.65	0.49, 0.82	12.50	5.76, 27.11
				DZ	326	0.07	−0.26, 0.41	1.33	0.37, 4.75
	M	2,921	25.4	MZ	701	0.53	0.42, 0.64	5.01	3.41, 7.37
				DZ	484	0.29	0.14, 0.44	2.30	1.48, 3.56
Alcohol abuse/ dependence	F	1,925	15.5	MZ	501	0.55	0.40, 0.69	6.14	3.53, 10.66
				DZ	326	0.30	0.09, 0.51	2.54	1.31, 4.93
	M	2,921	40.2	MZ	701	0.59	0.50, 0.68	5.60	4.01, 7.84
				DZ	484	0.33	0.20, 0.46	2.42	1.67, 3.51
Nicotine dependence	F	1,903	6.5	MZ	494	0.54	0.31, 0.78	9.26	3.45, 24.87
				DZ	317	0.35	0.05, 0.65	3.74	1.25, 11.20
	M	2,924	16.7	MZ	699	0.65	0.54, 0.76	9.78	5.98, 15.99
				DZ	485	0.40	0.24, 0.56	3.41	2.03, 5.72
Caffeine monthly use	F	1,920	—	MZ	499	0.41	0.34, 0.48	a	
				DZ	325	0.24	0.14, 0.34	a	

Disorder	Sex	N	%	Zyg	Pairs	r	CI	χ²	CI
Caffeine withdrawal	F	1,195	22.3	MZ	218	0.36	0.14, 0.58	2.83	1.43, 5.57
				DZ	137	-0.13	-0.45, 0.18	0.67	0.25, 1.80
Any illicit drug abuse/dependence	F	1,925	11.0	MZ	501	0.70	0.57, 0.83	13.37	7.01, 25.50
				DZ	326	0.19	-0.08, 0.46	1.94	0.79, 4.79
	M	2,935	22.3	MZ	704	0.77	0.70, 0.85	15.76	10.12, 24.53
				DZ	489	0.38	0.24, 0.53	3.06	1.95, 4.80
Cannabis abuse/dependence	F	1,925	7.8	MZ	501	0.72	0.58, 0.86	17.14	8.01, 36.71
				DZ	326	0.24	-0.08, 0.55	2.45	0.77, 7.78
	M	2,935	18.6	MZ	704	0.76	0.68, 0.84	15.36	9.63, 24.50
				DZ	489	0.38	0.23, 0.54	3.16	1.94, 5.15
Sedative abuse/dependence	F	1,925	1.8	MZ	501	0.59	0.24, 0.95	19.36	3.35, 112.04
				DZ	326	0.31	0.09, 0.53	b	
	M	2,935	3.2	MZ	704	0.59	0.32, 0.85	16.34	4.66, 57.23
				DZ	489	0.04	-0.39, 0.47	1.20	0.15, 9.44
Stimulant abuse/dependence	F	1,925	3.3	MZ	501	0.69	0.45, 0.92	24.23	6.84, 85.84
				DZ	326	0.37	-0.03, 0.77	5.03	0.99, 25.54
	M	2,935	7.8	MZ	704	0.69	0.55, 0.82	15.66	7.82, 31.37
				DZ	489	0.22	-0.02, 0.47	2.29	0.95, 5.54
Cocaine abuse/dependence	F	1,925	3.6	MZ	501	0.80	0.64, 0.95	40.76	13.56, 122.58
				DZ	326	0.16	-0.33, 0.65	2.15	0.26, 17.99
	M	2,935	5.7	MZ	704	0.63	0.45, 0.81	13.87	6.01, 32.02
				DZ	489	0.46	0.21, 0.70	6.07	2.35, 15.68
Opiate abuse/dependence	F	1,925	0.6	MZ	501	0.82	0.46, 1.00[c]	165.33	8.27, 3304.97
				DZ	326	0.65	0.34, 0.95	b	

(continued)

APPENDIX 5.1. (continued)

Disorder	Sex	N	Prevalence (%)	Zygosity	No. of pairs	Tetrachoric correlation	95% CI	Odds ratio	95% CI
Opiate abuse/ dependence (cont.)	M	2,935	2.0	MZ	704	0.21	0.06, 0.37	b	
				DZ	489	0.10	−0.06, 0.25	b	
Hallucinogen abuse/ dependence	F	1,925	0.9	MZ	501	0.68	0.25, 1.00[c]	49.30	3.82, 635.8
				DZ	326	0.58	0.29, 0.86	b	
	M	2,935	3.5	MZ	704	0.70	0.51, 0.88	24.18	8.78, 66.63
				DZ	489	−0.02	−0.15, 0.12	b	
Bulimia—narrow	F	2,163	2.8	MZ	599	0.55	0.27, 0.83	12.62	3.64, 43.72
				DZ	432	0.29	0.00, 0.58	4.11	0.48, 35.26
Bulimia—broad	F	2,163	5.7	MZ	599	0.51	0.29, 0.73	7.49	3.17, 17.66
				DZ	433	0.25	−0.09, 0.58	2.77	0.76, 10.07

Note. Odds ratio is odds of a twin being affected if the cotwin has the disorder versus if the cotwin does not have the disorder.
[a]Not calculated because based on continuous variable.
[b]Zero cell, or not available; correlations calculated using Mplus program with constraint of equal thresholds for twin 1 and twin 2.
[c]Estimate hit upper bound.

APPENDIX 5.2. Model-Fitting Information: Change in Fit Relative to Full Model for Male and Female Twin Pairs Analyzed Separately

Disorder	Model	df	LRT Females	LRT Males
Conduct disorder	AE	1	0.0	3.2
	CE	1	2.2	0.6
	E	2	12.0	40.1
Adult antisocial behavior	AE	1	0.0	2.9
	CE	1	2.2	0.6
	E	2	12.1	60.1
Alcohol dependence	AE	1	0.0	< 0.1
	CE	1	8.6	7.2
	E	2	32.4	81.7
Alcohol abuse/ dependence	AE	1	< 0.1	0.2
	CE	1	3.9	11.0
	E	2	45.6	132.9
Nicotine dependence	AE	1	< 0.1	0.4
	CE	1	1.9	8.9
	E	2	20.0	102.7
Caffeine monthly use	AE	1	0.8	a
	CE	1	6.9	
	E	2	154.5	
Caffeine withdrawal	AE	1	0.0	a
	CE	1	2.2	
	E	2	6.5	
Any drug abuse/ dependence	AE	1	0.0	0.0
	CE	1	11.3	26.4
	E	2	59.4	190.1
Cannabis abuse/ dependence	AE	1	0.0	0.0
	CE	1	8.1	21.4
	E	2	49.5	161.5
Sedative abuse/ dependence	AE	1	0.0	0.0
	CE	1	1.3	4.1
	E	2	4.7	11.8
Stimulant abuse/ dependence	AE	1	< 0.1	0.0
	CE	1	2.1	10.4
	E	2	20.4	53.3
Cocaine abuse/ dependence	AE	1	0.0	0.9
	CE	1	6.9	1.7
	E	2	36.3	40.7
Opiate abuse/ dependence	AE	1	0.0	0.0
	CE	1	1.4	0.0
	E	2	6.4	0.0

(continued)

Disorder	Model	df	LRT Females	LRT Males
Hallucinogen abuse/	AE	1	0.0	0.0
dependence	CE	1	0.9	6.7
	E	2	4.6	24.4
Bulimia—narrow	AE	1	< 0.1	a
	CE	1	1.8	
	E	2	12.3	
Bulimia—broad	AE	1	0.0	a
	CE	1	1.6	
	E	2	18.5	

Note. LRT is likelihood ratio test, representing the fit of this model compared to the full (ACE) model.
[a]Bulimia and caffeine use and withdrawal not assessed in male pairs.
*Best-fitting model by Akaike's Information Criterion (AIC; Akaike, 1987); if no *, full model is best (or the fits of AE and CE cannot be distinguished).

APPENDIX 5.3. Parameter Estimates from Full and Best-Fitting Models, for Females, Males, and Sexes Combined

Disorder	Group	Model	Test of Sex Differences[a]	a^2 (%)	95% CI	c^2 (%)	95% CI	e^2 (%)	95% CI
Conduct disorder	Females	Full		62	0, 84	0	0, 64	38	16, 71
		AE		62	29, 84	—		38	16, 71
	Males	Full		16	0, 58	32	0, 54	52	39, 65
		CE		—		37	20, 53	63	47, 80
	Combined	Full	1.3*	26	0, 60	25	0, 53	49	39, 62
Adult antisocial behavior	Females	Full		65	0, 91	7	0, 79	28	09, 64
		AE		73	38, 91	—		27	09, 62
	Males	Full		24	0, 63	19	0, 52	57	37, 79
	Combined	Full	2.1*	28	0, 67	22	0, 53	50	33, 70
Alcohol dependence	Females	Full		61	27, 76	0	0, 27	39	24, 58
		AE		61	42, 76	—		39	24, 58
	Males	Full		50	13, 64	4	0, 35	46	36, 57
		AE		54	44, 64	—		46	36, 56
	Combined	Full	0.5*	56	31, 64	0	0, 21	44	36, 51
Alcohol abuse/ dependence	Females	Full		50	0, 67	4	0, 46	46	33, 61
		AE		55	40, 67	—		45	33, 60
	Males	Full		53	21, 68	7	0, 34	41	32, 50
		AE		60	51, 68	—		40	32, 49
	Combined	Full	0.5*	52	25, 65	6	0, 29	42	35, 50
Nicotine dependence	Females	Full		52	0, 77	6	0, 58	42	23, 69
		AE		58		—		41	23, 65
	Males	Full		57	19, 77	11	0, 43	32	23, 44
		AE		69	58, 78	—		31	22, 42
	Combined	Full	0.8*	55	22, 74	11	0, 38	34	26, 45

(continued)

111

APPENDIX 5.3. *(continued)*

Disorder	Group	Model	Test of Sex Differences[a]	a² (%)	95% CI	c² (%)	95% CI	e² (%)	95% CI
Caffeine monthly use	Females	Full	b	22	5, 33	7	0, 21	72	67, 76
		AE		29	25, 33	—		71	67, 75
Caffeine withdrawal[c]	Females	Full	b	28	0, 48	0	0, 28	72	52, 94
		AE		28	6, 48	—		72	52, 94
Any drug abuse/ dependence	Females	Full		68	35, 79	0	0, 28	32	21, 47
		AE		68	53, 79	—			21, 47
	Males	Full		78	49, 84	0	0, 26	22	16, 30
		AE		78	70, 84	—		22	16, 30
	Combined	Full	1.9*	75	57, 81	0	0, 26	25	19, 32
Cannabis abuse/ dependence	Females	Full		70	26, 83	0	0, 03	30	17, 46
		AE		70	26, 83	—		30	17, 46
	Males	Full		76	44, 83	0	0, 29	24	17, 32
		AE		76	68, 83	—		24	17, 32
	Combined	Full	0.5*	75	50, 81	0	0, 22	25	19, 33
Sedative abuse/ dependence	Females	Full		53	0, 82	0	0, 66	47	18, 89
		AE		53	11, 82	—		47	18, 89
	Males	Full		57	3, 79	0	0, 39	43	21, 74
		AE		57	26, 79	—		43	21, 74
	Combined	Full	< 0.1*	55	13, 74	0	0, 33	45	26, 69
Stimulant abuse/ dependence	Females	Full		64	0, 86	0	0, 69	32	14, 61
		AE		68	42, 86	—		32	14, 58

Disorder	Group	Model	Change in LRT[a]	%	95% CI	%	95% CI	%	95% CI
	Males	Full		66	32, 79	0	0, 29	34	21, 49
		AE		66	51, 79	—		34	21, 49
Cocaine abuse/dependence	Combined	Full	< 0.1*	67	35, 77	0	0, 27	33	23, 46
	Females	Full		77	24, 90	0	0, 46	23	10, 44
		AE		77	56, 90	—		23	10, 44
	Males	Full[c]		39	0, 79	26	0, 66	35	21, 56
	Combined	Full	1.5*	66	17, 81	5	0, 47	30	19, 42
Opiate abuse/dependence	Females	Full		77	0, 98	0	0, 86	23	2, 81
		AE		77	19, 98	—		23	2, 81
	Males	Full		0	0, 48	0	0, 34	1.00	52, 100
	Combined	Full	3.2*	19	0, 68	6	0, 47	75	32, 100
Hallucinogen abuse/dependence	Females	Full		64	0, 92	0	0, 82	36	8, 94
		AE		64	6, 92	—		36	8, 94
	Males	Full		65	22, 82	0	0, 36	35	18, 59
		AE		65	41, 82	—		35	18, 59
	Combined	Full	< 0.1*	65	26, 80	0	0, 33	35	20, 57
Bulimia—narrow	Females	Full		51	0, 77	4	0, 66	45	23, 76
		AE		55	25, 77	—		45	23, 75
Bulimia—broad	Females	Full		50	0, 68	0	0, 54	50	32, 73
		AE		50	28, 68	—		50	32, 72

Note. If only full model shown, this was best fit model, or fits of AE and CE could not be distinguished.
[a]Change in LRT comparing MF equality and MF different models; all tests $df = 2$.
[b]Consistent with male–female equality (based on AIC).
*Not conducted, analyses based on female pairs only.
[c]Based on pairs using caffeine regularly.

CHAPTER SIX

Twin Model Assumptions

Every statistical analysis is based on assumptions about measurement and about the processes underlying the variables being measured. In this chapter we describe two additional assumptions made in twin studies: *random mating* and the *equal environment assumption* (EEA). If an assumption is found to be invalid, we say that there has been a failure of the assumption. Failure of the assumptions of the twin model can lead to incorrect genetic and environmental estimates. This possibility has been the basis for many critiques of the twin method. We thus give particular attention to these assumptions and consider the evidence concerning their validity in the VATSPSUD.

RANDOM MATING

Twin models assume random mating with respect to genetic background; that is, when choosing a mate, one does not select someone with a similar genetic history. The failure of this assumption is known as *assortative mating*. The effect of assortative mating for genetic background on twin study results is to underestimate the magnitude of genetic influences and overestimate shared environmental influences on a characteristic. The reason for this arises from the mathematical predictions of the twin model: If parents are genetically correlated, then the genes of their DZ twin offspring (and other non-MZ offspring) will be correlated in excess of the 0.50 predicted by genetic theory. This will reduce the observed difference between the similarity of MZ and DZ pairs, leading to a lower estimate of heritability.

We know that spouses (and other couples who produce offspring) do not select each other randomly. Couples tend to come from similar socioeconomic and educational backgrounds. However, the critical assumption for our twin models is not that couples come from different backgrounds but that they are uncorrelated for their genetic liability to the disorder of interest. This is difficult to study. When we assess the parents of twins, we are assessing their expressed trait (e.g., whether they've ever been depressed), not the underlying genetic liability that contributes to that trait and that cannot be directly measured. Even if couples have similar traits, this does not necessarily mean that the assumption is violated. It is likely that some of the similarity observed between spouses is due to the long-term influences of living together. That is, it is being a couple that leads to the similarity, not the other way around. Such "congruence" does not represent a violation of the assumption of random mating, because it would not alter the proportion of genes shared by DZ twins.

In our judgment, two major pieces of evidence justify ignoring the effects of assortative mating on the outcomes studied in VATSPSUD. First, although the mothers and fathers interviewed as part of the FFP study did tend to resemble one another in their rates of disorders (we studied MD, GAD, and alcoholism), the overall degree of resemblance was modest (Maes et al., 1998) and too low to cause a significant bias in our twin models.

Second, the effects of assortative mating on genetic and environmental effects in a population are actually rather complex. The largest concern is overestimating the impact of shared environment. However, as we saw in Chapters 4 and 5, we have actually found less evidence for shared environmental effects than we expected, suggesting that violations of this assumption are not a substantial problem in this study.

EQUAL ENVIRONMENT ASSUMPTION

The EEA requires that twins from MZ pairs and DZ pairs are equally similar for the environments relevant to the development of a particular trait. This assumption is necessary because the twin model assumes that the correlations of the shared environmental component for both types of pairs equal 1.0 (see Figure 3.2). If the shared environment of MZ pairs is actually more similar than that of DZ pairs, this will inflate the difference in correlations between MZ and DZ twins and produce an overestimate of genetic influences.

The EEA has long been of interest to both twin researchers and critics of the twin method. Three major methods have been developed to evaluate the validity of the EEA (Kendler, 1983), including direct measurement of environmental similarity based on variables obtained from twin report, indirect measurement of similarity of treatment based on physical similarity, and pair similarity based on true versus perceived zygosity. We applied each of these methods, as well as a fourth method of our own devising based on parents' reports of their approach to rearing twins. We describe the basis for each method and then describe the results of its application to the VATSPSUD.

Similarity of Environmental Exposures

The first method rests on observations that particular aspects of the childhood, adolescent, or adult environment—such as sharing playmates as children—are more similar for twins from MZ pairs than for those from DZ pairs (Kendler, Heath, Martin, & Eaves, 1986; Kendler et al., 1992a; Loehlin & Nichols, 1976; Rose, Kaprio, Williams, Viken, & Obremski, 1990). If these measured environments, acting directly or as indices of other aspects of environmental similarity, influence twin resemblance for traits (such as liability to develop MD), then this might represent a violation of the EEA. Most researchers find that MZ twins have a higher score on such measures of similarity than do DZ twin pairs. The untutored student might conclude from this that twin studies are in big trouble. However, this student would be missing a key step. Twin studies of psychiatric disorders would indeed be in some trouble if MZ pairs had more similar environments than DZ pairs *and* if we could show that these environments altered risk for a particular psychiatric disorder. To pick a silly example, imagine that twins from MZ pairs were much more highly correlated for eating peanut butter than were DZ pairs. This would jeopardize the validity of our twin studies only if it could also be shown that the consumption of peanut butter affected risk for MD. Even if such an effect were found for MD, there is no guarantee that a similar effect of peanut butter would exist for twin resemblance for anxiety disorders or alcoholism. There is no such thing as a "generic" violation of the EEA. Potential violations of the EEA must be evaluated disorder by disorder.

In the VATSPSUD, we used several standard measures of environmental similarity (see Sidebar 6.1). The typical way we analyzed these data was to predict the pair similarity for a particular trait or disorder from zygosity and measures of similarity of childhood environment. We have performed such analyses for all the disorders studied in the VATSPSUD. In the large majority of cases, the EEA was supported. That is, we did not find that twin pairs with more similar childhood environments were more similar for psychiatric outcomes.

In our early studies of the EEA, we also used what is an admittedly crude measure of similarity of adult environment—the frequency of pair contact, typically measured for the year prior to the interview. Our results for this measure have been more mixed. We found no evidence that twin pairs who were in frequent contact were more likely to be concordant for major depression, anxiety, or eating disorders. However, among both female and male twin pairs, we found (even after controlling for zygosity) a significant association between current frequency of contact and twin resemblance for alcohol

SIDEBAR 6.1. Assessment of Twin Environmental Similarity

In the VATSPSUD, we assessed childhood environmental similarity using four items first proposed by Loehlin and Nichols (1976). In our interviews with female twins, these questions were:

> "I'm now going to ask you several questions about how close you and your twin sister were as children. How often . . .
>
> 1. did you share the same room?
> 2. did you have the same playmates?
> 3. did you dress alike?
> 4. were you in the same classes at school?"

The response options were "always," "usually," "sometimes," or "never." Typically, we have summed these items to produce a single index. The questions were modified appropriately when administered to male and opposite-sex twin pairs.

In examining the four traditional questions on childhood environments, we realized that they could be improved on in at least three ways. First, we developed questions to assess similarity of adolescent environments. Three items assessed the degree to which twins shared peers and activities:

> "As teenagers, how often would . . .
>
> 1. you and your twin have the same friends?
> 2. you and your twin go around with the same group?
> 3. your twin go out with you if you went to the movies or a dance?"

As with the childhood items, the possible responses to these items were "always," "usually," " sometimes," or "never."

Second, we assessed, with two items, the twins' view of their relationship within the twinship. One was:

> "When you were growing up, were you emotionally closer to your twin than would be usual for ordinary sisters?"

The response options ranged from "a lot closer" to "just about as close as ordinary sisters." The second item was:

> "Some twins like to be as alike as possible in their dress, interests, and personality. Other twins like to be as different from one another as possible. When you and your twin were growing up, did you . . . ?"

The response options ranged from "always try to be as alike as possible" to "always try to be as different as possible."

(continued)

SIDEBAR 6.1. (continued)

Third, we assessed the way in which the twins perceived themselves as being treated by their social environment. We attempted to assess whether they were seen as individuals (the differences between twins in a pair were emphasized) or as a pair (they were commonly treated as "the twins," thereby emphasizing their similarity to each other). We inquired of the twins, in separate questions, the extent to which their parents, relatives, teachers, friends, and peers "nearly always" or "usually" emphasized "your similarity" or emphasized "your differences."

We included these items in the FF3 interview, getting complete information from 1,865 twins and both members of 821 pairs of known zygosity. We then conducted a factor analysis using these items, the four childhood items, and adult contact frequency. When we studied the characteristics of the items, we found that they clustered into three independent factors. *Childhood Treatment* was based on the four childhood environmental similarity items. *Cosocialization* included items assessing the degree to which the twins socialized with one another in adolescence and childhood, as well as their emotional closeness. *Similitude* included items that reflected the degree to which the twins' similarities, rather than their differences, were emphasized by parents, teachers, and friends *and* one item that assessed how much the twins themselves tried to be as alike as possible.[a]

We checked these factors by seeing how closely the two members of a twin pair agreed in their ratings of their relationship, then created scores for each factor and computed the pair correlations for the scores. We found reasonable agreement between twins. Pair correlations for the three factors were: Childhood Treatment, 0.62; Cosocialization, 0.63; and Similitude, 0.49 (all significant at $p < 0.0001$).

---

[a]The interpretation of similitude is somewhat difficult in EEA studies because high scores on this factor could be a result rather than a cause of the similarity of the twins' behavior.

---

dependence (Kendler et al., 1992a; Prescott et al., 1999). How should this result be interpreted? Do twins in more frequent contact develop more similar drinking habits and problems, or do twins with more similar drinking patterns have more frequent contact?

We suspect that both processes are at work. That is, a twin's drinking habits are probably influenced by the drinking habits of his or her cotwin. But it is also likely that twin pairs with very similar drinking habits are more likely to socialize together than are pairs in which one member likes to drink and the other abstains. Analyses of other traits suggest that, on average, similarity of behavior influences frequency of contact more than the other way around (Kendler, 1983; Morris-Yates, Andrews, Howie, & Henderson, 1990). However, we decided to take a "worst case scenario" and reanalyze our data assuming that all the causal effects go from contact to drinking and not from drinking to contact.[1] In so doing, we found that the estimated heritability of broadly defined alcohol dependence declined modestly, from 61 to 46%. This means that at the most violations of the EEA accounted for only one-fourth of the genetic variance estimated from a standard twin model.

As a further illustration of our approach to the testing of the EEA, we describe in detail our attempt to use measures of childhood and adult environmental similarity to predict similarity in our male–male pairs for the use and abuse of illicit substances (Kendler, Karkowski, Neale, & Prescott, 2000a). We used drug use because, given evidence that it can be strongly influenced by the social environment, it might be more vulnerable to violations of the EEA than psychiatric disorders such as MD or panic disorder. We examined four phenotypes defined by level of involvement (use, heavy use, abuse, and dependence)[2] for each of six substances (cannabis, sedatives, stimulants, cocaine, opiates, and hallucinogens) and a summary category of "any substance." We tested the effects of similarity of childhood environment (based on answers to the childhood environment questions from interviews or questionnaires) and frequency of contact as adults. This made for 7 substance classes times 4 phenotypes times 2 kinds of environment for a total of 56 independent tests of the EEA.

After adjusting for zygosity, the similarity of childhood or adult environments significantly predicted twin resemblance in 7 of the 56 tests. That is not a very impressive number given that 3 positive results would be expected by chance alone. The positive tests did not point to any particular level of use or class of substance. However, all the significant effects were in the predicted direction—an unlikely event by chance alone. We found that similarity of childhood environment predicted twin similarity for stimulant use, hallucinogen use, heavy use of cannabis, and heavy use of any substance. Frequency of contact as adults predicted twin resemblance for heavy use of cocaine, hallucinogen abuse, and sedative dependence. To evaluate the size of these possible biases, we conducted analyses designed to detect and correct for the effects of the EEA (Hettema, Neale, & Kendler, 1995).

We included in the twin model an additional measured variable that represents environmental similarity of the twin pair (see Figure 6.1). If environmental similarity affected liability (i.e., if the specified shared environment path, c_s, were significantly greater than zero) and if inclusion of this variable decreased the estimate of the genetic variance, this would suggest a failure of the EEA.

For each of the conditions for which we detected evidence of a possible violation, we conducted follow-up analyses, using our composite measure of childhood similarity or adult contact frequency. For nearly all of the analyses, the variance accounted for by environmental similarity was negligible (averaging 7%) and not significantly different from zero. The one exception was frequency of adult contact and heavy cocaine use. With the inclusion of this variable, the heritability of liability declined from 80 to 60%. Overall, these results do not provide impressive evidence in favor of major violations of the EEA for drug use, abuse, and dependence in our study.

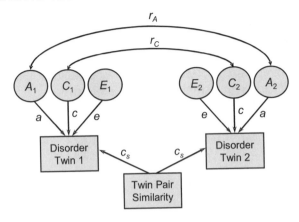

FIGURE 6.1. Twin model including measure of pair similarity.

One problem with these tests of the EEA is that "absence of evidence" is not "evidence of absence." In other words, by failing to find strong evidence for violations of the EEA, we have not produced definitive evidence that the EEA is valid. The results we obtained could arise from our having used inadequate measures of the relevant environment.

We therefore developed additional questions so that we could apply a stronger test of the EEA. These items focus on adolescent experiences because we thought these might be more important than childhood experiences in influencing risk for psychiatric or substance use disorders. We also decided to use a factor score approach so that the measures would be more reliable. The items clustered into three factors, which we termed Childhood Treatment, Cosocialization, and Similitude (see Sidebar 6.1).

We compared the scores on these factors in MZ pairs with those of DZ pairs. As expected, the factor scores for MZ twins were substantially and significantly higher than those for DZ twins on the Similitude and Cosocialization factors. To our surprise, the two twin groups did not differ in their reported levels of similarity of Childhood Treatment.

The critical analysis relevant to the EEA is whether the scores on these environmental factors predict pair similarity for psychopathology. We studied five psychiatric and two substance dependence disorders (MD, GAD, panic disorder, phobias, bulimia, nicotine dependence, and alcohol dependence) using two different models.[3] We had a total of 42 individual statistical analyses: 7 disorders by 3 factors by 2 statistical methods. To our surprise, none of the results was significant at the 5% level, even though two or three significant associations would be expected by chance alone. With our new and, we believe, improved measures, we were unsuccessful at showing possible violations of the EEA.

When a method obtains so many negative findings, the researcher ought to consider the possibility that something is really wrong with the approach.

To reassure ourselves that this was not the case, we included a phenotype that we knew was strongly influenced by peer group—smoking initiation (that is, the decision whether or not to become a regular smoker; Urberg, Shyu, & Liang, 1990). When we repeated the EEA analyses on smoking initiation, we indeed found a significant effect, not for Childhood Treatment or for Similitude but for Cosocialization—exactly the factor we would have predicted. The effects were not huge, but they were statistically significant using both of our methods. We again assumed a worst-case scenario: that all of the measured effect on smoking was due to EEA violation (i.e., that peers influence smoking, not that adolescents select their friends to be similar for smoking habits). As we saw with illicit substances, the results were underwhelming. The estimated heritability of smoking initiation declined from 83 to 73%.

Parental Treatment

We were sufficiently preoccupied with the validity of the EEA that we decided to take another approach to this problem (Kendler, Neale, Kessler, Heath, & Eaves, 1994b). Prior studies suggested that parents of MZ twins treat the twins more similarly than do parents of DZ pairs (Loehlin & Nichols, 1976; Scarr, 1968). If this is true, *and* if the kind of parental treatment for which MZ pairs are more highly correlated than DZ pairs significantly influences the risk for particular forms of adult psychopathology, then differential parental treatment would violate the EEA.

We asked all interviewed parents the following question:

> "We're interested in learning how you approached raising twins. Some parents of twins like to emphasize the similarity of their twins by doing such things as dressing them alike. Other parents of twins like to stress their differences. Would you say you: nearly always emphasized their similarity, usually emphasized their similarity, usually emphasized their differences, or nearly always emphasized their differences?"

Although parents varied widely in their reported approach to rearing twins, there was a strong association between our assigned zygosity and the reported approach to raising twins in both mothers and fathers. Both parents were more likely to emphasize the similarities in MZ twins and the differences in DZ twins. We then applied our EEA structural equation model (SEM; Figure 6.1) to these data, now treating parental ratings of their approach to twin rearing as the specified shared environment. For the four disorders tested (MD, GAD, phobias, and problem drinking), we found no evidence that twin resemblance was explained by similarity of maternal or paternal treatment. Again, we found no support for EEA violations.

In sum, despite our best efforts, our studies employing measured similarity of the environment yielded little evidence of EEA violations. It appears that concerns about the EEA in the literature, at least with respect to psychiatric disorders, are not well supported empirically.

Physical Resemblance

A large body of evidence suggests that physical attractiveness influences a wide range of social interactions (Patzer, 1985) and thus may be relevant for psychological functioning. Some critics of the twin method have claimed that the greater physical resemblance of twins from MZ pairs may cause resemblance for psychological traits.

Given the striking degree of physical resemblance of MZ twins, one would expect MZ pairs to be more correlated for attractiveness than DZ pairs. If, for example, being attractive increases self-esteem and thereby reduces the risk for depression, this could be a violation of the EEA.[4] To test the EEA by this method requires some measure of the degree of physical resemblance of the twin pairs. Using this measure, the simple task is then to ask, separately for MZ and DZ pairs, whether pair similarity for a particular disorder is predicted by physical similarity of the pair.

When we interviewed our twins face-to-face, we took photographs (with permission), initially for the purpose of zygosity determination. However, we also realized that we could use them to test the EEA (Hettema et al., 1995). Along with our close colleague Jack Hettema, we developed a reliable system for rating pair physical resemblance from these photographs. We rated all 882 pairs of female–female twins for whom we had usable photographs from both twins. As might be expected, the average similarity scores were higher in MZ than in DZ pairs, but variation was seen within each zygosity group.[5]

Using the structural model described earlier (Figure 6.1), we then included physical similarity as a specified form of shared environment in the twin models for five disorders: MD, GAD, phobia, alcohol dependence, and bulimia. For four of the disorders (MD, GAD, phobia, and alcohol dependence), we found no evidence for violations of the EEA. The c_s path could be set to zero without a significant worsening of model fit. However, for bulimia, the results were ambiguous and differed depending on how bulimia was measured. In one analysis we found no evidence for EEA violations, but in another the results suggested that nearly all twin resemblance could be explained through the c_s path.

Our conclusion is that for four of the disorders, the results are consistent with the EEA. For bulimia, our results were ambiguous, and it is possible our heritability estimates are biased upward.

Perceived versus True Zygosity

Probably the most clever method for testing the EEA was initially proposed by Scarr (1968). It is based on the proposition that similarity of twins may be influenced by the expectations of twins and their parents that MZ pairs will be more similar than DZ pairs. This method involves comparing trait similarity in twin pairs as a function of their "real" zygosity and their "perceived" zygosity. This method is possible because a substantial proportion of twins are actually misinformed as to their true zygosity. Many but not all of these errors arise because parents are provided incorrect information at birth. As described in Chapter 3, 20–30% of MZ pairs—those that split early in development—have two placentas and two inner and outer sacs in the womb. Obstetricians not highly familiar or experienced with twin pregnancies sometimes conclude that such pairs are DZ and so inform the parents. The opposite error also occurs. As we noted in Chapter 3, by chance, DZ embryos can implant so close together in the wall of the uterus that during development their placentas grow together. If not carefully examined in a laboratory, these fused placentas look like a single placenta and can lead an obstetrician to conclude that the twins, if they are the same sex, must be MZ.

To test the EEA by this method, we compare four types of twin pairs—real MZ twins who think they are MZ, real MZ twins who think they are DZ, real DZ twins who think they are MZ, and real DZ twins who think they are DZ. These four types form a particularly interesting natural experiment. If the EEA is valid, then pair similarity for a trait should be determined completely by actual zygosity and not be influenced by perceived zygosity. In contrast, if pair similarity is influenced by perceived zygosity, then this suggests a failure of the EEA.

This method of evaluating the EEA has one distinct advantage over the other approaches we utilized. Whereas the other methods require the investigator to assess particular sources of trait similarity in twins (physical appearance, dressing alike as children, actions of parent), this method provides a global test for *all* potential environmental influences that are dependent on attitudes and expectations associated with zygosity.

In our female–female sample, we asked each twin whether, in her opinion, she and her cotwin were definitely identical, probably identical, probably fraternal, definitely fraternal, or she was not sure what kind of twins they were (Kendler, Neale, Kessler, Heath, & Eaves, 1993b). We then compared these responses to our objective zygosity determination, which (at this stage in the VATSPSUD) was based on self-report measures, photographs, and, when there was uncertainty, DNA analyses. In our 1,030 FF pairs with clearly assigned zygosity, we found that in 477 of the 590 pairs (80.8%) classified as MZ, both twins agreed that they were definitely or probably identical. In 395 of the 440 (89.8%) pairs classified as DZ, both twins agreed that they were definitely or probably fraternal. We then fit our structural model for testing the EEA (Figure 6.1)—this time with perceived zygosity as the specified shared environment. For all five disorders we tested (MD, GAD, phobias, bulimia, and problem drinking), we could set the c_s path to zero. These results mean that, in our data, once true zygosity was taken into account, perceived zygosity did not contribute further to twin resemblance. Twin pairs who were really MZ but thought they were DZ were approximately as similar as other

MZ pairs. Pairs who were really DZ but believed they were MZ were as similar as other DZ pairs.

Whereas most large twin studies obtain information only from the twins themselves, we had information from our interviews with the parents of the female–female twin pairs. We asked the same question of the parents regarding the zygosity of their twin offspring. Compared with our objective assignment of zygosity, mothers and fathers were correct about the zygosity of their twins 84 and 79% of the time, respectively. Using mothers' perceived zygosity and then fathers' perceived zygosity as indices of a specified shared environment, we fit models for four of our more common disorders: MD, GAD, phobias, and problem drinking. The results were very similar to those based on twins' beliefs. In none of the 8 analyses (4 disorders times 2 parents) did we detect evidence that parental perceived zygosity had an impact on twin resemblance.[6]

SUMMARY

It is quite reasonable to be concerned about biases in twin studies of psychiatric and drug abuse disorders. Twin studies are not controlled experiments, and therefore biases can certainly creep in. In our view, the most likely biases in studies of reared-together twins are due to violations of the EEA. Such biases are of particular concern because they lead to overestimations of heritability.

Consistent with other studies, we found evidence that some aspects of the environment of members of MZ pairs are, on average, more similar than those of members of DZ pairs. However, using four different methods (twin ratings of similarity of childhood, adolescent, and adult environments; similarity of parental treatment; ratings of physical similarity from photographs; and comparisons of true versus twin-perceived and parent-perceived zygosity), we found no consistent evidence for significant EEA violations. We were unable to show that the kinds of environmental experiences for which MZ pairs are more similar than DZ pairs have anything to do with subsequent risk for psychiatric or substance use disorders.

A few findings suggested possible violations of the EEA. However, when we corrected for these effects, the result was only a modest decline in heritability estimates. Our results are generally consistent with those of other twin studies, which also find little support for any widespread or consistent violations of the EEA.[7]

One explanation for the lack of findings is that our methods have poor power to detect EEA violations. Therefore, in our study of parental perceived zygosity and approaches to rearing, we performed formal power analyses (Kendler et al., 1994b). The power depended on the prevalence of the disorder. For the more common disorders of MD and alcoholism, we had greater than 70% power to detect effects of violations of the EEA that accounted for as little as 5% of the variance in liability.

What can we conclude from our efforts? We would be surprised if the EEA were found to be precisely correct. Violations probably occur. Our guess is that they are more frequent for traits involving social behavior (such as drug use) than for disorders such as depression and anxiety. However, we also think it is unlikely that the EEA produces large-scale biases in the results we have obtained from the VATSPSUD. We cannot rule out the possibility that we have simply not measured the right kind of environment. But for us, the smattering of positive results compared with the large number of negative findings and the absence of any consistent picture of violations across a range of methods speaks volumes. The heritability estimates presented in this book may not be precisely correct, and some of them might be slightly inflated due to EEA violations that are below the level our methods can detect. However, on the basis of the data reviewed in this chapter, we would argue that the estimates from our twin analyses are substantially correct.

NOTES

1. In this early study (Kendler et al., 1992a), we used a rather simplistic method of randomly excluding from the analysis high-contact MZ and low-contact DZ pairs until the two groups of twins were matched in level of contact. Later, we made these corrections statistically and obtained similar results.

2. *Use* meant any lifetime use. *Heavy use* was defined as using the substance more than 10 times in a month. (See Sidebars 5.2 and 5.6.)

3. In the first, or *pairwise*, approach, we predicted concordance for the disorder in twin pairs from the mean factor score of the twin pair, controlling for the effect of zygosity. This model asks, separately, within MZ and DZ twins, whether—correcting for any relationship between factor scores and affection status (whether neither, one, or both were affected)—twin pairs who scored more highly on these factors were more likely to be concordant for the disorder. In the second, or *individual*, method, we predicted the probability of the cotwin being affected from the twin's factor score, the twin's affection status, and the interaction between them. For example, evidence for a violation of the EEA would be found if one twin's affection status was a significantly better predictor of her cotwin's affection status when the twin reported high frequencies of social contact with the twin during adolescence.

4. In the largest study of its kind, we found no relation between level of beauty (rated from photographs) and level of depressive symptoms in our sample of female–female pairs (McGovern, Neale, & Kendler, 1996). However, even if such an association did exist, it would not be precisely correct to call it a violation of the EEA. This is better described as an evocative genotype–environment interaction in which "genes for beauty" affect level of social support or praise and thus influence risk for depression. This is not really, then, a "bias" in the estimate of heritability but represents an unusual "outside the skin" pathway through which genes might influence risk (see Chapter 14).

5. We formed a rough 1–7 scale, from most to least similar in appearance. Rater 1 scored all 882 pairs, and raters 2 and 3 scored 100 pairs each. Finally, rater 1 scored the same 100 pairs some weeks later, long after he could remember the scores he had assigned to particular pairs. Our test–retest reliability among the three raters was good ($r = 0.68$), and the test–retest reliability of rater 1 was excellent ($r = 0.77$). For our structural models, we most commonly utilized a dichotomy or a trichotomy of pairs based on their degree of similarity (Hettema et al., 1995). The correlation between zygosity (being MZ) and our dichotomous measure of similarity was 0.78.

6. As might be expected, a similar relationship was found between parental perceived zygosity and the parents' approach to raising twins. This made us curious about the origins of parental treatment of twins. Did parental treatment relate to the parents' ideas about the zygosity of their children or to their true zygosity? In mothers, perceived zygosity strongly predicted rearing approach, whereas true zygosity did not. In fathers, both perceived zygosity and true zygosity significantly predicted rearing behavior.

7. Kendler (1983) reviewed the extant literature—then nine studies—concluding that they provided no consistent evidence of violations of the EEA. The literature since then has grown considerably. Most studies continue to support the EEA (e.g., Heath, Jardine, & Martin, 1989; Klump, Holly, Iacono, McGue, & Willson, 2000; Morris-Yates et al., 1990; Xian et al., 2000). However, a few studies have emerged that raise concerns about this assumption (e.g., Clifford, Hopper, Fulker, & Murray, 1984; Kaprio, Koskenvuo, & Rose, 1990), although the assumptions of at least one of these studies have been questioned (Lykken, McGue, Bouchard, & Tellegen, 1990).

PART III

ENVIRONMENTAL RISK

CHAPTER SEVEN

Childhood Experiences and Risk for Psychopathology

W e now switch perspectives. In Part II, we were psychiatric geneticists trying to quantify the magnitude of the etiological role of genetic factors in common psychiatric and substance use disorders. In Part III, we take the perspective of psychiatric epidemiologists. Our goal is to understand the association between key *environmental risk factors* and these psychiatric and substance use disorders. In Part II, we considered our sample as essentially a large collection of twin pairs and analyzed twin-pair similarity to estimate genetic and environmental contributions to risk. In Part III, we view the participants as an epidemiological cohort—a large, representative sample of adults born in Virginia. Here we use a variety of analyses, attempting first to quantify the association between environmental risk factors and the risk for psychiatric and substance use disorders. Then we begin to struggle with a central theme of this book—how, in the study of environmental risk factors, can we move from *correlation* to *causation*?

We consider environmental risk factors in two groups. In Chapter 8, we explore the effects of *proximal* risk factors—those occurring in the 1-year period preceding the interview. In this chapter, we examine *distal* risk factors—events or experiences from childhood and adolescence—and their associations with the lifetime occurrence of the disorders assessed in the VATSPSUD. We attempt to answer three questions:

1. Is parenting received in childhood associated with psychopathology experienced in adulthood?
2. Is loss of a parent during childhood a risk factor for the development of psychiatric disorders?
3. Is childhood sexual abuse associated with adult psychopathology?

IS PARENTING RECEIVED IN CHILDHOOD ASSOCIATED WITH ADULT PSYCHOPATHOLOGY?

Our studies of parenting in the VATSPSUD have attempted to address four questions: What aspects of parenting are associated with adult psychopathology? Do these associations differ for different types of disorders? Do the parenting styles of mothers and fathers interact to influence risk for psychopathology? Are these associations truly causal or merely correlational?

There is a long history behind the assumption that the way children are raised has a profound long-term impact on their psychosocial development (Maccoby, 1992). The focus on the relationship between parental rearing behavior and mental health is a more recent phenomenon but has generated a large literature (Parker & Gladstone, 1996; Perris, Arrindell, & Eisemann, 1994). Before describing our results, we review five issues raised by this research that influenced our work.

One central theme of prior literature is figuring out how many meaningful dimensions of parenting exist. As might be expected, many scales have been developed over the years to measure parenting behavior. In an incisive review of the early literature, Maccoby and Martin (1983) observed a broad consensus for one parenting dimension that reflects the level of warmth or lovingness communicated to the child by his or her parents' words and actions. This dimension has received a variety of names, including "love versus hostility," "acceptance versus rejection," and "warmth" (e.g., Perris et al., 1994). Another dimension identified by Maccoby and Martin (1983) that has less consensus reflects the level of control and authority that the parents attempt to impose upon the child. Names for this dimension have included "autonomy versus control," "restrictive versus permissive," "strictness," and "protectiveness." They noted that evidence has accumulated that this second dimension can be separated into two relatively distinct factors that reflect level of control and the degree of "autonomy giving." Several other dimensions for parenting behavior have been proposed, but there is much less consensus about them. As described in Sidebar 7.1, for the VATSPSUD we selected a scale for parenting that contains the three most agreed-upon dimensions (Coldness, Protectiveness, Authoritarianism).

A second focus of prior literature is addressing whether the association between parenting and subsequent psychopathology is mainly a result of the direct effect of individual dimensions (e.g., low parental warmth increases risk for adult depression) or whether the relationships are more complex, reflect-

SIDEBAR 7.1. Assessment of Parenting in the VATSPSUD

We focused on the parenting received by the twins as recalled by the twins, their cotwins, and their parents (Kendler, 1996b). The measure we used to assess parenting is a shortened form of the Parental Bonding Instrument (PBI; Parker, Tupling, & Brown, 1979; Parker, 1989, 1990), a widely studied and validated scale. The PBI was designed to assess two dimensions quite similar to those identified in the prior literature by Maccoby and Martin (1983): warmth and overprotection. However, analyses conducted by us and by other researchers have shown that the overprotection items are better grouped into two scales reflecting parental *Protectiveness* and *Authoritarianism*. High scores on the Protectiveness scale reflect an overprotective and controlling approach to parenting, whereas high scores on Authoritarianism indicate a parental style that discourages autonomy and independence. For consistency with the other scales, we reversed the direction of the warmth scale, renaming it *Coldness*, with high scores reflecting low levels of warmth and caring in the parent–child relationship.

Examples of these items (using wording from the version that asked twins about the parenting they received from their mothers) are:

- Coldness—My mother: "was emotionally distant from me" and "enjoyed talking things over with me" (reverse).
- Protectiveness—"was overprotective of me" and "tended to baby me."
- Authoritarianism—"was consistent in enforcing rules" and "let me dress in any way I pleased" (reverse).

We defined the age range covered by the PBI as up to the twins' 16th birthdays. We changed the pronouns in the items as needed to permit responses from parents, twins, and cotwins. Twins and parents were given four response options to each item, which ranged from "a lot" to "not at all."

Each twin answered four sets of PBI items for the ways she perceived herself as having been raised by her mother and by her father and for the ways she perceived her cotwin as having been raised by their mother and by their father. Each parent completed two sets of PBI items reflecting his or her perceptions about raising each twin.

The analyses we describe are based on 787 families for whom we have complete data on the PBIs from both twins and at least one parent (see Kendler, Myers, & Prescott, 2000b, for more detail). Our analyses are of the female twin pairs, because we did not interview parents of male and opposite-sex twins about the parenting they provided. In these analyses we combined the reports on parenting from the twin, the cotwin, and the mother or father. For example, for the level of mother's coldness to twin 1, we combined the reports of the mother describing how she raised twin 1; of twin 1 describing how she was raised by her mother; and of twin 2 describing how she perceived twin 1 was raised by her mother. We assumed that the combined report of multiple informants would reflect more accurately the true parenting because it would be less influenced by error or bias than the report of any single informant.

The scores of the PBI scales are arbitrary and without any inherent meaning. To allow us to compare results across the three parenting dimensions, we standardized the PBI scores. We took every rating and put it on a normal distribution so that scores of -1.0 and $+2.5$ would mean, respectively, that the score was 1 standard deviation below the mean or $2\frac{1}{2}$ standard deviations above the mean.

ing an interaction either between parenting dimensions or between the parenting received from the mother versus that from the father. For example, one influential theory postulates that the most pathogenic form of parenting results from a combination of low levels of warmth and high levels of control (Parker, 1983). Alternatively, other studies suggest that the pathogenic effect of having one cold and distant parent can be largely offset by having a warm and loving relationship with the other parent (Werner, 1987). Our study was able to investigate the presence and nature of such interactions.

A third issue, too infrequently addressed in the prior literature, is whether there is any specificity in the association between dimensions of parenting and risk for particular psychiatric and drug abuse disorders. The literature on the parenting–psychopathology link has focused overwhelmingly on depression. Little attention has been given to addressing whether the kind of parenting that increases risk for depression also affects the liability to anxiety disorders or substance use or whether different patterns of parenting predispose to different kinds of disorders. Our study was designed to address these questions.

Also too infrequently studied is a fourth issue—whether parenting received from fathers is of similar importance to that received from mothers. Perhaps due to the nearly exclusive focus of psychodynamic schools on the mother–child relationship, father–child relationships remain understudied.

Fifth, and perhaps most important, few studies of the association between parenting behavior and psychopathology have investigated the reason for these associations. In particular, previous studies have too quickly assumed that "correlation equals causation" and that parenting directly causes psychopathology. However, there are alternative explanations. Figure 7.1 illustrates three possible explanations for the association between parenting and psychopathology (in this case, depression), only one of which (a) is causal. Parental coldness could be associated with offspring depression because of a true causal relationship—being raised by rejecting parents might negatively affect self-esteem and vulnerability to stress, thus directly increasing risk for developing depression (Figure 7.1a). But Figures 7.1b and 7.1c show two alternative explanations worth considering. In Figure 7.1b, a set of genetically influenced traits affect both parenting style and risk for depression. These traits might make parents less capable of being loving and warm and, when passed on genetically to their children, increase the risk of depression in those children.

Another plausible explanation is illustrated in Figure 7.1c: that characteristics of children influence the behavior of their parents. Early research on parent–child relationships focused on the unidirectional nature of the relationship (i.e., parent → child). But, influenced by a well-known article by Bell (1968), research conducted more recently has acknowledged the inherent bidirectionality of the parent–child relationship. Certain childhood traits (e.g., a highly irritable temperament) may make it more difficult for parents to respond to a child with warmth and understanding and also increase that child's risk for later episodes of depression (Figure 7.1c). As we shall see,

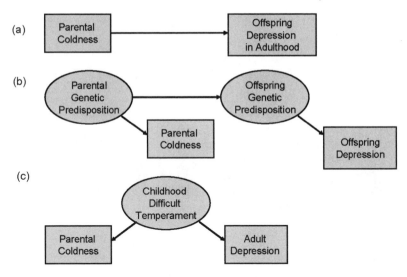

FIGURE 7.1. Alternative explanations for an association between parenting received in childhood and adult depression. (a) Causal model; (b) indirect influence via genetic factors; (c) parenting and depression influenced by childhood characteristics.

studying twins and their parents can help us choose among these alternative explanations.

In the VATSPSUD, we studied three dimensions of parenting—Protectiveness, Authoritarianism, and Coldness—based on an abbreviated version of the Parental Bonding Instrument (PBI; see Sidebar 7.1). We began by examining the association between each of the three dimensions and the seven psychiatric and substance use disorders assessed in the VATSPSUD. We examined these associations separately for maternal and paternal parenting. Based on prior results showing that the prevalences of the disorders differ among women of different ages, we included age at interview as a covariate in these analyses.

The results are shown in Figure 7.2a. We quantified the magnitude of the parenting–psychopathology associations by using odds ratios (ORs). Because the PBI scores are standardized, the ORs reflect the change in risk expected for a change of 1 standard deviation in the parenting score. So the OR of 1.26 for maternal coldness and depression means that for every 1 standard deviation increase in the mother's coldness, the risk for MD increases by 26%. We found that each of the parenting dimensions is associated with the internalizing disorders. The relationship with bulimia and the substance use disorders is less consistent, but parental coldness appears to be important.

We do not want to overinterpret these results. Our analyses have a major limitation in that they include only two variables in what is certainly a complex causal system. As shown in Figure 7.1, other variables could account for the association between parenting and adult psychopathology. For example, if

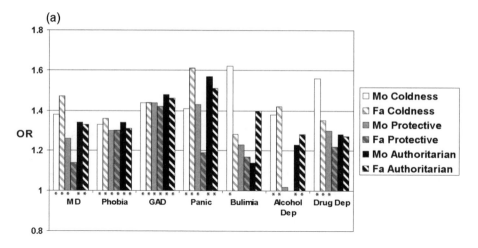

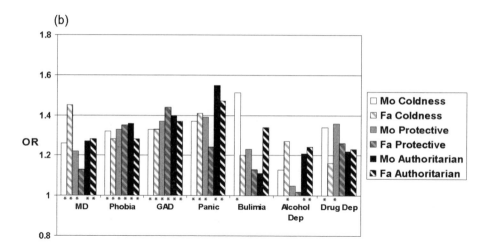

FIGURE 7.2. Odds ratios (OR) for the association between parenting dimensions and lifetime psychiatric and substance use disorders among adult twins. MD = major depression; GAD = generalized anxiety disorder; Dep = dependence; Mo = mother; Fa = father. (a) Without adjusting for covariates; (b) after adjusting for covariates; *significantly greater than 1.0 ($p < 0.05$). Data from Kendler, Myers, and Prescott (2000b, Table 1).

the association between parenting and twin psychopathology were largely noncausal and mediated through parental psychopathology (as depicted in Figure 7.1b) or through childhood temperament (Figure 7.1c), then the parenting–psychopathology association would disappear when these additional variables were added to the analyses.

To try to determine whether the association between parenting and later outcome is likely to be causal, we conducted a second series of analyses, adding measures that reflect six domains associated with parenting behavior: demographic features, family characteristics, parental symptoms and personality, parental lifetime psychopathology, child vulnerability, and childhood temperament. Including these variables in the analysis allows us to test specifically for the noncausal paths illustrated in Figures 7.1b and 7.1c. If their inclusion decreases the OR for the parenting–psychopathology association, this is evidence that the association is noncausal. The results are shown in Figure 7.2b and discussed subsequently.

We can reach four major conclusions from this study. First, the magnitude of the associations between parenting behavior and psychopathology, although usually statistically significant in our large sample, is modest. For example, moving from an average level of maternal coldness to 1 standard deviation above the mean (which is equivalent to moving from a score higher than obtained by ~50% of the population to a score higher than ~84% of the population) increases the lifetime risk for most disorders by 20–60% (i.e., OR of 1.2 to 1.6).

Second, the effects of dysfunctional parenting are not specific to a particular diagnosis. In general, the associations are strongest for the internalizing disorders of major depression and the three anxiety disorders (GAD, panic disorder, and phobias). The associations are weaker between parenting and bulimia, alcoholism, and drug dependence, but this could be due to methodological factors.[1]

Third, the addition of other family risk variables (Figure 7.2b vs. 7.2a) produces only a modest reduction in the relationships between parenting and offspring psychopathology. These results increase our confidence that the association between parenting behavior and psychiatric and substance disorders in the offspring is at least partly causal and not the result of the mechanisms illustrated in Figures 7.1b and 7.1c.

Fourth, the strength of association is similar for parenting by mothers and by fathers. As least for girls, obtaining poor-quality parenting from their fathers appears to be as important as poor parenting from their mothers.

Interactions among Parent Dimensions

These initial sets of analyses address many of the important questions we began with about the relationship between parenting and risk for psychopathology. However, as noted earlier, one question inadequately addressed in the prior literature is the importance of interactions between dimensions of parenting. Parker and colleagues (Leon & Leon, 1998; Parker, 1979, 1983; Rodgers, 1996) have suggested that a parenting style termed "affectionless control," characterized by both high levels of coldness and high levels of control, is particularly pathogenic—especially for depression. In our study, this hypothesis would predict positive interactions between Coldness and either Protectiveness or Authoritarianism in influencing risk for psychiatric disorders. Other interactions might be important for risk for other disorders but have received less attention.

We therefore examined, separately for each disorder and separately for mothers and fathers, all the possible two-way interactions between the three parenting dimensions. The results are strikingly unimpressive. The number of significant interactions is slightly more than would be expected by chance (given that we did so many analyses), and none of them are the same across mothers and fathers (further suggesting that these may be chance results). Our results do not support the hypothesis that certain key combinations of parenting (e.g., high Coldness and high Protectiveness) are especially pathogenic for children.

We also wanted to examine whether the parenting received from the mother and the father interact with each other in predicting risk for psychopathology in their offspring. Both clinical experience and some research findings (Werner & Smith, 1989) suggest that a good relationship with one parent can offset the pathogenic impact of a bad relationship with the other parent. This hypothesis predicts a *positive* interaction between high levels of maternal and paternal coldness in predicting psychopathology in offspring. That is, having a cold, unloving relationship with both parents is predicted to have more than twice the negative effect of such a relationship with one parent. Our results do not support this hypothesis. No significant positive interactions were seen for parental coldness for any of the seven disorders examined. However, there is modest evidence that above-average levels of parental protectiveness and authoritarianism in both parents is associated with higher than expected risk for several disorders.

Interpretations

As described in Chapters 4 and 5, the results from our traditional twin modeling suggest no evidence that shared family environment affects risk for most of the disorders studied in the VATSPSUD. Now we are claiming to have found significant, albeit modest, associations that we suspect are causal between parenting behavior and risk for these same disorders. How can we explain these apparently contradictory findings?

In fact, these two sets of findings are entirely consistent. One reason for this is a conceptual one: Although twins have the same parents and (are assumed to) receive the same type of parenting from them, they may react to the parenting in different ways. If the twins' reactions are guided in part by genetically influenced characteristics (e.g., temperament), then parenting effects would show up in twin models as genetic, not shared environmental, effects. Another reason is statistical: Our standard twin modeling is not a sensitive method for detecting small shared environmental effects, particularly in the presence of moderate degrees of heritability. Based on the results of our parenting analyses, the aggregate effect summed across all three parenting dimensions and across both parents would create an overlap in liability between siblings of between 1 and 4%. Our twin sample is not large enough to detect effects of this size.[2]

IS PARENTAL LOSS A RISK FACTOR FOR PSYCHIATRIC DISORDERS?

Two major descriptive traditions within psychology and psychiatry have focused on children's loss of a parent as a critical risk factor for subsequent psychiatric disorders. Psychoanalytic theory suggests that depression frequently arises as a result of stressful experiences in adulthood, reactivating the trauma of early parental loss (Breier et al., 1988). Attachment theory, deriving from the seminal work of Bowlby (1980), postulates an evolutionarily derived instinctive pattern of attachment behavior in infancy and childhood, the disruption of which can have substantial and diverse long-term consequences.

Four key issues in the literature have influenced our work. First, very few studies have explored the relationship between parental loss and risk for a broader spectrum of disorders (Tennant, 1988). Motivated by the work of Freud and other psychoanalysts, most studies of parental loss have examined only depression. Our understanding of parental loss as a risk factor would differ considerably if its effects were specific (influencing risk for depression only) rather than more general (increasing risk for a whole range of disorders). Our study design enabled us to address this issue.

Second, there are two major causes of parental loss: death and divorce. These may represent quite different risk factors because parental separation is often accompanied (and preceded) by parental strife and other aspects of family dysfunction, whereas this is not often the case with the death of a parent. We therefore studied separately the loss of parents due to death and to marital breakup (see Sidebar 7.2).

Third, relatively little attention has been paid to the importance of the timing of parental loss and the increased risk of illness. Nearly all studies of the impact of losing a parent have examined whether a given outcome (e.g., MD) has or has not ever occurred (Tennant, 1988) but not the time course of increased risk for onset of disorders in relation to the loss. Therefore, we studied the time course of the change in risk after loss of a parent. In particular, we wanted to know whether parental loss is associated with a lifelong increased risk of illness or if parental loss produces a temporary "spike" of increased risk that returns to baseline over some period of years.

Fourth, as we address repeatedly in this book, the tricky issue of causality has rarely been adequately addressed in the literature on parental loss.

SIDEBAR 7.2. Defining Parental Loss

Parental loss was defined as a physical separation from a mother, father, or substitute parent figure occurring prior to the twins' 17th birthdays. Long-term separations, such as those due to military service, were not counted as long as the parent returned to the family at the conclusion of the separation. We counted as divorce a few cases of long-term marital separation that occurred without a legal divorce. If twins experienced more than one type of loss, we used the age at the first loss event.

For these analyses, our assessment of MD explicitly excluded episodes that could be normal grief reactions (i.e., lasting less than 3 months and following the death of a family member or close friend).

Although loss of a parent itself could contribute directly to increased risk for subsequent psychopathology (similar to parental coldness, as in Figure 7.1a), there are also indirect mechanisms (similar to those depicted in Figures 7.1b and 7.1c). Parents may have genetically influenced traits that increase the risk of death or divorce and that, when passed on to their children, increase their risk for psychopathology. Alternatively, a child may have certain traits (e.g., high levels of CD) that cause sufficient family strife to increase both the risk of parents' divorce and the child's risk for later psychopathology. In Chapter 15 we take another critical look at the causal nature of the relationship between parental loss and psychopathology in the offspring by combining information from twins and their interviewed parents.

In VATSPSUD we studied the association between parental loss and risk for seven disorders. The results are portrayed in Figure 7.3.[3] Loss of a parent was associated with a significantly increased risk of MD, GAD, panic disorder, AD, and drug abuse/dependence, but not with risk for phobias or bulimia. The lack of an association with bulimia might be caused by a reduction in statistical power due both to the relative rarity of the condition and to the fact that this disorder was assessed only in female twins. The results shown in Figure 7.3 are different from those presented in Figure 7.2, so the findings cannot be compared directly. Parenting quality is something one experiences over many years; our results reflect the effects of parenting on risk for disorders accumulated over the entire lifetimes of the twins. By contrast, loss of a parent is temporally discrete: It happens at one particular time. The results shown in Figure 7.3 reflect the risk for a disorder in the year of loss of the parent. If we analyze the effects of parental loss using the same methods that we did for parenting quality, the magnitudes of all these effects are modest: They correspond to an increase in lifetime risk of 30–70%, quite similar to those seen in Figure 7.2.

We also found that there are differences associated with a parent's death versus parents' divorce. Parent death is quite specific, significantly increasing risk only for MD. Although we are not major fans of psychoanalytic theory, we must admit that this finding is consistent with the prediction from Freud's famous essay "Mourning and Melancholia" (Freud, 1917/1957). By contrast,

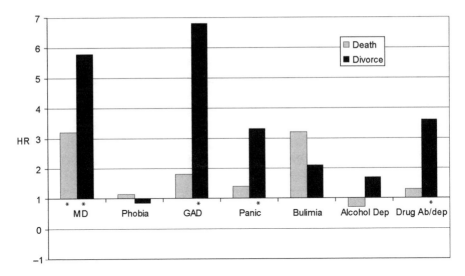

FIGURE 7.3. Hazard ratios (HR) for the association between type of parental loss and the same-year onset of psychiatric and substance use disorders among male and female twins; *significantly greater than 1.0 ($p < 0.05$). MD = major depression; GAD = generalized anxiety disorder; Ab/dep = abuse/dependence.

loss of a parent due to divorce is largely nonspecific, increasing risk for mood, anxiety, and substance use disorders.

What can we learn about the relationship between loss and risk of illness by examining the time course of increased risk? We first tested whether the increase in risk of illness after parental loss that we depicted in Figure 7.3 was permanent or whether the risk decreased over time. Figure 7.4 portrays these two scenarios. A constant change in risk after parental loss is depicted as a solid line. The dashed line shows the expected pattern if there is a decay of risk. In this case, an initial "jump" in risk occurs during the year after the loss of the parent, followed by a decline, reflecting the speed with which the risk returns to baseline.[4]

The results of our analyses are summarized in Figure 7.5. For four of the five analyses in which we detected a significant effect of parental loss by death or divorce (see Figure 7.3), the impact of the loss decays over time. The decay is relatively slow for all disorders, ranging from 21 years for GAD to 49 years for panic disorder. Because these participants had lost parents when they were 16 or younger, this means that the increase in risk for these disorders associated with parental loss persists into middle adult life. Only with alcohol dependence is there a permanent increase in risk associated with parental loss. For MD, the one disorder for which we could meaningfully make the comparison, the impact of death on risk is much shorter-lived than the impact of divorce. The estimated times for return to baseline risk are 13 years for death and 35 years for divorce.

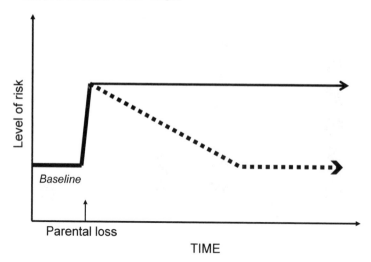

FIGURE 7.4. Alternative models for the time course of the effect of parental loss on risk for psychiatric disorder.

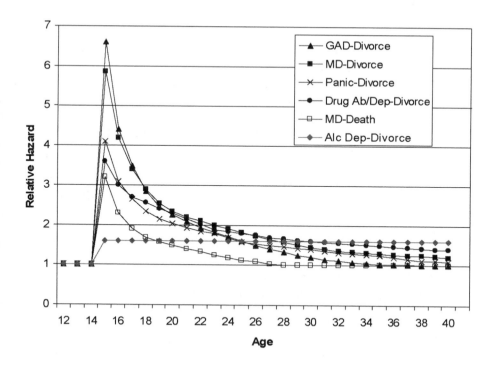

FIGURE 7.5. Results from analyses of the time course of the significant effects of parental loss on risk for psychiatric disorder. GAD = generalized anxiety disorder; MD = major depression; Alc = alcohol; Ab/dep = abuse/dependence.

What do these results tell us about the relationship between loss and risk of psychopathology? We tentatively suggest the following interpretation. By far the shortest time to recovery is seen for MD and parent death. Here, we suspect that parent death acts like a true highly traumatic discrete event. In contrast, the risk for MD, GAD, and panic disorder following loss of a parent due to divorce is increased for a considerably longer period, 20 to 35 years. We may be seeing the longer term impact of the marital and family dysfunction that is often associated with parental divorce. For drug abuse/dependence, the increased risk associated with parental divorce does not return to baseline for 55 years, and for alcohol dependence it never returns to baseline. Here we suspect a mixed picture, including direct effects of parental and family discord, as well as indirect factors. In Figure 7.6 we depict what may be the source of the indirect association between parent divorce and offspring substance abuse, occurring because both are influenced by the parent's liability to substance abuse.

How do our findings relate to the literature? As noted earlier, many studies have found an association between loss of a parent and depression (e.g., Lloyd, 1980; Tennant, Smith, Bebbington, & Hurry, 1981; Tennant, Hurry, & Bebbington, 1982; Tennant, 1988), with far fewer studies looking at other disorders (e.g., AD; Hope, Power, & Rodgers, 1998). Of note, most studies have not detected an increased risk for MD after parent death (Agid et al., 1999; Birtchnell, 1980; Crook & Eliot, 1980; Tennant, 1988). Indeed, when we applied standard statistical models to our sample, we did not detect an association between parent death and increased risk for MD. The increased risk for depressive onsets may be modest and detectable only by statistical methods that focus on the time course of excess risk, as we have done here.

The most comparable study in the literature was done by Kessler and colleagues. Using data from the NCS (Kessler, Davis, & Kendler, 1997), they examined parental death and divorce separately. As we did, they found parental divorce to be associated with a wide variety of mood, anxiety, and substance use disorders. However, they found no consistent association between parental death and risk for MD or any other psychiatric or substance use disorder, a result that differs from our finding for parental death and MD.

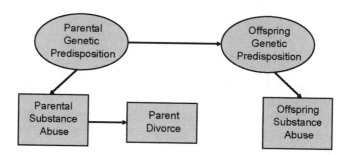

FIGURE 7.6. Indirect association between parental divorce and offspring substance abuse.

IS CHILDHOOD SEXUAL ABUSE
ASSOCIATED WITH PSYCHIATRIC DISORDERS?

Another childhood experience with implications for later psychopathology is sexual abuse. Careful estimates of prevalences in the general population are difficult to obtain, but studies of women from Europe, North America, New Zealand, and Australia have suggested that in these populations, 20–35% had received some kind of unwanted sexual attention during childhood and 5–15% had experienced severe forms of sexual abuse, such as attempted or completed intercourse (Fergusson & Mullen, 1999). A large amount of research documents an association between childhood sexual abuse (CSA) and adult psychopathology. The rates of CSA reported by women undergoing psychiatric treatment are much higher than the rates for the general population. In epidemiological samples, women who report CSA are more likely to have significant symptoms of depression, anxiety, eating disorders, and substance abuse. The impact of CSA among men is less well studied.

As with quality of parenting, the assumption of most research is that CSA is a direct risk factor for future psychopathology (Figure 7.7a). However, CSA often occurs in the setting of other potential risk factors for psychopathology, including parental psychopathology and family dysfunction, some or all of which might increase risk for psychopathology (Figure 7.7b).

An important issue in CSA research is whether reports of abuse are valid and reliable. We assessed CSA using a self-report method because in a prior survey respondents had indicated that they would prefer to answer CSA ques-

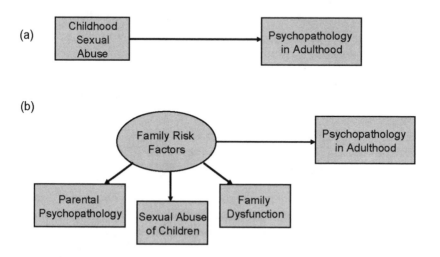

FIGURE 7.7. Alternative explanations for an association between childhood sexual abuse and adult psychopathology.

tions by self-report rather than by interview. We believe that our use of questionnaires increased participants' willingness to disclose information about this difficult topic. It is likely, however, that some portion of cases was missed because women did not wish to reveal their experiences.

A total of 427 women (30.3% of the sample) reported one or more episodes of some form of CSA (Kendler et al., 2000c). Sexual invitation, sexual kissing, fondling, and exposing had similar prevalences, ranging from 17–21%. Sexual touching and intercourse were less common, reported by 10.6 and 8.4% of the sample, respectively.

The prevalences of CSA found in our study are in the same range as those reported by other researchers, suggesting that if there is underreporting in our study it is occurring at rates similar to those seen in other samples (Fergusson & Mullen, 1999). We found that cotwin reports confirmed CSA in many cases, but not all. This is not too surprising, because about one-third of the women in our sample who reported CSA also reported that they had told no one about it. Thus many twins may be unaware of their sisters' experiences.

As in our analyses of parenting quality, the goal here was to understand the association between CSA and adult psychopathology.[5] We subdivided CSA into three categories based on the most severe form of CSA a twin reported (see Sidebar 7.3). The prevalences of each form were: nongenital CSA, 7.8%; genital CSA without intercourse, 14.1%; and intercourse, 8.4%.

Figure 7.8a presents the increase in lifetime risk for psychiatric and substance use disorders associated with the different levels of CSA based on self-report. Rates are relative to those among women with no CSA.

Several conclusions can be drawn from these results. First, the association between CSA and psychopathology is stronger than we saw for the other distal environmental risk factors examined in this chapter (parental loss and parenting). Second, a relatively clear "dose–response" curve is seen. For all the disorders, the risk for psychopathology is stronger for the most severe form of CSA (intercourse) than for the nongenital forms. Third, the impact of CSA is not specific—it is associated with increased risk for all the forms of psychiatric and substance use disorders we examined.

Because we are concerned with possible noncausal reasons for the CSA–psychopathology association, we repeated these analyses, controlling for possible confounding family factors. These included: quality of parents' marriage, parent–child relationship (based on the PBI scales), family financial status, measures of whether family members got along, frequency of church attendance, parental education, parental disciplinary practices, and prolonged parent–child separations prior to age 16. In addition, as a partial control for genetic predisposition for psychopathology, we included parental psychopathology based on our interviews with the parents. By including these variables, we attempted to determine whether CSA has a direct effect on risk of disorder (Figure 7.7a) or is only an index of other family risk factors (Figure 7.7b).

SIDEBAR 7.3. Assessment of Childhood Sexual Abuse

As part of our FF4 interview, we included a self-report questionnaire that assessed CSA based on a questionnaire developed by Mullen and colleagues (Mullen, Martin, Anderson, Romans, & Herbison, 1993). The sample includes 1,411 twins who returned mailed questionnaires with complete information about CSA. For 903 of these women, we also had reports about their CSA experiences from their cotwins. We assessed prevalence of different types of CSA using the following items:

"Before you were 16, did any adult, or any other person older than yourself, involve you in any unwanted incidents like . . .
  a. inviting or requesting you to do something sexual?
  b. kissing or hugging you in a sexual way?
  c. showing their sex organs to you?
  d. touching or fondling your private parts?
  e. making you touch them in a sexual way?
  f. attempting or having sexual intercourse?"

The possible responses to these items were: "never," "once," and "more than once." In addition to asking the twin these questions about herself, we asked her the same questions about her cotwin, adding the response option "not sure."

We divided CSA into three categories based on the most severe form of CSA a twin reported. We termed these: *nongenital CSA* (items a, b, and c), *genital CSA without intercourse* (items d and e), and *intercourse* (item f).

The results from these analyses are shown in Figure 7.8b. These results are based on about half the sample sizes of the prior analyses because they required personal interviews with both parents. Overall, the results are similar to those without the covariates (Figure 7.8a). This suggests that little of the association between CSA and psychopathology is mediated through parental psychopathology and family environmental variables (Figure 7.7b), giving us greater confidence that the association may be a direct causal effect of experiencing CSA (Figure 7.7a). We reconsider this issue using a different and potentially more powerful method in Chapter 15.

SUMMARY

We emphasize the following four findings from this chapter:

1. The risk for adult psychiatric and substance use disorders is significantly correlated with a history of having experienced (a) poor parenting, (b) parental loss, and (c) CSA.
2. Overall, the association of psychopathology with parenting and

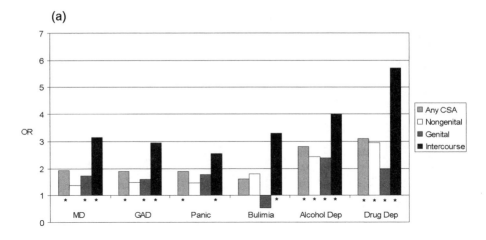

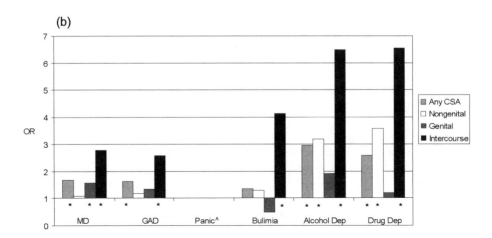

FIGURE 7.8. Odds ratios (OR) for the association between self-reported childhood sexual abuse (CSA) and psychiatric and substance use disorders among female adult twins. MD = major depression; GAD = generalized anxiety disorder; Dep = dependence. (a) Without covariates; *significantly greater than 1.0 ($p < 0.05$). Data from Kendler et al. (2000c, Table 2). (b) After adjusting for other family risk factors and parental psychopathology; *significantly greater than 1.0 ($p < 0.05$); ^ too few cases to estimate. Data from Kendler et al. (2000c, Table 5).

parental loss is relatively modest. The correlation is stronger, however, for CSA, which in its severest form is associated with three- to sixfold increases in risk of illness.

3. With one key exception, these risk factors are generally nonspecific in their impact. Parental death stood out in having a specific association with a single disorder—MD.

4. Evidence presented here and augmented by that reported later in the book suggests that much of the association observed between these environmental factors and risk for adult psychiatric and substance use disorders is causal. That is, disturbed parenting, loss of a parent in childhood, and CSA appear to be true environmental risk factors for adult psychopathology.

The findings in this chapter support key themes of this book. From the perspective of psychiatric geneticists, we saw in Chapters 4 and 5 that genetic factors were important true risk factors for psychiatric illness. Now the approaches of psychiatric epidemiology show that environmental risk factors also play an important causal role. Rigorous efforts to control for possible confounding factors do not make the effects of these environmental risk factors go away. To be comprehensive, etiological models for psychiatric illness must consider both sets of risk factors.

NOTES

1. In our first model (with age as the only covariate), the ORs for bulimia, alcohol dependence, and drug dependence were of the same magnitude as those for the other disorders. Much of the reduction in the OR for the second model was due to the inclusion of an item on teenage rebelliousness as reported by parents. Because early drug and alcohol use may have contributed to this parental perception, it is possible that inclusion of this item in the model represents an "overcorrection" of the results.

2. For example, using our standard ACE twin model, if a disorder has a true heritability of 30%, with 10% of the variance due to shared environmental factors, 80% power to detect that shared environmental effect would require ~50,000 twin pairs (Neale et al., 1994a)!

3. These analyses were conducted using Cox survival models with time-dependent covariates. When there was no statistical evidence for a decay of risk, we fit a simple "proportional hazards" model that gives a single estimate (in the form of a hazard ratio, or HR) of the change in risk of illness after parental loss. Another feature of this model is that any onset of a disorder prior to parental loss is censored and plays no role in the analyses. This model could be examined only for disorders with a meaningful age at onset. Thus we did not examine adult antisocial behavior, in which age at onset is not typically a meaningful concept. Some of the results were previously published in Kendler et al., 2002c.

4. When we found evidence for a decay of risk, we included two estimates: the instantaneous hazard ratio, reflecting the increase in risk that occurs in the year after parental loss, and the decay constant, which reflects the speed with which the increased risk returns to baseline.

5. We did not include phobias in this study because for many women the onset of phobia preceded the CSA, and we were interested in the association between CSA and risk for later psychopathology. In defining GAD, we used a 1-month rather than 6-month minimum duration of illness. See original report (Kendler et al., 2000c) for details of covariates.

CHAPTER EIGHT

Adult Experiences and Risk for Psychopathology

In Chapter 7, we examined the association between distal risk factors and lifetime psychopathology. In this chapter, we deal with *proximal* risk factors (events that occurred during the 1-year period preceding our interview) and their associations with the onset of episodes of MD and GAD during the same time period. We examine two major proximal risk factors: stressful life events and quality of social relationships.

STRESSFUL LIFE EVENTS

The research we present on stressful life events (SLEs) addresses the questions: How strongly does the occurrence of an SLE predict the onset of a depressive or anxiety episode? Does the type of event matter? What other aspects of life events are most salient with respect to risk for subsequent psychopathology? Do different kinds of events or aspects of events relate differently to the risk for anxiety versus depression? To understand the context for these questions and why our work may seem fixated on methodological details, it may be helpful to have a summary of prior research in this area.

The hypothesis that SLEs can lead to psychiatric illness goes back hundreds of years, but serious scientific study of the relationship between stress and psychopathology in natural settings began only in 1967 with the publication by Holmes and Rahe (1967) of their Social Readjustment Rating Scale. Since that time, many studies have been performed attempting to understand the degree and nature of the association between the experience of life stress and the development of psychiatric disorders.[1]

The Social Readjustment Rating Scale is a self-report checklist of common experiences that require readjustment in one's accustomed pattern of life. Four problems were quickly seen with this approach to measurement of stress. First, the definition of experiences was broad and included items that could reflect psychiatric symptoms, such as changes in sleeping or eating habits and sexual difficulties. Second, many of the experiences did not have a clear time of onset but were chronic problems better described as "difficulties" than "events." Third, the questionnaire format relied on the respondent to be the sole judge of what constituted an event, making the measure subject to differences among people in their perception of what constitutes an event. No objective third party (such as a trained interviewer) was involved in the rating process. Fourth, the checklist recorded only whether the event had or had not occurred in a given time period (e.g., the past year) and not the date of the event. Valuable information was thereby lost regarding the temporal relationship between stress and the onset of psychopathology.

These difficulties were perceived by the next generation of life-event researchers, particularly Brown (e.g., Brown & Harris, 1978), Dohrenwend (1978), and Paykel et al. (1969), who suggested a number of methodological improvements. Event lists were proposed that eliminated items reflecting symptoms or chronic difficulties. Interview-based measures were developed that dated the occurrence of the event and attempted to "objectify" event ratings.

Despite these methodological advances, several active areas of concern remain, three of which we discuss here. First, even within a single category of events, severity can vary widely. Two approaches have been developed to deal with this event heterogeneity, but each has limitations. The first method is to have respondents rate the severity of the event. However, this is likely to exaggerate the association between events and psychopathology. In what has been called "seeking after meaning," we humans are prone to rate as more severe those events that upset us more. A second approach is to have an objective rater (such as an interviewer) gather more information about the event that can be used to rate event severity independently of the person's reaction to it. This method poses practical difficulties of collecting objective information about event severity and training raters not to be biased by the reaction of the respondent to the event.

A second problem, raised in response to the first rating scale proposed by Holmes and Rahe (1967), is that only some of the bad things that happen to us in life are truly independent of our own actions. These are sometimes called "fateful" events. However, for a large proportion of events, it is quite difficult to determine how much our behavior contributed to that event. Human nature often leads us to believe that being fired by a supervisor or having conflict with a spouse is the other person's fault. But the reality is likely to be more complex and interactive. Thus it is probably best not to rely on self-report but instead to collect objective information from the respondent and then rate the event on its degree of independence or dependence.

The third methodological issue is that the severity of an event probably does not capture all that is relevant about the risk it poses for subsequent psychiatric illness. In addition to being rated by severity, events can also be meaningfully grouped into potentially important categories based on the type of event (e.g., illness, relationship difficulties) or based on particular themes. Paykel and colleagues proposed studying "entrance events" and "exit events" (Paykel et al., 1969). Brown has proposed that events be rated on four dimensions: loss, humiliation, entrapment, and threat (Brown, Harris, & Hepworth, 1995).

In the VATSPSUD, we adapted and developed measures of stressful life events in an attempt to address all of these methodological issues. We assessed a large number of SLEs in our interviews (see Sidebar 8.1). Figure 8.1 depicts the frequency of occurrence of 15 categories of SLEs based on the third wave of interviews with our female twin pairs. The occurrence of these events ranged widely, from assaults, which were very rare (occurring in only 0.09% of all months), to network crises, which were reported for 4.2% of all months.

We first tested for the relation between occurrence of an event and risk for an episode of MD.[2] All but two of the events, serious legal problems and being robbed, are significantly associated with an increased risk of MD onset during the same month in which the event occurred. Figure 8.2 portrays the ORs for the onset of MD in the month of SLE occurrence. Most of the events are associated with an increase of 2 to 7 times the baseline risk. For example,

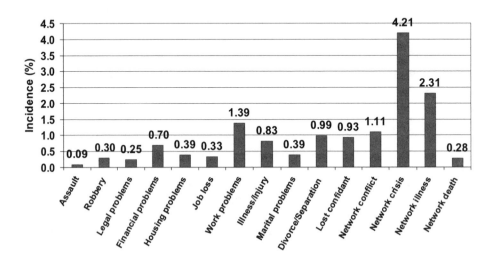

FIGURE 8.1. Stressful life events per month among female adult twins. Data from Kendler, Karkowski, and Prescott (1998).

SIDEBAR 8.1. Types of Stressful Life Events

In this chapter, we focus on SLEs that were assessed during personal interviews. The interviewer read a list of possible events, instructing the twin to respond positively if "any of these events happened to you during the past 12 months." Because of differences in length and structure of the different interviews used in the VATSPSUD, the individual SLE items were not always identical. However, we created 15 categories of SLEs that were the same across all the waves: 11 categories of "personal" events and 4 classes of "network" events, which concerned members of the respondent's social network.

PERSONAL EVENTS

Assault (assault, rape, or mugging)
Robbery
Legal problems (trouble with police or other legal trouble)
Major financial problems
Serious housing problems
Job loss (laid off from a job or fired)
Serious difficulties at work
Serious illness or injury
Serious marital problems
Divorce/separation (including broken engagement or breakup of another serious romantic relationship)
Loss of confidant (separation from loved one or close friend other than spouse/partner)

NETWORK EVENTS

Interpersonal conflict (serious trouble getting along with an individual in the network)
Crisis (a serious personal crisis experienced by someone in the network)
Illness (serious illness of someone in the network)
Death (of an individual in the network)

In some analyses, we divided the network into *close* and *other*. *Close* members of the network include the twin's spouse or cohabiting partner, children, parents, cotwin, and other nontwin siblings. *Other* members of the network include the categories of "other close relative" and "someone else close to you."

If the twin responded positively to an event, the interviewer dated it to the month in which it occurred. Our interviewers made an effort to rate only events that were a clear departure from the ongoing pattern of people's lives. Thus an individual with a marriage that was consistently bad for the entire year prior to interview would not be rated on an SLE for "serious marital problems." The intent was to examine the effects of particular events rather than levels of life stress in general.

Items referring to marriages or spouses were also asked about cohabiting partners. We used the phrase "living together in a marriage-like intimate relationship" to define partnerships and did not distinguish between same- and opposite-sex partnerships.

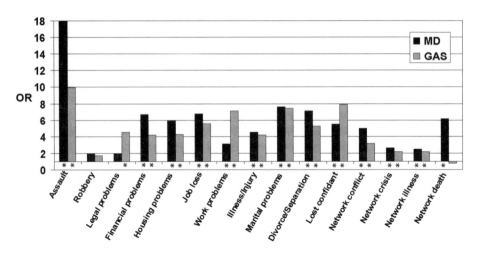

FIGURE 8.2. Odds ratios (OR) for major depression (MD) and generalized anxiety syndrome (GAS) among female twins associated with occurrence of a life event in the same month; $*p < 0.05$. Data from Kendler, Karkowski, and Prescott (1998, Tables 1 and 4).

network illness has an OR of 2.5, indicating that the risk of MD is 2.5 times greater among twins who reported an illness of someone in their personal network compared with twins who did not. The highest risk is observed for the most rare event, assault, which has an OR of 17.9.

We also examined the duration of elevated risk for depressive onsets in the months after the SLE. The time course differs widely across event categories. Some SLEs, such as job loss and network events, increase risk for a depressive onset only in the month of their occurrence. Other events, including financial, legal, and interpersonal problems, produce longer periods of risk. One explanation is that events that increase risk of MD for only a single month tend to be temporally discrete. You lose your job on a specific day, and if you are going to become depressed, it happens right away, not after a delay. By contrast, most events that produce a delayed risk for MD may reflect smoldering problems that flare up and then die down but do not entirely go away.

Figure 8.2 also depicts the ORs for the onset of generalized anxiety syndrome (GAS; see definition in Sidebar 8.2) in the month of occurrence of the SLE. Thirteen of the 15 SLEs (all but robbery and network death) are significantly associated with an increased risk of GAS onset in the month of event occurrence. Unlike with MD, nearly all of the anxiogenic effects of these events occur in the month of the event. Only two types of events are associated with occurrence of GAS episodes in subsequent months: Interpersonal conflict with a member of one's social network is associated with a modestly

SIDEBAR 8.2. Diagnostic Definitions Used in SLE Studies

• *Major depression (MD)*: based on DSM-III-R criteria (see Sidebar 4.1), except that we did not exclude episodes that followed the death of someone close to the respondent (i.e., what might be considered normal grief).

• *Generalized anxiety syndrome (GAS)*: based on DSM-III-R GAD criteria (see Sidebar 4.4) except that, as with MD, we required only a 2-week minimum duration of illness. We used this definition so that our analyses could focus on the differences between the symptoms of GAS and MD rather than on differences in duration of the two syndromes. We did *not* use the diagnostic hierarchy, which would exclude the diagnosis of GAS if it coincided with a depressive episode.

• *Pure MD*: during the MD episode, the participant never met criteria for GAS.

• *Pure GAS*: during the GAS episode, the participant never met criteria for MD.

• *Mixed MD/GAS*: during one episode without any 2-week remission, the participant met criteria for both MD and GAS.

See Chapter 4 for further details on assessment of depression and anxiety syndromes.

---

increased risk of GAS in the subsequent month, and marital difficulties are associated with increased risk for up to 3 months after the event.

We were interested in knowing whether any of the events have a specific risk for MD versus GAS. Using the same data set, we calculated the ratio of the ORs predicting the onset of MD and GAS in the month of the event occurrence. As is evident in Figure 8.2, only network death has high specificity for MD (ratio = 7.6, meaning that death of a network member was 7.6 times more likely to result in an episode of MD than in an episode of GAS). Five events have modest specificity for MD (ratios from 1.3 to 2.0): assault, serious financial problems, serious housing problems, divorce/separation, and network conflict. Three events have modest specificity for GAS (MD:GAS ratios < 0.8): legal problems, work problems, and loss of confidant. The remaining six lack specificity for MD versus GAS. These results suggest that SLEs have at most modest specificity for depression versus anxiety. However, our results do not take into account individuals who experienced syndromes with a mix of depressive and anxiety symptoms. Later in the chapter we return to this issue using more exact methods.

Severity and Number of Events

To deal with the problem of heterogeneity within event categories, we adapted Brown's severity measure of "long-term contextual threat" (LTCT, see Sidebar 8.3 and Brown, 1989). Across all events we studied, the risk for MD in the month of event occurrence significantly increases with greater LTCT. The observed risks for a depressive onset are shown in the left side of

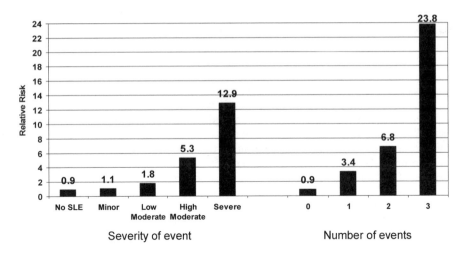

FIGURE 8.3. Relative risk for onset of a major depressive episode among female twins by severity of a life event (SLE) and number of life events in the same month. Risk is scaled relative to the average risk in the sample. Data from Kendler, Karkowski, and Prescott (1998).

Figure 8.3. The risk for an onset of MD approximately doubles with each increasing level of LTCT. Although most of the pathogenic effects of SLEs are restricted to those with high threat ratings, even SLEs rated as having minor or low moderate levels of LTCT significantly increase the risk for a depressive episode.

We also studied the effects of experiencing multiple events during the same month. The right side of Figure 8.3 shows the observed risk of an MD episode associated with experiencing between zero and three events. Risk for MD increases substantially with more events. Nearly a quarter of women who experienced three events in the same month developed a depressive episode.

Independence versus Dependence of Events

A certain proportion of the bad things that happen to us in life are truly independent of our own actions. Examples of such "fateful events" include the death of a parent from cancer, job loss due to closing of a factory, or a car accident in which an 18-wheeler jumps the divide and smashes into a whole row of cars going the opposite direction. However, for a substantial proportion of events, such as relationship conflicts or financial crises, our actions help to create the event. In some of our interviews we rated the degree to which events were independent of or dependent upon the respondent's behavior (see Sidebar 8.3).

SIDEBAR 8.3. Life Event Ratings

In our later interviews (FF3, FF4, MF2), in addition to recording the occurrence of SLEs, we rated two additional dimensions: *severity of threat* and *dependence/independence*, based on the work by Brown and colleagues.[a]

LONG-TERM CONTEXTUAL THREAT

To capture the variability in SLEs, we adapted Brown's severity measure of "long-term contextual threat" (LTCT; see Brown, 1989), using a 4-point scale: minor, low moderate, high moderate, and severe. "Threat" refers to the degree to which adapting to the event will require changes to the core aspects of the person's life plans or self-concept. "Long term" is defined as lasting at least a week, so a high-threat event that resolves very quickly would get a lower LTCT rating. The "contextual" part of LTCT indicates that ratings are based on what most people would be expected to feel about an event given a particular context and personal history, taking no account either of what the respondent says about his or her reaction or about any psychiatric or physical symptoms that followed it.

Threat ratings were developed to deal with the problem that events are quite heterogeneous in their psychological impact based on the circumstances in which they occur. Here are two examples of deaths of parents that would differ in their LTCT ratings.

> Jill is a 24-year-old graduate student whose 52-year-old father died suddenly of a heart attack while mowing the lawn. Jill had a warm and loving relationship with her father. He was the main breadwinner for the family of five children and was paying Jill's tuition and living costs at school. After his death, Jill dropped out of school, moved back home, and got a job so she could help her mother raise her younger siblings.

> George is a 54-year-old factory worker whose 81-year-old mother recently died in her sleep. She had suffered from Alzheimer's disease for 7 years. George had visited his mother weekly at her nursing home, but she had not recognized him for 2 years and had not spoken at all for the previous 10 months. Recently, she lost control of her bladder and bowel functions. Several times after visiting her, George told his wife, "My mother was a proud woman. She would have hated to see herself like this."

Although both of these events would be rated as "death of parent," from a psychological perspective they reflect quite different levels of stress. In addition to her psychological adjustment, the loss of her father had a major effect on Jill's life. In contrast, George was relieved at his mother's death; from his perspective, "My real mother died a long time ago."

EVENT INDEPENDENCE VERSUS DEPENDENCE

In our later interviews, we adapted Brown's procedures to characterize the degree to which the respondent's behavior contributed to the SLE (see Brown, 1989).[b] After

(continued)

SIDEBAR 8.3. *(continued)*

inquiring about the context and origin of the specific event, interviewers rated each individual life event as *definitely independent, probably independent, probably dependent*, or *definitely dependent*. For SLEs involving interpersonal difficulties, interviewers were instructed to assume that the events were dependent unless convincing evidence was presented to the contrary. This was done to compensate for the ubiquitous human trait of describing relationship problems as "the other person's fault."

---

[a]See Brown and Harris (1989) for descriptions of the original approach to the rating of life events by Brown and colleagues. Their method of rating LTCT and dependence was to have the interviewer present a description of the event and its context to a committee of experienced raters who would each rate levels of LTCT and dependence. Given the sample size of our study, this approach would have required more resources and person-power than we had available. Therefore, we adapted Brown's ratings to be done by the interviewer on the spot. This took extensive training, as well as lots of quality-control checks, to ensure, as much as possible, that the interviewers were being objective and not allowing the participants' emotional responses to influence the ratings. The structure of our interview helped with this task, as SLEs were always asked in the early phases of the interview prior to assessing psychiatric symptoms. The test–retest reliability for LTCT was $\kappa = 0.41$, while interrater reliability was $\kappa = 0.67$ (Kendler et al., 1998).

[b]As with the LTCT ratings, we adapted the committee-based assessment methods of Brown and colleagues and had our interviewers make the ratings (see Brown & Harris, 1989). Test–retest and interrater reliabilities for dependence were $\kappa = 0.63$ and $\kappa = 0.79$, respectively (Kendler et al., 1999b).

Using a statistical method called event history analysis, we explored the relationship between our dependence/independence dimension and the risk for onset of MD.[3] Across different categories of SLEs, dependent events are more strongly associated with the occurrence of a depressive onset than are independent events. However, definitely or probably independent SLEs still strongly predict the occurrence of an onset of MD (OR = 2.9).

Psychological Dimensions of Events and Episode Type

Measures of severity do not capture all that is relevant about events with respect to the risk they pose for subsequent psychiatric illness. In addition to grouping events into categories (such as personal or network) or levels of long-term contextual threat, we can also group or rate them by particular themes. We applied a system also developed by Brown (1989) to rate the level and subcategories of entrapment, danger, loss, and humiliation (see Sidebar 8.4).

Our study of psychological dimensions is based on the female twins participating in our FF3 interview who reported events that met criteria for high moderate or severe LTCT. We first examined these higher threat events and their associations with pure MD, pure GAS, and mixed syndromes (see

SIDEBAR 8.4. Psychological Dimensions of Life Events

In our FF3 and MF2 interviews we conducted very time-intensive ratings of four psychological dimensions: loss, humiliation, entrapment, and danger.[a] These ratings were made according to rating guidelines (see Brown, 1996) based on descriptive information written in the interview, the narrative summary written by the interviewer, and audiotapes of the interview. For each SLE that met LTCT ratings of high moderate or severe, trained raters (not the interviewers) scored 4 dimensions, using a 5-point scale (ranging from 0 = *not present* to 4 = *severe*). For all of the categories but danger, we scored additional subcategories. Raters ignored emotional reactions and remained blind to whether onsets of psychiatric symptoms occurred during the rating period.[b]

Loss: Diminution of a sense of connectedness or well-being, potentially covering every aspect of life, including a real or anticipated loss of a person, material possessions, health, respect in the community, employment, or a cherished idea about oneself or someone close to oneself. Subcategories: death, respondent-initiated separation, other key loss, lesser loss.

Humiliation: Feeling devalued in relation to others or against a core sense of self, usually with an element of rejection or sense of role failure. Subcategories: other-initiated separation, other's delinquency, put-down.

Entrapment: Ongoing circumstances of marked difficulty of at least 6 months' duration that the subject can reasonably expect will persist or get worse, with little or no possibility that a resolution can be achieved as a result of anything that might reasonably be done. Subcategories: long-term sustained, long-term worsened, failed positive event.

Danger: The level of potential future loss, including both the chance that a given traumatic event will recur or a possible sequence of circumstances in which the full threat or dire outcome has yet to occur.

---

[a]This practice differed from that used by Brown and colleagues, who rated humiliation and entrapment only for events with high ratings of loss or danger. See Brown et al. (1995); Brown (1996).

[b]Interrater reliability estimates (weighted κ) obtained for a sample of ratings were: loss, 0.77; humiliation, 0.87; entrapment, 0.92; and danger, 0.79. When both raters agreed on a nonzero dimension score, the weighted κ estimates (and sample size) for the categories were: loss, 0.91 ($n = 348$); humiliation, 0.99 ($n = 107$); and entrapment, 0.92 ($n = 47$).

Sidebar 8.2). Individuals who experienced such an event have 10 times higher risk for developing a pure MD episode, 4.5 times higher risk for a pure GAS episode, and 6.6 times the risk for developing a mixed depression/anxiety episode in the same month, compared with individuals experiencing no event.

We then looked at the psychological dimensions and whether they were associated with differential risk for the development of depression and anxiety episodes. Figure 8.4 summarizes the results for the effect of events in the month of their occurrence.

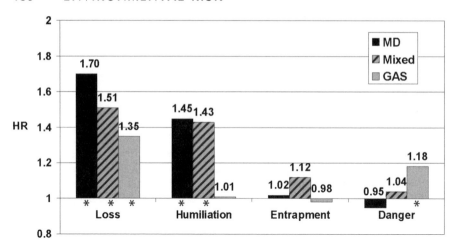

FIGURE 8.4. Hazard ratios (HR) in the month of event occurrence for pure depression (MD), pure generalized anxiety syndrome (GAS), and mixed syndromes as a function of life event ratings on the dimensions of loss, humiliation, entrapment, and danger. The baseline for the calculation of the hazard ratio was risk for episode onset in months containing a serious stressful life event; *significantly different from chance (1.0) at $p < 0.05$. Data from Kendler, Hettema, Butera, Gardner, and Prescott (2003c), Table 2).

Loss

The concept that loss is the central feature of depressogenic experiences can be traced back at least to Freud (1957). It was first introduced into SLE research by Paykel and colleagues (1969), who created a category of "exit events" that were predicted to be particularly potent at predisposing to depression.

As hypothesized, even among individuals with high-threat events, high ratings of loss are associated with significantly increased risk for pure depressive episodes in the same month as an event (HR = 1.7; see Figure 8.4) but not 1, 2, and 3 months after event occurrence.

We then looked at the associaton between risk and subcategories of loss (see Sidebar 8.4). We used the hazard ratio (HR) statistic to index the increase in risk associated with experiencing an SLE. Because all the participants included in these analyses had experienced some form of SLE, the risk (hazard) for developing a disorder was scaled relative to the "lesser loss" event category. For example, we found an HR of 3.0 for pure MD following a death, meaning that the risk of developing MD is 3 times greater for a participant who had someone close to her die compared to the risk for someone who experienced lesser loss. Risk for pure MD episodes is also substantially increased by the loss subcategories of *respondent-initiated separation* (HR = 3.2) and *other key loss* (HR = 2.6), relative to the category of *lesser loss*.

The associations between loss and risk for mixed episodes are similar to those for pure depression. The only substantial difference is that *respondent-initiated separation* is associated with onset of pure MD but not mixed episodes.

We found some evidence consistent with the prediction that loss is specific for depression. Overall, high ratings of loss are associated with onset of pure GAS episodes, but analyses of the loss subcategories indicate that pure GAS episodes are significantly predicted, in the month of event occurrence, only by *other key loss*. Two other subcategories of loss associated with depressive onset, *death* and *respondent-initiated separation*, do not increase risk for pure anxiety episodes.

Humiliation

Both evolutionary theory and observations of animal behavior have postulated that reduction of status or rank in group settings—forcing the individual into a subordinate position—is the essential depressogenic attribute of events (Gilbert, 1992). In humans, humiliation in a public setting is among the most potent possible experiences of subordination. Our results support this view. High-threat events rated high in humiliation are associated with increased risk for onset of pure depressive and mixed depression/anxiety episodes in the same month in which the event occurred (Figure 8.4). However, there is no evidence for an increase in pure anxiety episodes.

Risk for pure depressive episodes varies with the type of humiliation. Compared with those high-threat events with no evidence of humiliation, the risk of a pure depressive onset is substantially increased for events involving *other-initiated separation* (HR = 3.1), with a weaker but still significant effect seen for *put-down* (HR = 1.7) but not for *other's delinquency*.

Entrapment

Research in both humans and animals has suggested that helpless entrapment may be a key feature of depressogenic experiences. Individuals in such circumstances may be unable to alter their situations and may, thereby, develop a state of learned helplessness (Seligman, 1975).

Contrary to these predictions, we found that events with high ratings of entrapment were not significantly associated with increased risk for pure depression, pure anxiety, or mixed syndromes in the same month (Figure 8.4). However, these types of events did increase risk for mixed depressive/anxiety syndromes in the month following the event (HR = 1.33; results not shown in Figure 8.4). When we examined entrapment subcategories, this association was due primarily to events characterized by *long-term sustained entrapment*.

Danger

Danger reflects the anticipation of future adversities. Prior research suggests that such anticipation may particularly predispose individuals to develop anxiety symptoms (Finlay-Jones & Brown, 1981). For example, loss of a job may increase risk for depression, but the threat of job loss (e.g., hearing that 20% of the employees at one's workplace will be laid off in the next month due to budget problems) is more likely to predispose to anxiety.

Our results replicated these findings. Events with high ratings on danger are not associated with increased risk for pure MD episodes but are associated with increased risk for pure anxiety episodes in the same month (HR = 1.18 in Figure 8.4) and up to 3 months following the event (HR = 1.5).

Consistent with the notion that the impact is due to delayed effects, we found an increased risk for mixed episodes with onsets occurring in the month *following* an SLE rated high in danger (HR = 1.5) but not significant evidence for onsets occurring in the same month.

Combinations of Loss and Humiliation

Loss and humiliation have similar associations with risk for pure MD and for mixed depression/anxiety episodes. We explored the risk for these syndromes predicted by combinations of the loss and humiliation subcategories. The highest risk of onset (21.6%) occurs for events characterized as other-initiated separation and other key loss. By contrast, events involving other-initiated separation and lesser loss carry a much lower risk for onset (2.6%). Events characterized as other key loss also have risks of about 10% if they are accompanied by humiliation subcategories of other's delinquency or put-down. Four other combinations carry risks for depressive onsets of about 10%. Two of these are "pure" loss events with zero ratings for humiliation: death and respondent-initiated separation.

The most interesting of these results is that by far the greatest risk for MD is seen for events that were rated high on both loss and humiliation. The risk is more than twice that seen for traumas that (like death of a close relative) are pure loss events. These results suggest that environmental experiences that involve loss of status and elicit "psychobiological programmes of defeat and submission" (Gilbert, 1992, p. 207) appear to be more depressogenic than those that involve solely loss.

Causality

As we have stated previously, correlation does not equal causation. We have clearly shown that SLEs and onsets of disorder are strongly correlated in time. What evidence do we have that the association is causal? As epidemiologists, we can use data from the VATSPSUD to address this question in two ways. (In Chapter 15, we examine how the use of genetically informative samples helps us to address causality in other ways.)

First, we looked at measurement issues. As described earlier, the strongest association between SLEs and onsets is seen for the month in which the event occurred. This raises the possibility that the onset of disorder caused the event, and not the other way around.

We asked about the SLEs in one section of the interview, before we assessed psychiatric symptoms that had occurred during the past year. At the end of this latter section, we inquired of twins with depressive onsets in the past year whether anything had happened to precipitate the episode. Using data from the first two waves of our study (Kendler et al., 1995a), we examined interviews from 96 twins who had reported a serious SLE and a depressive onset in the same month. Most (84%) of the time twins responded with the same previously reported SLE. In another 11%, they reported a different SLE that co-occurred in the same month in an understandable sequence of events that included the serious SLE. We replicated these results for a later wave (Kendler et al., 1998), in which a review of 102 similar cases revealed none in which the depressive onset plausibly caused the SLE. Thus, although our results do not provide a definitive answer to the question of causality, in a very high proportion of cases in which a severe SLE and an onset occurred in the same month, the twins themselves believed the SLE had occurred before and had had a causal influence on the depression and not the other way around.

Our second approach to addressing causality was to use our measures of dependence/independence. With dependent SLEs, the relationship between the event and the subsequent onset of anxiety or depression is causally ambiguous. It is possible that some aspect of the respondent's own behavior, such as his or her temperament or prodromal symptoms of the disorder, caused the SLE and predisposed to the onset of illness. In contrast, the causal relationship is much clearer for independent SLEs, because these fateful events could not plausibly be the result of the respondent's behavior.

As noted previously, we found that after adjusting for event severity, dependent SLEs are more closely associated with depressive onsets than are independent SLEs. This suggests that there is some degree of noncausal association between dependent events and MD. Our reasoning is as follows. We can plausibly assume that for independent SLEs, the entire relationship with depression is due to the fact that SLEs increase risk for MD (i.e., SLE → MD). For dependent SLEs, part of the relationship is also causal (i.e., SLE → MD), but part of the relationship is probably noncausal and due to traits (such as neuroticism) that increase risk both for SLEs and for MD. Our finding that (after controlling for event severity) dependent SLEs were indeed more strongly associated with MD than independent SLEs suggests that the difference is due to these noncausal mechanisms. However, the finding that events rated as probably or definitely independent are also strongly associated with risk for depression suggests that a substantial proportion of the association between SLEs and MD is causal. We will return to this critical issue, using a quite different approach, in Chapter 15.

SOCIAL SUPPORT

Social support can be broadly defined as the degree of caring and sustenance an individual obtains from his or her social environment. Interest in the nature of human social relationships and their impact on health has a long tradition in the field of mental health and the disciplines of sociology, social psychology, and public health. Indeed, a vast body of research has demonstrated that the quality of social relationships predicts general health and mortality (House, Landis, & Umberson, 1988), psychiatric symptoms (Kessler, Kendler, Heath, Neale, & Eaves, 1992), and emotional adjustment to stress (Monroe & Steiner, 1986).

Several aspects of social support have been identified. One of these has been called *social integration*—the feeling of being part of a community. Two other aspects are *emotional support*, the provision of assistance with psychological needs, and *instrumental support*, the provision of material needs such as transportation, money, or physical assistance (Antonucci, 1985).

We combined these dimensions to create a global measure of social support (see Sidebar 8.5) and tested whether low levels increased the risk for the onset of episodes of MD or 1-month GAD (used in these analyses rather than GAS). However, we were concerned about the direction of causal effects. If we found that low social support was associated with MD (or GAD), how could we be sure that the low social support was causing the disorder and not that the disorder was causing lower social support? This is a realistic concern, because it is known that individuals in episodes of a disorder find it difficult to participate in social interactions and often reduce their level of social contact. Furthermore, the social network of individuals with high levels of depression and anxiety can experience "support fatigue." That is, early in episodes of illness, individuals often elicit increased support as people try to help them cope. But if episodes persist, social support often declines, as friends and acquaintances get burned out and find it hard to be around individuals who are so frequently dysphoric.

We took two steps to try to assure ourselves of the direction of causal effects. First, we used our longitudinal data. We examined whether levels of social support at one wave could predict the risk for MD (or GAD) at a future wave. Because the waves were always separated by at least a year, we knew that depressive or anxiety episodes assessed at a later wave could not be influ-

SIDEBAR 8.5. Measuring Social Support

For the analyses reported in this chapter, we assessed social support using a self-report questionnaire administered to the FF sample and as part of the first wave of interviews with the MM/MF sample. This instrument included 24 items that assessed frequency of social contact and degree of emotional and instrumental support received from the social network.

The first five items recorded the frequency of social contact with the cotwin, friends, and other relatives and attendance at meetings of "clubs or other organizations" and "church or other religious services." Another item assessed the presence and number of confidants.

The remaining 18 items assessed the quality of social support received from six classes of relationships: spouse or partner, cotwin, children, parents, other relatives, and friends. Three questions were asked for each relationship:

> "How much does X listen to you if you need to talk about your worries or problems?"
>
> "How much does X understand the way you feel and think about things?"
>
> "How much does X go out of his or her way to help you if you really need it?"

In exploring the structure of the items, we found that we could use a single factor as a measure of global social support. We standardized levels of social support so that change in risk for MD or GAD was expressed in terms of standard deviation units. Because we scored social support in the "reverse" direction, an OR of greater than 1 means that low levels of social support indicate an increased risk for developing a disorder.

encing social support measured at the earlier wave. This approach is illustrated in Figure 8.5a.

We found that a lower level of global social support at an earlier interview predicts moderately increased risk for developing future episodes of MD and GAD. Compared with women with an average level of social support, those who had 1 standard deviation lower than the average have about a 40% increased risk for developing an episode of depression in the year prior to a future interview (OR = 1.41; 95% CI = 1.27, 1.57). A similar result is seen for GAD (OR = 1.40; 95% CI = 1.26, 1.55).

A second concern was that the association between low social support and future risk for MD and GAD could also be an artifact of having had past episodes, which both decrease social support *and* increase risk for future episodes. Therefore, in a second set of analyses, we *controlled* for history of depression (or anxiety, as appropriate) in the year prior to the time 1 interview and then tested whether social support was still predictive of future episodes. This model is depicted in Figure 8.5b. As expected, the direct effect of social support decreases somewhat, but for both MD and GAD, social support significantly predicts risk for future episodes even after controlling for

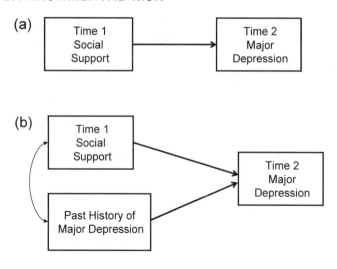

FIGURE 8.5. Models for social support and depression.

history of past episodes. The OR for MD is 1.27 (95% CI = 1.14, 1.42) and for GAD is 1.33 (95% CI = 1.20, 1.49).

We can conclude two things from these results. First, low social support appears to be a true risk factor for the development of episodes of MD and GAD. However, overall the effect is smaller than that seen with SLEs and CSA (see Chapter 7). Second, without proper controls, it would be easy to overestimate the predictive power of social support. For MD, as an example, it appears that part of the association between social support and future risk for MD is indirect and the result of prior depression, predicting both poor social support and future depression.

Our results are consistent with most but not all studies that suggest that social support has a moderate direct effect on risk for psychiatric disorders (Cohen & Wills, 1985; Henderson, 1998). Some studies suggest that low levels of social support increase risk—most typically for depression—only in the context of life stress. This is sometimes called the *buffering model* of social support (Cohen & Wills, 1985). In the VATSPSUD, we do not see much evidence for this model. We have found that high levels of social support do not seem to protect individuals from the depressogenic effects of SLEs (Wade & Kendler, 2000).

In these analyses, we emphasized the traditional view of social support as something that "happens" to individuals. Although we studied how episodes of MD or GAD might affect support levels, our approach may have failed to capture all the ways in which individuals might be responsible for their own social environments. In an influential article with a provocative title that begins "Social Support as an Individual Difference Variable . . . ," Sarason and colleagues (Sarason, Sarason, & Shearin, 1986) argue that the conceptualization of social support as a solely environmental variable that acts on the person is mistaken. Instead, individuals help to create their social support through stable aspects of their temperament and behavior.

SUMMARY

In this chapter, we examined the impact of proximal environmental risk factors and showed that social support and several dimensions of SLEs are associated with increased risk for MD and GAD in the last year. As we saw in Chapter 7 with childhood experiences, these results are consistent with adult experiences having a causal influence on the risk for psychopathology. However, there is reason to postulate that noncausal processes are involved as well. We explore this issue further in Chapter 13, where we examine genetic influences on SLEs and social support.

NOTES

1. See Brown & Harris, 1989; Dohrenwend & Dohrenwend, 1984; Holmes & Rahe, 1967; Kessler, 1997; Paykel, 1994; and Thoits, 1983, for reviews of the association between SLE and depression. See Kendler et al. (1995a) for information about our assessment of the reliability of SLE ratings.

2. These analyses used the statistical technique of discrete time survival analysis, which examines each "person-month" of observation as to which if any SLEs occurred in that month and whether episodes of MD or generalized anxiety syndrome (GAS; see Sidebar 8.2) started in that month. Analyses using the FF sample are based on data from the FF3 interview on 1,898 twins with 24,648 person-months of exposure. Analyses combining the FF3 and MF2 data include 7,322 twins with 98,592 person-months. See Allison (1982) and Laird and Olivier (1981) for details of analyses and Kendler, Karkowski, and Prescott (1998) and Kendler, Hettema, Butera, Gardner, and Prescott (2003c) for further details of the statistical methods.

3. These life history analyses used the standard method of logistic regression applied to person-months to examine whether event occurrences predict onsets and, if so, with what kind of time lag. Across all SLEs in this sample, LTCT and dependence ratings were positively correlated (Spearman rank, $n = 2,971$, $r = 0.23$, $p < 0.0001$), meaning that dependent events had higher threat ratings than independent events. Therefore, when examining the relationship of event dependence and risk for MD, we adjusted statistically for LTCT levels. The original analyses are reported in Kendler, Karkowski, and Prescott (1999b).

A CLOSER LOOK AT GENETIC AND ENVIRONMENTAL INFLUENCES

CHAPTER NINE

Sex Differences

In Part II of this book, we adopted the typical perspective of a psychiatric geneticist interested in determining the heritability of psychiatric and substance use disorders. In Part III, we put on the hat of the psychiatric epidemiologist and examined the association between several putative environmental risk factors and their association with these same disorders. In Part IV, we break out of these rather conventional perspectives and start to demonstrate the richness of our design and analytic methods. In the four chapters in this section, we address a diverse series of topics, each of which is quite important to understanding pathways of risk. We hope the reader finds that the conceptual "wall" between the genetic and environmental perspectives starts to break down in this section as we consider the joint actions of genes and environment. This wall will, we hope, dissolve completely in the final section of this book.

TYPES OF SEX DIFFERENCES

Clinical and epidemiological studies have repeatedly demonstrated that *rates* of psychiatric and substance use disorders differ in men and women. As we described in Chapters 4 and 5, our study replicates these findings. However, we were also interested in exploring some deeper and more intriguing questions about sex differences. Our goal in this chapter is to address whether the genetic and environmental *sources* of variability in risk are different for men than for women. This is a change from the focus of much of the research on sex differences, which addresses questions about "mean differences" in rates of disorders (e.g., do men have higher rates of substance abuse?) or in risk factors (e.g., do women have better social support?).

Two distinct kinds of questions can be asked about the sources of sex differences in genetic risk for psychiatric and substance use disorders.[1] The first and simpler question is *quantitative*: Are genetic factors more important in the etiology of a particular disorder in males or in females? This is the question that we addressed systematically in Chapters 4 and 5, when we described the results from twin analyses of internalizing and externalizing disorders. These analyses included four groups of twin pairs (male MZ, male DZ, female MZ, and female DZ) and addressed whether the etiological role of genetic and environmental risk factors for these disorders differed for males and females. Although the estimates were rather different for some disorders (including CD and abuse of or dependence on some illicit substances), none of the differences reached statistical significance. As we noted in Chapter 4, this may be due in part to limited statistical power.

The second, subtler, and (we think) more interesting question is *qualitative*: Are the genes involved in the etiology of a disorder the same or different in men and in women? The analysis of qualitative sex differences is more complex than the analysis of quantitative differences. Therefore, we have chosen to devote a separate chapter to these results, rather than including them in Chapters 4 and 5.

To understand the nature of this question, a brief background in sex-limited and sex-modified genetic effects will be helpful. Geneticists who concern themselves with issues such as producing chickens that will lay more eggs or cows that will produce more milk have pondered this problem for some time. How, for example, would you select sires for a herd of dairy cows? You cannot measure milk production in bulls and take the highest producer to sire a herd because bulls, like males of all species, do not lactate. However, males do have genes that influence lactation. By measuring the milk production of a bull's female relatives (i.e., mother and sisters), one can infer the bull's milk-producing genotype. This is an example of a *sex-limited genetic effect*, in which genes influence a phenotype in one sex but are "silent" in the other. Examples in humans would be the genetic predispositions to cancer of the uterus or prostate, which can be manifested only in, respectively, females and males, because the other sex does not possess the relevant organ.

Sex limitation does not apply to psychiatric and substance use disorders because both men and women are susceptible to all these disorders. Rather, the related concept of *sex-modified gene expression* is relevant. Here, the genetically influenced phenotype is present in both males and females, but gene expression is modified by the biological and cultural differences between the sexes.

One human trait that demonstrates sex-modified gene expression is chest circumference. In males, chest circumference is influenced by one major set of genes, those that govern the size of the body's bone structure. In contrast, among females, chest circumference is influenced by two sets of genes: those that govern the size of the body's bone structure and those that influence the size of the breast. Many studies have shown that the genes that have a strong influence on general body size are much the same in men and women. However, genes for breast size will not be manifested in men. Therefore, in relatives of different sexes, the genes for chest circumference will be partially correlated (due to genes for body size that affect both sexes) and partially uncorrelated (due to genes for breast size that act only in females). Thus, when trait similarity is lower among pairs of opposite-sex relatives than among pairs of same-sex relatives, geneticists suspect the presence of sex-modified gene expression.

How can twin research use these methods? MZ twins are of no help. Although long wished for by twin researchers, opposite-sex MZ twin pairs do not occur. DZ pairs, on the other hand, come in three varieties—MM, FF, and MF. As you may recall from Chapters 1 and 2, we decided to include MF or opposite-sex (OS) pairs in the second stage of the VATSPSUD because we were interested in exploring sex differences. Although they frequently have been excluded from other twin studies (which typically focus on same-sex pairs), qualitative sex differences can only be studied by including OS DZ pairs. Indeed, OS pairs are probably nature's *best* experiment for the study of sex effects in humans. In such pairs, two individuals—one male and one female—are conceived at the same time, develop in the same womb, are born at the same time, and are reared in the same family.

Coming back to our example of chest circumference, we would expect higher correlations among male DZ pairs (who share genes for general body size) and among female DZ pairs (who share genes for both general body size and breast size) than we would expect among OS DZ pairs (who share genes for general body size but *not* for breast size).

The degree of resemblance between genetic risk factors for men and women is expressed by a statistic called the *genetic correlation* (r_g). This correlation can vary from zero (risk factors are completely different) to unity (risk factors are completely overlapping). The twin-pair correlations for three levels of r_g are shown in Figure 9.1. Although the figure depicts hypothetical data, the values are in the range we observe for disorders studied in the VATSPSUD. The MZ correlations are about twice as great as the same-sex DZ correlations, indicating that familial resemblance is due to genetic factors. There is some evidence of quantitative sex differences, because the correlations are higher for FF than MM pairs. The key piece of information for evaluating qualitative sex differences comes from the opposite-sex pair correlation. If this correlation falls midway between that of the male and female DZ correlations, r_g will equal unity, meaning the genetic risk factors in men and women are completely overlapping. If the OS correlation is zero, r_g would be estimated to be zero, meaning the genetic risk factors in men are entirely independent of those in women. The third pattern (the black bars in Figure 9.1) shows an example in which the genetic risk factors are divided equally into those that affect both males and females and those that are sex specific; here, r_g would be estimated to be 0.5.[2]

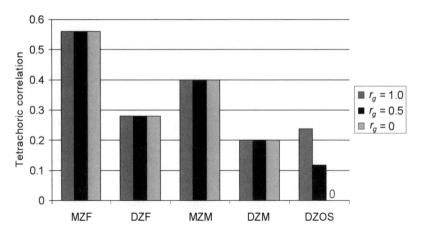

FIGURE 9.1. Twin-pair similarity for traits with different degrees of sex-modified gene expression. r_g = genetic correlation; MZF = monozygotic female; DZF = dizygotic female; MZM = monozygotic male; DZM = dizygotic male; DZOS = dizygotic opposite sex.

MAJOR DEPRESSION

As elsewhere in this book, we first focus on MD. After we describe in detail our analyses testing for qualitative sex differences in MD, we review the results for other disorders.

Our first approach to modeling sex differences in risk for lifetime MD was relatively straightforward. We began by examining the tetrachoric correlations in all five groups of twin pairs (Kendler, Gardner, & Prescott, 1999a; Kendler & Prescott, 1999a). Twin-pair similarity was lower in the OS DZ pairs (0.10) than in the two groups of same-sex DZ pairs (0.17 in FF and 0.12 in MM pairs).[3] These values are consistent with the existence of qualitative sex differences.

We used the twin-pair correlations for MD to test three hypotheses: (1) that the same genetic factors operate in males and females (r_g = 1.0); (2) that entirely different genetic factors operate in males than in females (r_g = 0); and (3) that genetic factors operating in males and females partially overlap (r_g takes a value between zero and one). By a small margin, the fit of the partially overlapping model (3) was superior to that of the same-factors model (1), and both fit better than the no-overlap model (2). The estimate for r_g was 0.52. This means that the genetic risk factors that predispose to MD in men and women have both substantial overlap (52%) and substantial differences. However, even with the sample sizes we obtained in VATSPSUD, the figure has a substantial sampling error attached to it and is better thought of as a rough guideline rather than a precise value.

The finding of qualitative sex differences in MD, though intriguing, stood on slim statistical grounds, so we looked for a way to confirm or disconfirm it. We had obtained lifetime histories of MD on two separate occasions from our MM/MF sample and on three occasions from our FF sample. In order to reexamine sex-dependent models for MD, we combined twins' reports about their lifetime histories of MD from two waves of interviews (Kendler, Gardner, Neale, & Prescott, 2001a). The major advantage of using information from multiple interviews is that it allows us to remove the effects of measurement error (see Chapter 12). Theoretically, this procedure should substantially improve our power to discriminate between competing models. We again fit the same three models to DSM-III-R criteria for lifetime MD and could now reject the hypotheses that r_g was equal to 1 or to 0 by a more comfortable statistical margin. The estimate of r_g was 0.55, very close to the value obtained in the earlier analysis. Although our two studies were not independent of one another (because the data analyzed in the first set of analyses were included in the second set), these results confirmed our initial findings and put them on a stronger statistical foundation.

These analyses also produced an interesting result about quantitative sex differences for MD. As reported in Chapter 4, our initial separate analyses of MM and FF pairs yielded higher heritability estimates in females (0.41) than in males (0.31). However, the results did not differ significantly from one another. When we reexamined this question in our second set of analyses (using two waves of assessment and including OS pairs), the heritability estimates were very similar to those we had obtained originally—but the additional information allowed us to reject equal heritability in the two sexes.

In summary, our results suggest that there are both quantitative and qualitative sex effects for MD. Genetic risk factors were more important for depression in women than in men. Furthermore, they were also partially distinct in the two sexes.

The literature on the impact of sex on genetic risk for MD is far from clear. With respect to quantitative differences, results from other twin studies are mixed. One major study reported higher heritability in females than in males (Bierut et al., 1999), but other studies have not found significant differences (Kendler, Pedersen, Neale, & Mathe, 1995b; McGuffin et al., 1996). However, the low power to detect these effects means that negative findings from these smaller twin studies are hard to interpret.

Even less is known about qualitative sex effects on genetic risk for MD. Most but not all prior family studies have found higher levels of resemblance for MD in pairs of same-sex relatives than in opposite-sex relatives (Faraone, Lyons, & Tsuang, 1987; Merikangas, Weissman, & Pauls, 1985; Reich et al., 1987). The major twin study from Australia that found quantitative sex differences (Bierut et al., 1999) chose not to report results for sex-specific gene effects because of low power. A study of lifetime MD in more than 15,000 pairs of twins from the Swedish Twin Registry produced results strikingly similar to those obtained in the VATSPSUD. In this study, higher heritability was found in women (42%) than in men (29%), with an estimated genetic correlation between the two sexes of 0.63 (Kendler, Gatz, Gardner, & Pedersen, 2006).

If gender differences in genetic risk factors for MD do exist, how might they arise? Because men and women are exposed to different social and psychological factors of etiological relevance for MD (Bebbington, 1996), it is possible that differences in exposure evoke distinct genetically based variation in the two sexes. Alternatively, biological factors, including levels of gonadal hormones during early development (Collaer & Hines, 1995) and the variable hormonal environment of the menstrual cycle and pregnancy (Seeman, 1997), could elicit distinct sets of genetic factors in women and in men (Garcia et al., 1989). In particular, some evidence suggests that there are genetic factors that specifically predispose women to depression in the postpartum period. Such genes, like those affecting breast size, would be expressed in women but not expressed in men, causing the genetic correlation in liability to MD to fall below 1. Although these are speculations, they are deserving of careful research, as they suggest that genetic factors contribute, perhaps in important ways, to differences in risk for and prevalence of MD in men and women.

ANXIETY DISORDERS

The story of sex effects in panic and generalized anxiety disorder can be briefly told. We found no evidence for quantitative or qualitative effects in either condition (Hettema et al., 2001b; Kendler, Gardner, & Prescott, 2001b). However, we put only modest stock in these negative results because of the problems with low power associated with these analyses, especially for panic disorder because of its rarity. It is probably best to say that with respect to panic disorder, sex effects on genetic risk factors are unknown.

For our analyses of sex differences in phobias, we broadened the definition to include irrational fears. As you may recall, our diagnosis of phobias had two requirements: (1) the presence of significant irrational fear and (2) objective behavioral changes associated with that fear (see Sidebar 4.5). As described in Chapter 4, the majority of individuals who reported these fears did not describe significant behavioral effects of their fears and thus did not meet the second criterion for phobias. (The exception was for agoraphobic irrational fears, for which a majority did report interference.) Using the three-level definition (no fear, fear without interference, phobia) gave us greater statistical power to detect sex differences.

The results were heterogeneous for the different categories of phobias. For three types (agoraphobia, situational phobia, and blood–injury phobia), the best-fit model suggested qualitative but not quantitative sex effects. That is, heritability in males and females was estimated to be the same (analogous to what we found in Chapter 4), but there was evidence that the genetic factors were not completely overlapping in the sexes. The genetic correlations estimated from the best-fit models were low: 0.24 for agoraphobia, 0.40 for situational phobia, and 0.35 for blood–injury phobia. Because these had wide confidence intervals, the particular values should not be taken too seriously. They do suggest, however, that for these phobia subtypes, the genetic risk factors in men and in women are even less correlated than they are for major depression.

The results for animal phobia were different. For this disorder the best-fit model was one with equal heritability in men and women and a genetic correlation of 1. That is, we found no evidence for quantitative or qualitative sex differences.

The results for social phobia (which, as discussed in Chapter 4, was notably different from the other phobia types) were harder to interpret. They suggested that social phobia was the result of genetic factors in males and of family environment in females.

There are really no other good studies examining the impact of sex on the pattern of genetic risk factors for anxiety disorders. Other large twin studies have apparently chosen not to devote resources to assessing these common and in some cases disabling syndromes. We do not feel on firm enough ground to speculate about the sources of sex differences in risk for these disorders, nor are we confident that sex effects do not exist for panic disorder and GAD. The most we can conclude is that our results on fears and phobias are suggestive. Sex may alter how genes influence our liability to at least some classes of anxiety disorders. Further enlightenment in this area must await additional research.

ANTISOCIAL BEHAVIOR

As we described in Chapter 5, there are large sex differences in the prevalence of antisocial behavior (ASB). At all ages, males are more likely than females to exhibit these characteristics. The results from our analyses based on same-sex twin pairs indicated that there are significant quantitative sex differences in the relative proportions of genetic and environmental influences on ASB (Figure 5.2).

The results remained similar after we included opposite-sex DZ pairs in the analyses.[4] For childhood ASB (CD occurring before age 15), we found significantly more genetic influence among males than among females. For adolescent ASB (CD occurring between ages 15 and 17), we found no sex differences in genetic influences. For adult ASB, the genetic influence was greater among females than among males. Thus it appears that for females genetic influences increase over time, whereas for males they decrease. This raises the question of whether childhood and adult ASB are due to the same or different sets of genetic and environmental factors. We return to this issue in Chapter 10, in which we examine how genetic influences change over time.

Our analyses of qualitative sex differences suggested that the genetic factors that influence ASB in males and in females are largely overlapping. For childhood and adolescent ASB, the estimated values for r_g were very close to 1.0. For adult ASB, the estimate was 0.62, suggesting that there may be some qualitative sex differences. However, this estimate did not differ significantly from 1.0, perhaps because the low prevalence of adult ASB in women (< 4%) limits the statistical power.

There is relatively little literature on sex differences in genetic influences on ASB. The twin study most comparable to ours, of Australian adult twins from the general population, found somewhat lower heritability for conduct disorder in females than in males (43 and 65%, respectively; Slutske et al., 1997). However, these values were not significantly different—perhaps, again, because of the low prevalence of ASB among females.

ALCOHOLISM

In our study of twin similarity for alcoholism described in Chapter 5, we examined several different definitions, including a narrow definition (DSM-IV alcohol dependence), a broad definition (DSM-IV alcohol abuse or dependence), and a multiple-threshold definition (unaffected, abuse only, and dependence with or without abuse). As in our analyses based on same-sex pairs (Figure 5.3), we found virtually no evidence for quantitative sex differences (Prescott et al., 1999).

However, we did find significant evidence for qualitative sex differences. The results are summarized in Figure 9.2. For each of these definitions, the twin-pair similarity of opposite-sex pairs was lower than that of same-sex DZ

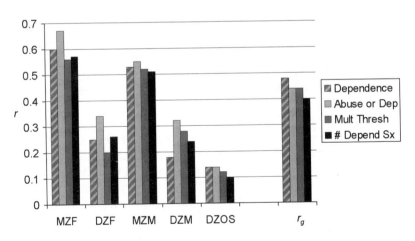

FIGURE 9.2. Twin-pair similarity and estimated male–female genetic correlations for alcoholism. r = correlation; r_g = genetic correlation; dep = dependence; mult thresh = multiple threshold; # depend sx = number of dependence symptoms. Data from Prescott, Aggen, and Kendler (1999, Table 2).

pairs. The estimated values of r_g were very similar for all of the definitions we examined. They ranged from 0.40 for number of DSM-IV alcohol dependence symptoms to 0.48 for DSM-IV alcohol dependence. All of the values were significantly greater than zero and less than unity.

These results indicate that, although genetic influences on risk for alcoholism are equally important for females and males, these genetic factors only partially overlap in the two sexes. Some twin and family studies provide hints of possible qualitative and quantitative differences in genetic risk factors for alcohol problems in men versus women (McGue, Pickens, & Svikis, 1992; Prescott et al., 2005a; Prescott, Kuhn, & Pedersen, 2005b), but others do not (Heath et al., 1997). The lack of consistency among studies may be due to differences in methodology and limited sample sizes, so at this stage it is difficult to reach any definitive conclusions.

If qualitative sex differences in genetic risk for alcoholism do exist, how might they arise? Several studies suggest that alcoholism is a heterogeneous set of disorders. Subtypes of alcoholism may differ in the degree to which they are genetically influenced. One subtype, characterized by early age of onset and antisocial behavior, is much more common among males than females and has been found in some studies to be particularly heritable (Cadoret, Troughton, & O'Gorman, 1987; Cloninger, 1987b; McGue et al., 1992). Another subtype, about equally common in men and women, is characterized by later onset, symptoms of depression and anxiety, and, perhaps, less genetic influence. Our twin analyses of multiple disorders (described in Chapter 11) found that alcoholism has genetic overlap with other externalizing disorders and, to some degree, with the internalizing disorders. This finding suggests that the genetic factors underlying antisocial alcoholism differ from those underlying other subtypes. Such a pattern could produce the evidence we see for qualitative sex differences. For example, if one set of genes predisposes to the male-preponderant antisocial alcoholism and another set predisposes to a more female-preponderant alcoholism with depressive or anxiety symptoms, lower correlations would be produced between male–female twin pairs than among same-sex pairs.[5]

NICOTINE DEPENDENCE

Our analyses of sex differences for nicotine dependence used two definitions—one a score based on the Fagerstrom Test for Nicotine Dependence (FTND; Heatherton et al., 1991) and the other a dichotomous measure (abbreviated here as ND) based on the closely related Fagerstrom Tolerance Questionnaire (FTQ; see Sidebar 5.4). This work was conducted in collaboration with our colleague Hermine Maes (Maes et al., 2004). For both measures, we found very little evidence for quantitative sex differences. As we described in Chapter 5, the same-sex correlations were very similar for males and females, and we could not reject the hypothesis of equal genetic influences. The twin-pair correlations among opposite-sex pairs (0.30 for ND and 0.35 for FTND) were very similar to those observed among male DZ pairs (ND = 0.36, FTND = 0.35) and female DZ pairs (ND = 0.38, FTND = 0.40). Thus our results do not provide any evidence for qualitative sex differences. Contrary to our finding with alcoholism, the genetic influences on nicotine dependence appear to arise from the same sources for males and females.

There is very little literature on sex differences in genetic influences on nicotine dependence. Most other twin studies that have assessed tobacco-related traits have used amounts consumed (e.g., number of cigarettes smoked) or duration of smoking. These studies have generally not found evidence for sex differences in heritability (Madden, Pedersen, Kaprio, Koskenvuo, & Martin, 2004).

ILLICIT SUBSTANCE ABUSE AND DEPENDENCE

As we noted in Chapter 5, because of the low prevalences of illicit substance use disorders in the VATSPSUD, we had limited power to detect quantitative sex differences. Even for opiate abuse/dependence, in which the heritability estimates were quite different for males and females (0 and 77%, respectively), we could not conclude that these are significantly different.

We conducted formal analyses of quantitative and qualitative sex differences for cannabis and cocaine, two substances for which we thought we might be able to detect such differences because these substances had relatively higher rates of use and abuse/dependence compared with most of the other illicit substances we examined. We also used multiple-threshold definitions in an attempt to gain more statistical power. The heritability estimates were similar to those obtained previously (Figure 5.7). The estimated genetic effects were: for cannabis, 73% in males and 49% in females; for cocaine, 40% in males and 74% in females. Despite the addition of more than 1,000 OS twin pairs to the analysis, these quantitative sex differences did not reach statistical significance. However, it is possible that there are true differences but that our analyses were underpowered to detect them. In contrast, we found no evidence of qualitative sex differences. The estimated values for r_g were 0.98 for cannabis and 1.0 for cocaine, exactly what would be expected if the genetic factors for males and females completely overlapped.

Only two other twin studies have published results from analyses of illicit substance use disorders in male and female twins (Gynther, Carey, Gottesman, & Vogler, 1995; van den Bree et al., 1998). Both of these were based on small clinical samples and did not have the statistical power to address either quantitative or qualitative sex differences in genetic influence. Thus, although there are some hints that men and women may differ in the magnitude of genetic influences on substance use disorders, the evidence is far from conclusive.

SUMMARY

Psychiatric epidemiologists have long been interested in the impact of sex on psychiatric and substance use disorders. This is not surprising, because it is rare to find a disorder for which sex is not a strong predictor of risk. The vast majority of psychiatric epidemiological studies conducted in the United States and around the world in the past 20 years have found that women are substantially more prone to develop internalizing disorders and men are much more prone to develop externalizing disorders. Often these effects are strong and among the most reproducible of known risk factors.

By contrast, sex effects are much less "on the radar screen" for psychiatric geneticists. If there is anything that we can conclude from this chapter, it is that this attitude is likely to be held in error, at least for some important disorders (in particular, MD and alcoholism). We are a bit more confident of this conclusion because, in studies of simpler organisms (such as fruit flies and rodents), it is by no means rare to find genetic effects that affect behavior differently in males and females (Kendler & Greenspan, in press).

Men and women differ in important ways both in their social roles and in their biology. Thus it is not surprising that expression of some genetic risk factors would be moderated by these differences.[6] We will take up another important topic in sex differences in Chapter 11, where we will examine the evidence for sex-dependent expression of alcoholism and depression and ask, might the genetic risk factors that predispose to depression in women increase the risk for alcoholism in men?

NOTES

1. The same methods outlined here can be applied to examining sex differences in shared environmental risk factors. Our discussion focuses on sex differences in genetic effects largely because we found so little evidence for shared environmental effects on risk for the disorders we examined in VATSPSUD. Standard twin studies do not provide power to determine whether a reduced correlation in opposite-sex (versus same-sex) DZ twins is a result of qualitative sex effects on genetic or on shared environmental factors. However, we believe we are on firm ground in our analyses in assuming that genetic effects are responsible for these sex effects, because our analyses of the same-sex twin pairs revealed so little evidence for the importance of the shared environment.

2. We follow the traditional convention of using the term r_g to refer to the genetic correlation, with a scaling of -1.0 to $+1.0$, rather than the term r_A used elsewhere in the book, which is expected to equal 0.50 for opposite-sex twins. Of interest to the more quantitatively inclined, when $r_g = 1$, the correlation in the OS pairs should equal the square root of the product of the correlations of the MM and FF DZ pairs.

3. The results differ a bit from those presented in Chapter 4 because they are based on the third rather than the first wave of interviews from our FF sample.

4. This work was conducted in collaboration with our colleague Kristen Jacobson. These results were published in Jacobson, Prescott, and Kendler (2002) and are described in more detail in Chapter 10.

5. Heterogeneity of subtypes may also help to explain why some early adoption and twin studies concluded that genetic factors were less important for females than for males. Many of these studies were based on twin pairs identified because one of the twins was hospitalized for a psychiatric or substance use disorder. However, the reasons for entering treatment often differ for men and for women, particularly in early studies, when substance abuse treatment was associated with a great deal of stigma for women. Twin studies using volunteer samples or population-based registries have found genetic influences to be of equal importance in men and women (Heath et al., 1997; Prescott et al., 2005b).

6. We have not, in these discussions, considered the possible role of genes on the X chromosome contributing to sex differences. As readers may recall from their last basic biology class, all female mammals have two X chromosomes, receiving one from their mother and one from their father. Males have only one X chromosome, which they always get from their mother, and one Y chromosome, which they always get from their father. X chromosomes are rather large and contain more genes than the small Y chromosome. In all the cells in a female's body, one of the X chromosomes is randomly "silenced." This means that, in both males and females, cells have only one functional X chromosome. If disorders are due to genes on the X chromosome, they have a distinctive pattern of resemblance in relatives. Most strikingly, risk in fathers and sons is uncorrelated because they do not share an X chromosome. Also, because one X chromosome is randomly silenced in women, MZ twin sisters resemble one another less than MZ twin brothers do. The patterns of family resemblance observed in our sample and other twin studies do not closely resemble the pattern predicted for X-linked inheritance. We therefore consider other mechanisms—such as sex-limited gene expression—to be more plausible explanations for the sex differences we observed.

CHAPTER TEN

Genetic and Environmental Influences on Stability and Change

The twin models presented in this book thus far have not dealt directly with the critical issue of *time*. In this chapter, we ask: How does the impact of genetic and environmental risk factors on psychiatric and substance use disorders vary over time? As with the sex differences discussed in Chapter 9, the changes in these risk factors can be of two kinds—*quantitative* and *qualitative*. Quantitative change means that the same genetic or environmental risk factors operate over time, but their importance varies. Qualitative change means that across time new sets of risk factors become operative.

Although the popular concept of genes often seems to imply that they are "set" or "immutable" in their impact, this is far from the case. As we have learned more about the actions of genes, it has become clear that the genome is a highly dynamic system. The expression of individual genes is constantly being turned "on" or "off" or "up" or "down" in response to the internal signals of development, physiological changes, and environmental experiences.

When considering development, we typically think of childhood and adolescence, with puberty as the paradigmatic example. However, developmental changes continue to occur throughout adult life. The brain is not fully "grown up" until at least the late 20s. Male baldness, the graying and then whitening of hair, the putting on of weight in middle adulthood, and the cessation of menstruation in women at menopause are all examples of the developmental processes that continue into middle and late adult life. Twin studies have consistently shown substantial heritabilities for these developmental changes—genetic factors play an important role in influencing the individual differences in the timing of these developmental milestones of adult life (Fabsitz, Carmelli, & Hewitt, 1992; Kirk et al., 2001; Snieder, MacGregor, & Spector, 1998).

Studying twins through time can also clarify the time course of the effects of environmental risk factors for psychopathology. Some experiences may have such a profound effect on the individual that they convey an increased risk for psychopathology for years or even decades.[1] Other experiences may have a much shorter effect, increasing risk of illness for only days or weeks. Such effects can be discriminated in models that examine twins at two or more points in time. In this chapter, we consider the evidence for genetic and environmental influences on stability and change in MD, ASB, and alcohol consumption.

STABILITY AND CHANGE IN MAJOR DEPRESSION IN WOMEN

We begin by considering the influences on stability and change in risk for MD among female twin pairs. This study was based on episodes of MD in the year prior to interview, as reported at the first and second FF interviews (Kendler, Neale, Kessler, Heath & Eaves, 1993e). By design, the second interview occurred at least 12 months after the first. On average, the interval between these interviews was 17 months, which meant that we asked the twins about the occurrence of MD episodes during two *nonoverlapping* time periods. For convenience, we refer to these two interviews as time 1 and time 2.

Given the relatively short time period between these two interviews, we predicted that the genetic risk factors for MD should not change measurably. That is, we expected a high correlation between the genetic risk factors as assessed at time 1 and at time 2. A more interesting question was what we would see for the correlation between the environmental risk factors.

As we discussed earlier in this book, environmental risk factors for adult psychiatric disorders can be grouped into two sets. One set, which we have called *distal*, includes important adverse events usually experienced in childhood or adolescence that produce enduring long-term increases in risk. In Chapter 7 we reviewed the evidence for three such risk factors: premature loss of a parent, poor parental rearing behavior, and CSA. If most of the environmental risk for MD comes from distal experiences, we should see a high correlation between the environmental risk factors for time 1 and time 2. This would occur because an individual at high risk for MD at time 1 due to a childhood trauma would still be at high risk from that trauma when interviewed again 1 or 2 years later.

The second set of risk factors, which we have called *proximal*, includes recent environmental adversities (i.e., those experienced close to the time of the onset of a disorder). As we described in Chapter 8, a feature of these kinds of adversities, which include stressful life events (SLEs), is that most of them result in only a transient increase in risk of illness. The risk for an onset of MD is increased for only a few months after the occurrence of most types of SLEs. If proximal experiences were the predominant source of environmental risk for MD, then we would expect a low correlation of the environmental risk factors across time.[2] For example, imagine that a twin has experienced a bad SLE during the year prior to her time 1 interview that markedly increased her liability to MD. When we interview her again at time 2 (at which point more than 12 months would have passed since the occurrence of the SLE), her susceptibility to MD would be back down to her baseline level because her increased risk from that prior SLE would have entirely dissipated.

The results are summarized in Figure 10.1. We spend some time here explaining these results. They show how critical information about the action of genetic and environmental risk factors over time can be derived from a simple pattern of correlations in twins.

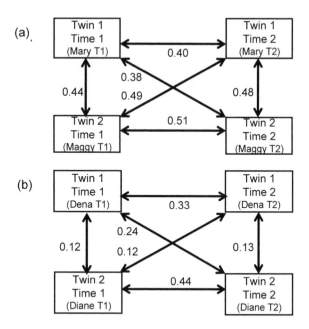

FIGURE 10.1. Observed tetrachoric correlations for major depression among female twin pairs during two 1-year intervals. (a) MZ pairs; (b) DZ pairs. Adapted from Kendler, Neale, Kessler, Heath, and Eaves (1993e, Figure 2). Copyright 1993 by the American Medical Association. Adapted by permission.

The figure shows the correlations for the liability to MD over time among MZ (Figure 10.1a) and DZ (Figure 10.1b) twin pairs. For each type, we have three kinds of correlations. It will take a bit of effort to keep these straight, but it will be worth the effort! The first of these are *cross-twin within-time* correlations. This type of correlation reflects the degree of resemblance between the two members of a twin pair assessed at approximately the same time. This is the typical pair correlation utilized in the twin models described in Chapters 4 and 5. The second type of correlation is *within-twin cross-time*. This type represents the within-person stability of the liability to MD between the time 1 and time 2 assessments. The third correlation—and the most informative about the sources of change—is *cross-twin cross-time*. This reflects, for example, the correlation in liability to MD for twin 1 at time 1 with her cotwin (twin 2) at time 2.

Consider a hypothetical pair of MZ twin sisters: Mary, twin 1, and Maggy, twin 2. Imagine that our job is to predict, from Mary's risk for time 1 MD, Mary's own risk for time 2 MD and Maggy's risk for time 2 MD. Because Mary and Maggy share all their genes, the stable genetic factors that influence Mary's risk for time 1 MD would be reflected equally well in Mary's or Maggy's time 2 MD. However, this is not the case for enduring environmental effects. Imagine that Mary had had a major environmental trauma in childhood that produced an enduring increase in her risk for MD but that Maggy had not experienced this trauma. In this case, Mary's time 1 MD would better predict her own time 2 MD than it would predict Maggy's time 2 MD. This would occur because the correlation between Mary's risk at time 1 and her risk at time 2 reflects both enduring genetic and environmental effects, whereas the correlation of Mary's risk at time 1 with Maggy's risk at time 2 reflects *only* the enduring genetic effects.

With this background, let's look at the data. We expected the within-twin cross-time correlations to be comparable across all the twins (twin 1 and twin 2 from MZ and DZ pairs), and this was indeed the case. The values ranged from 0.33 to 0.51 (the differences are consistent with statistical variation). These results tell us that, across time, an individual's risk for MD is moderately stable.

The cross-twin within-time correlations for past-year MD were substantially higher among MZ twin pairs than for DZ pairs both at time 1 (0.44 vs. 0.12) and at time 2 (0.48 vs. 0.13). These results tell us that past-year MD is relatively heritable. Given the results for lifetime MD (Chapter 4), this is not too surprising.

The key is the cross-twin cross-time correlations. Looking first at the MZ twins in Figure 10.1a, twin 1's risk for time 1 MD is correlated with her own risk for time 2 MD at 0.40, about the same as the correlation with twin 2's risk at time 2 (0.38). Similarly, twin 2's risk at time 1 is correlated about the same with her own risk at time 2 (0.51) as with the risk of twin 1 at time 2 (0.49). This is the pattern of results that would be predicted if enduring genetic effects were largely or totally responsible for the stability of risk for MD over time, with enduring environmental effects playing little or no role.[3] It is also worth noting that the cross-twin cross-time correlations in DZ twins, seen in Figure 10.1b, are about half those of the within-twin cross-time correlations (and the cross-twin MZ correlations). This is what would be predicted by a model in which genetic factors were largely or completely responsible for the longitudinal stability of risk for MD.

We then submitted the data to formal model-fitting using the model illustrated in Figure 10.2. Here we are interested in estimating the cross-time correlations of the genetic (r_A), shared environmental (r_C), and unique environmental (r_E) factors. As with other analyses with MD, no evidence was found for shared environmental factors that contribute to liability to MD. In the full model, the genetic correlation was nearly 1 and the unique environmental correlation nearly 0. In the best-fit model, shown in Figure 10.2, the genetic correlation was constrained to unity and the unique environmental correlation to zero.

Implications

There are three major implications of these results. First, the difference between the temporal patterns for genetic and environmental risk factors could not be more striking. *Whereas the genetic risk factors for MD were entirely stable across time, the environmental risk factors were entirely occasion specific in their effect.* In the case of MD, genes appear to provide a stable

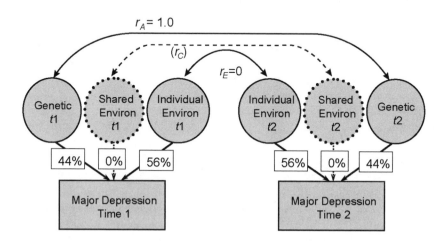

FIGURE 10.2. Results from best-fitting two-wave twin model for major depression in women. Adapted from Kendler, Neale, Kessler, Heath, and Eaves (1993e, Figure 3). Copyright 1993 by the American Medical Association. Adapted by permission.

background level of liability that is relatively constant, at least through the middle years of adult life. These results illustrate the advantages of longitudinal analyses: The differences in the temporal nature of the genetic and environmental risk factors would have gone undetected had we examined the twins only once.

Second, in aggregate, environmental risk factors are etiologically important for MD, but their impact on liability to MD is short-lived, probably lasting for just a few months. Note that we can reach this conclusion without actually measuring the events themselves. These analyses powerfully demonstrate how genetically informative designs can provide key insights into the actions of environmental risk factors.

Third, the heritability of "1-year" MD is 44% (see Figure 10.2), reassuringly similar to that found for lifetime MD (41% for DSM-III-R MD in women; see Figure 4.3).[4] At this point, some readers may be scratching their heads. We devoted all of Chapter 7 to showing that experiences in childhood produce a lasting impact on risk for a range of psychiatric and substance use disorders, including MD. Now we appear to be saying the opposite. What gives?

Of the three distal risk factors examined in Chapter 7, two (parental loss and poor parenting) tend to make twins similar rather than different in their risk.[5] For this reason, they appear in our models as *shared* rather than *unique* environment. Our model-fitting analyses of past-year MD indicate no evidence for shared environmental effects. However, as we noted in Chapter 7, unless we had a twin sample many times larger than the VATSPSUD, we would not expect to be able to detect a shared environmental effect of this size using traditional twin models (which assess the environment through latent variables rather than directly).

The third risk factor, CSA, which was moderately correlated for twins within a pair, would sometimes contribute to shared and sometimes to unique environmental effects. When severe CSA occurred to one twin but not to the other, its effect on risk was substantial and might have been expected to show up in our analyses as an enduring environmental effect. However, it did not, probably because of the relative rarity of severe CSA. Recall that not only are SLEs much more common in aggregate than CSA, but also that the more severe ones have a much stronger immediate association with onset of MD than does the enduring increased risk that we see with severe CSA.[6] Thus our interpretation is that the reason that, in our models, the aggregate impact of unique environmental effects on MD showed no strong continuity of risk over time is that the effects of SLEs (that show up in our models as time-specific environmental effects) dominated the rarer and typically less potent early risk factors (that would appear in our models as enduring environmental effects).[7] If this study were repeated with a larger sample size, we would predict that the correlation in individual-specific environmental effects on MD over time would be detectable but modest, probably in the range of 0.10–0.20.

Figure 10.3 illustrates the temporal effects of genetic and environmental risk factors on MD suggested by these results. The figure depicts the liability to MD over time for three hypothetical individuals, Laura, Mimi, and Helen, who have three different levels of genetic risk for MD. We assume that an individual's liability at a particular time is the sum of her baseline genetic risk and the effects of recent stressors. (Her baseline risk would also be influenced, to a modest degree, by exposure to early environmental traumas.) If the total liability exceeds a theoretical threshold (the dashed line in the figure), the individual develops an episode of MD.

Suppose that over the time period portrayed, each of the three women experiences one mildly stressful and one highly stressful life event. Each of these events, for short periods of time, increases the women's liability to MD. For Laura, the low-risk individual, neither event precipitates a major depression because, even when under high stress, her total liability remains below the threshold. For Mimi, who has intermediate genetic liability, only the severe event causes her to develop MD. But for Helen, who has high genetic risk, even a mild life event is severe enough to cause her to cross the threshold and develop a depressive episode. Although it is a much simplified heuristic, this model does capture the clinical implications of these analyses.[8] We should emphasize that, although we have depicted the genetic effects as stable across the time period shown here (in middle adulthood), genetic liability may experience larger fluctuations during other developmental periods, such as puberty and menopause.

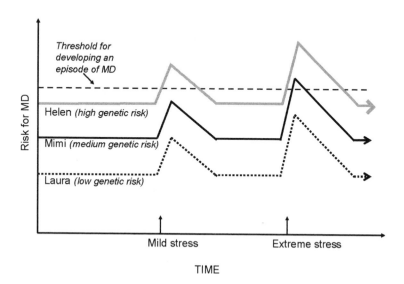

FIGURE 10.3. Schematic representation of the longitudinal interplay of genetic and environmental factors in creating risk for major depression (MD).

INFLUENCES ON THE DEVELOPMENT OF ANTISOCIAL BEHAVIOR

In Chapter 5, we described the twin-pair results for CD and AASB. Although these disorders are conceptualized as manifestations of the same construct, we obtained somewhat different patterns of results in our twin analyses. These findings were similar to those from other twin and adoption studies (Cloninger & Gottesman, 1987; Lyons et al., 1995; Miles & Carey, 1997) in suggesting more shared environmental influence on CD than on AASB and more genetic influence on AASB than on CD. We speculated that the shared environmental effects for CD might be due to the fact that twins often share the same friends and social settings during early adolescence, whereas later in adolescence and into early adulthood they go their separate ways, encountering new environments and opportunities to express their genetic liability.

What our earlier results do not address is whether the genetic factors that influence CD and AASB are the same or different. Our colleague Kristen Jacobson conducted several analyses to address the genetic influences on antisocial behavior across development (Jacobson et al., 2002).

These analyses were based on data collected by self-report questionnaires administered as part of our fourth interview wave of FF pairs and our second interview with MM and MF pairs. We asked twins to report the frequency with which they had engaged in ASBs during three age periods: before age 15, from age 15 to 17, and at 18 and older. The measures for CD and ASB differ to reflect age-relevant behaviors (see Sidebar 5.1). Our analyses were based on a model that included three possible sets of genetic and environmental factors (A, C, and E). One set influences early adolescent ASB and also carries forward to influence ASB later on in life. A second set reflects new genetic and environmental influences that arise after age 15. The third set is included to estimate genetic and environmental influences that are specific to adulthood.

Figure 10.4 portrays hypothetical results from such an analysis. The top figure (10.4a) depicts a case in which the genetic and environmental variance estimates are stable over time. If we were to conduct a standard twin analysis of the data at these three times, we might conclude (erroneously) that there was no change occurring in the genetic and environmental factors. However, in this example, the genetic influences (shown in black) and shared environmental influences (shown in dark gray) endure over time, but there is new variation in the individual-specific influences (shown in light gray shades) at stages 2 and 3.

In the second figure (10.4b), both the relative amounts of variation and the sources of this variation are changing over the stages.[9] The total amount of genetic variance increases from 25 to 35%. The genetic variance at stage 2 is due to a combination of 15% enduring genetic influences (those that continue from stage 1) and new genetic sources that enter after stage 1 ($A2 =$

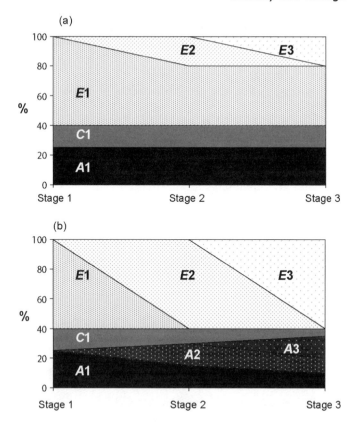

FIGURE 10.4. Hypothetical results for genetic and environmental influences for a trait over three developmental stages. (a) Total genetic and environmental influences are stable over time. Genetic influences (A) and shared environmental influences (C) endure over time; individual-specific influences (E) are largely enduring, with some new variation in stages 2 and 3. (b) Genetic variance increases and is in part due to new sources over time. Shared environmental influence decreases and has no new sources over time. The amount of individual-specific environmental variance is stable but comes from completely new sources at each stage.

15%). At stage 3, the genetic variance is due to 10% enduring from stage 1, 10% enduring from stage 2, and 15% new genetic variance (A3). The shared environmental variance is due to the same source throughout (C1), but its influence decreases over time (from 15 to 5%). The individual-specific variance estimate is 60% at all three stages, but it arises from completely different factors at each stage.

The concept of "new" genetic variance emerging over time might at first seem strange. But recall that the human genome is dynamic. It might help to imagine an example in which we were studying height in children from the ages of 5 to 15. It would be perfectly plausible to find one set of genes that influence height throughout these years but another set of genes whose effects emerge at puberty. The reason is that individuals have different-sized "growth spurts" at puberty, in part because of genetic differences in the hormonal changes they undergo and in the growth patterns in response to these hormonal alterations.

Now let's turn to our actual results. Figure 10.5a summarizes the results for males. As we saw in Chapter 5, among males there is little evidence of genetic influences on ASB in early adolescence; the estimated genetic variance is just 6%. Shared environmental factors account for 28%, and the remaining 64% is attributable to individual-specific environmental effects and measurement error. By late adolescence the pattern has changed, with the total genetic

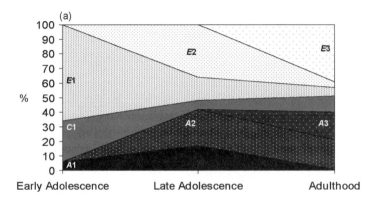

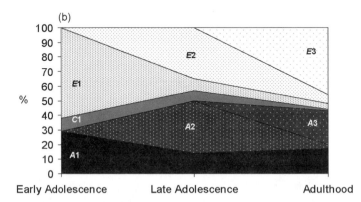

FIGURE 10.5. Estimated proportions of genetic and environmental variance for adolescent and adult antisocial behavior in (a) males and (b) females. Adapted from Jacobson, Prescott, and Kendler (2002, Figure 3). Copyright 2002 by Cambridge University Press. Adapted by permission.

variance increasing to 42%. Most of this (25%) is attributed to new genetic effects (A2), with the rest due to the genetic factor contributing to early adolescent ASB (A1). Conversely, the influence of the shared environment has shrunk to just 6%, and all of this is attributed to the same shared environmental factors that influence early adolescent ASB (C1). There is no evidence of new shared environmental influences (i.e., C2 does not differ from 0% and thus is not shown in the figure). In contrast, it appears that the individual-specific environment is changing. Of the 52% E effects, 36% are estimated as being new (E2) and only 16% as continuing from early adolescence. This suggests that environmental influences on ASB (such as those of peers not shared by twins) remain important but are not the same over time. This might reflect the changes in peer groups that arise when boys move from middle school to high school.

Interestingly, although the total genetic and environmental proportions remain virtually the same from late adolescence to adulthood, our analysis indicates that new genetic and individual-specific environmental influences arise in adulthood. Of the 40% of genetic variance seen for ASB in adulthood, almost none (1%) is due to the genetic factors that influence ASB in early adolescence; 20% is shared with late adolescent ASB; and 19% is new to adulthood. Similarly, of the 49% individual-specific environmental variance, most (39%) is estimated to arise in adulthood (E3), with only small amounts carrying forward from early (E1 = 6%) or late (E2 = 4%) adolescence. As with late adolescence, there is no evidence for new shared environmental factors. The 11% shared environmental variance is attributed to the same factor that influences early adolescent ASB.

The results for females are shown in Figure 10.5b. As we saw in Chapter 9, there is stronger evidence for genetic influences on early adolescent ASB in females (A1 = 29%) than in males. Otherwise, the results are broadly similar to those seen for males. The genetic factor carries forward to a small degree, but there is evidence of new genetic variance occurring both in late adolescence (A2 = 36% of the total 50% genetic variance) and in adulthood (A3 = 23% of the total 43%). The shared environmental influences are small in early adolescence (C1 = 9%) and decrease over time, with no evidence for new shared environmental effects. As with the males, the individual-specific variance ranges from about 40 to 60%, and this is largely occasion specific, that is, the individual-specific factors that influence ASB do not appear to persist over time.[10]

We can draw two important conclusions from these analyses. First, as suggested by the cross-sectional results from our sample and other studies, the relative importance of shared environmental factors declines across adolescence, whereas genetic factors increase in importance. Second, these changes are due in large part to important new genetic and environmental influences that arise during late adolescence and adulthood and affect antisocial behavior at distinct developmental stages.

STABILITY AND CHANGE IN ALCOHOL CONSUMPTION IN WOMEN

In our final example of this chapter, we consider the genetic and environmental influences on alcohol consumption among women. We studied alcohol consumption rather than past-year episodes of alcoholism, which were infrequent among women and not assessed in our early interviews. Although the results presented in Chapter 5 provide little evidence for shared environmental effects on risk for alcoholism, there were several reasons that these factors might be important for alcohol consumption. First, the fact that several twin studies, including our own, have found that both MZ and DZ twin pairs are strongly correlated for the age at which they begin to use alcohol suggests the importance of family or peer influences on this important alcohol-related variable (we consider this in more detail in Chapter 15). Second, because drinking patterns are to some degree socially acquired, we might expect that frequency of drinking (e.g., whether one is a weekend or a daily drinker) might be a familial–environmental characteristic.

We analyzed reported drinking in the year prior to the first and third interviews conducted with the female twin sample. Here we present results for two measures: *drinking frequency*, the number of days in a typical month in which one or more alcoholic drinks were consumed; and *drinking quantity*, the typical number of drinks consumed on a drinking day. This work was based on 496 MZ and 351 DZ female twin pairs who had used alcohol sometime during the assessment period (Prescott & Kendler, 1996).[11]

The average drinking frequency for the sample was 3.4 days per month ($SD = 5.3$), but with a wide range (0–30 days). The average drinking quantity was 1.4 drinks per drinking day ($SD = 1.3$), with a range of 0 to 13 drinks. Over time, the twins tended to reduce both their frequency of drinking and the quantity they consumed. The average per-year change in the sample was a decrease of –0.1 drinking days per month and –0.06 drinks per occasion. However, the type of change was quite variable among the sample, with some individuals increasing, some decreasing, and some remaining stable.

The approach we used differs somewhat from that employed in the prior two examples. Because we were assessing drinking in adulthood, we did not use the "developmental" model portrayed in Figures 10.4 and 10.5. In addition, because our outcome measures were continuous rather than categorical (as with the MD example, for which we assessed the presence or absence of MD during the preceding year), we were able to estimate genetic and environmental influences on stability and change. We applied our twin model to study average drinking frequency and quantity (i.e., the average across time 1 and time 2) and change in drinking frequency and quantity (calculated as the time 2 minus the time 1 values).

The results are summarized in Figure 10.6. For drinking frequency averaged over the two interviews, there was substantial genetic influence (41%;

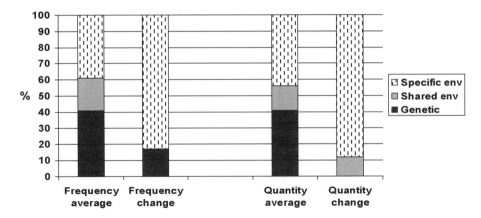

FIGURE 10.6. Estimated proportions of variance for stability and change in alcohol consumption among females. Env = environment. Data from Prescott and Kendler (1996, Table 5).

95% CI = 33, 49) and also evidence for shared environmental influences (20%; 95% CI = 12, 28), with the remainder attributable to individual environment (39%; 95% CI = 36, 41). The pattern, however, was quite different for the sources of change in frequency across the two interviews. Individual-specific factors were responsible for the great majority of the change in drinking frequency (83%; 95% CI = 77, 89), with only a small influence of genetic factors (17%; 95% CI = 13, 21) and no evidence for shared environment.

The results for the average drinking quantity across the two interviews were similar to those for frequency, with variance proportions of 41% genetic (95% CI = 31, 51), 15% shared environment (95% CI = 6, 24), and 44% individual environment (95% CI = 41, 47). Variation in how drinking quantity changed across the two occasions, however, was due predominantly to individual-specific effects (88%; 95% CI = 82, 94). To the degree that there is familial resemblance for change in drinking quantity, however, it was attributable to shared environmental effects (12%; 95% CI = 1, 23) and not to genetic factors.

In summary, we saw distinct sources of individual differences in the kinds of factors that influenced stability versus change in drinking patterns. We found moderate genetic influences on the average level of drinking quantity and frequency across the two interviews. By contrast, changes in patterns of alcohol consumption appeared largely to result from influences unique to each individual twin, with only relatively small genetic or shared environmental effects. Using a different approach from that used in our first example with multiple assessments of MD, we found that these analyses again showed the value of adding time to twin models.

Effects of Age and Cohort

Like other samples with a broad age range, the VATSPSUD showed significant differences in alcohol and drug use associated with different birth cohorts. Men and women who were born in the 1950s (and thus were teenagers in the late 1960s and early 1970s) tended to show higher use of psychoactive substances than those born either earlier or later. Another influence on substance use is ease of access to the substance. Some evidence suggests that whereas Prohibition in the United States had little long-term effect on the drinking patterns of individuals who were already drinkers, those who came of age while alcohol was illegal were less likely to become regular drinkers. The legal drinking age in Virginia changed from 18 to 21 in 1980, a time when many individuals in the VATSPSUD were adolescents.

Age-related changes in drinking patterns are also associated with developmental stage. A typical pattern is an experimental phase followed by increasing drinking during adolescence, peak drinking in young adulthood, and then reductions over time coinciding with taking on new roles and responsibilities (Johnstone, Leino, Ager, Ferrer, & Fillmore, 1996).

Because of the impact of developmental stage, the direction and amount of change observed across the 5-year interval between our two assessments at the FF1 and FF3 interviews might be expected to differ for individuals from different historical cohorts. Thus we repeated our analyses, allowing different results for the different age groups.

We first tested for cohort differences by dividing the sample into two groups based on whether the legal drinking age was 18 or 21 at the time the participants turned 18 and by looking to see whether these groups differed in their drinking patterns. We found little evidence for an effect of legal drinking age on drinking frequency or quantity.

To test for age differences in drinking patterns, we divided the sample into six age groups based on their ages at the wave 1 interview: under 21, 21–25, 26–30, 31–35, 36–40, and 41 and older. Figure 10.7 summarizes the results of the twin analyses by age groups. Unlike categorical variables, for which we present the results as proportions of variance (i.e., they add up to 100%), when we use continuous variables (such as number of days or drinks) we can estimate whether the absolute amount of genetic and environmental variance changes across groups. For all four measures, we scaled the values so that the total variance was 100% at age 30. The values for other ages are shown as percentages relative to the age-30 values.

The pattern of results was different for each of the measures. For average drinking frequency, the total variance increased across age, so that the frequency with which women drink was more variable among older than younger women. As shown in Figure 10.7, the genetic and shared environmental variances were estimated to be the same across age groups. For simplicity, the figure shows the results for the youngest, middle, and oldest groups. The observed group differences were due to increases in individual-specific vari-

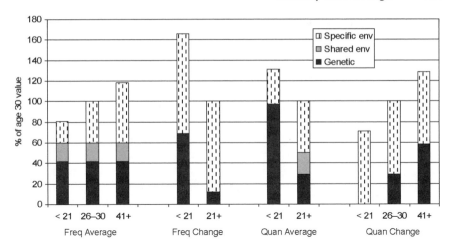

FIGURE 10.7. Estimated sources of variance in stability and change in alcohol consumption among females in different age groups. Quan = quantity; freq = frequency; env = environment. Data from Prescott and Kendler (1996, Table 5).

ance. This suggests that as the twins in a pair get older and go their separate ways, they encounter different environments that influence drinking frequency in varying ways.

The results for change in drinking frequency differed between women younger and older than age 21, but the groups over 21 did not differ significantly from each other, so we combined them in Figure 10.7. The younger women were more variable in how they changed. Furthermore, this change was under stronger genetic influence in the younger than in the older women. We might speculate that change in drinking frequency among these women (who are drinking illegally) is mediated by other genetically influenced characteristics. For example, women with more risk-taking personalities might show a greater increase in drinking over this period. The results for average quantity were similar to those for change in frequency, with younger women being more variable in how much they drank. Genetic factors were much more important for the youngest group of women, accounting for 74% of the variance in level of consumption. Among women over 21, genetic factors accounted for 29% of the variance and shared environmental factors for 21%.

Yet another pattern was observed for change in drinking quantity. Here the total variation increased over age, indicating that older women in their 40s and 50s were more variable in their patterns of change, with some women increasing and others decreasing the quantity of alcohol they consumed. However, the greater variability across age was estimated as due to increasing genetic variation, which accounted for as much as 45% of the total variance in the oldest group.

What can we conclude from these results? First, we observed a lot of variation across age groups, particularly between women under and over age 21. This is a time at which drinking patterns are in flux and vary with the changes in lifestyles that occur during this period (attending college, joining the workforce). A large proportion of the variation in change in drinking was attributed to individual-specific effects. This is not surprising, as drinking patterns are likely to be influenced by environmental factors not shared by twins, such as life roles, peer groups, or drinking habits of boyfriends and husbands. In Chapter 15 we consider the effects of certain life events (including marriage, divorce, and motherhood) on the pattern of alcohol consumption.

The results also suggest some general conclusions about age differences in genetic effects. First, we cannot make simple generalizations; the importance of genetic factors may increase or decrease over age. Second, different age groups show different amounts of variability. This means that, even if genetic effects are equally important at different ages, the apparent heritability can differ.[12] For example, in the case of average drinking frequency, the genetic factors were equally important for different age groups, but because the individual-specific environment increased over age, the genetic proportion (heritability) decreased from about 50% in the under-21 age group to about 33% in the over-40 age group.

SUMMARY

The goal of this chapter has been to explore temporal variation in the impact of genetic and environmental risk factors on psychiatric and substance use disorders and traits. Our results indicate that these risk factors are often dynamic in their effects. Static models (those that do not consider time or development) can capture only part of the impact these risk factors have on disease liability.

A few general themes are noteworthy. First, classes of risk factors can differ dramatically in their temporal stability. In looking at onsets of depressive episodes, we found that genetic risk factors were completely stable, whereas environmental risk factors were entirely occasion specific in their effects. Among women, the impact of shared environmental experiences on antisocial behavior that is evident in early adolescence completely disappears by adulthood (Figure 10.5b). In contrast, the genetic risk factors for antisocial behavior that are first seen in early adolescence continue to be important into adulthood.

A second theme is that over time, "new" genetic and environmental risk factors (i.e., those not present at earlier time periods) can become important. For example, among both males and females, we found evidence for genetic influences on ASB that became active only in adulthood (Figures 10.5a and 10.5b).

Third, as we saw with alcohol consumption, genes and environment can play quite different roles in influencing stability of a trait versus changes in that trait. As if things were not already complicated enough, we also found evidence that the causes of stability and change in alcohol consumption themselves differed as a function of birth cohort.

Finally, in all of our examples, there was a trend for the effects of genes to be more enduring and of comparatively greater importance in influencing trait stability, whereas environmental effects were typically more time limited in their action and more important in causing change.

NOTES

1. In Chapter 7, we saw that loss of a parent was associated with an increased risk of onset for most disorders that lasted for years to decades. Although those analyses could not definitively address whether the parental loss *caused* the onset, they were suggestive—especially for loss due to death. In that chapter, we also showed that the effect of CSA on risk of illness—which was likely causal—persisted at least into adulthood.

2. To the extent that individuals help create life events, there might be correlations over time in individual-specific risk. See Chapter 13.

3. In considering the analysis of environmental effects over time, we must also consider measurement error. Such error will show up in our models as unique environmental effects that will be time specific in their effect.

4. The relationship between the heritability of lifetime and 1-year MD actually involves several subtle issues. Two are especially noteworthy. First, errors of memory are probably fewer for MD assessed in the past year than over an entire lifetime. As pointed out in Chapter 12, reducing error tends to increase estimated heritability. Second, when assessing MD over as short a time period as a year, it is possible that individuals with a high liability to illness may not have an episode because of insufficient time or the absence of an environmental precipitant. This kind of error will tend to reduce the heritability of 1-year versus lifetime MD. Our estimate of the heritability of 1-year MD is only slightly greater than for lifetime MD, suggesting that these two processes may have roughly balanced one another.

5. Parenting received is not always experienced the same way by members of a twin pair, so this form of risk factor could contribute to unique environmental effects.

6. See Figures 7.8 and 8.3.

7. As noted earlier, measurement error will also contribute to the occasion-specific unique environmental effects.

8. This pattern of findings—that genetic effects are relatively stable over time whereas environmental effects are largely occasion specific—is by no means unique to this study. Such a pattern has been seen for a rather wide variety of psychiatric and psychological traits (e.g., Eaves, Long, & Heath, 1986; Larsson, Larsson, & Lichtenstein, 2004; van den Berg, Posthuma, & Boomsma, 2004).

9. Because the CD and AASB measures were based on different items, we could not measure whether the total genetic and environmental variance changed over

time (as we did in the studies of alcohol consumption), only whether the proportions changed. The estimates shown here differ somewhat from those reported in Chapter 5. This is due to different sample sizes and inclusion of males from opposite-sex twin pairs in the analyses described here.

10. As with the prior analyses, some proportion of the occasion-specific E variance is due to measurement error.

11. We excluded abstainers because they artificially increased the level of stability and because it is not clear that it is appropriate to assign them "zero" on the drinking scale. As is typical for alcohol consumption, the values were positively skewed, so the analyses were conducted on log-transformed scores.

12. This can occur because, as pointed out in Chapter 3, heritability is nothing more than the ratio of genetic variance to total variance in a particular population.

CHAPTER ELEVEN

The Genetics of What?
Comorbidity, General versus Specific Effects, and Risk Indicators

Until now, when we have studied genetic and environmental influences using twin models, we have examined one psychiatric or substance use disorder at a time. The goal of these analyses has been to understand the sources of variability among people in their risk for developing these disorders. We are attempting to estimate how much of the variation in risk is due to genetic differences and how much is due to differences in environmental exposure and experiences. An implicit assumption of these analyses is that the DSM diagnostic categories are the "right" unit of analysis. That is, our prior analyses assumed that the DSM definitions and distinctions between disorders correspond to the "true" structure of genetic and environmental risk factors. In this chapter we use twin data to evaluate this assumption.

Another aspect of our models is that genetic and environmental risk factors are assumed to influence an unmeasured "liability." This liability may represent a concatenation of processes leading from genes and environment to behavior. In the latter part of this chapter we describe how data from twins can be used to help define liability and to identify subclinical characteristics that may be more closely related to the action of genes than are the clinical disorders themselves.

The models that we present in this chapter get increasingly complex, but we ask the reader to bear with us. As we move beyond the simple and static descriptive twin models (such as our old friend the *ACE* model), the explanatory power of our models increases, but with greater clinical relevance comes greater intricacy. We believe this is a worthwhile trade-off.

STUDYING THE SOURCES OF COMORBIDITY

In the first half of this chapter, we take a multivariate approach, which involves examining two or more disorders at a time. When this is done in a genetically informative population such as twins, it becomes possible not only to examine the sources of variance in risk for individual disorders but also to understand the sources of *covariance* between different disorders. By covariance, we mean the tendency for the risk for one disorder in a population to be positively correlated with the risk for another disorder. Put another way, these methods allow us to distinguish between risk factors that are unique to individual disorders and those that are shared across multiple disorders.

The covariance in risk among disorders is another way of expressing the more common concept of *comorbidity*. Although comorbidity has several definitions, we use it to mean that during his or her lifetime an individual experiences two or more disorders at greater than chance expectation. Since the advent of structured psychiatric diagnostic interviews, studies of comorbidity have been a growth industry. A wide variety of epidemiological studies have shown that comorbidity within psychiatric disorders, within substance use disorders, and across psychiatric and substance use disorders is more the rule than the exception (Boyd et al., 1984; Kessler et al., 1994b).

Although epidemiological studies can document the magnitude of comorbidity (or covariance in risk), they typically cannot provide insight into the causal mechanisms. Here twin studies can help. Figure 11.1 illustrates one kind of twin model for comorbidity. As in our basic twin model (Chapter 3), the risk for each disorder is partitioned into genetic, shared environmental, and individual-specific factors. Risks for the two disorders are correlated through three paths: correlated genetic risk factors (the path labeled r_A), correlated shared environmental risk factors (r_C), and correlated individual-specific

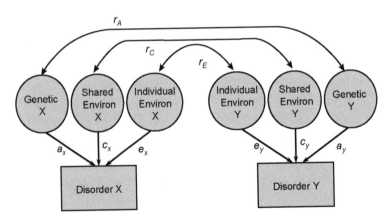

FIGURE 11.1. A bivariate twin model to estimate the sources of overlapping liability for two disorders.

environmental risk factors (r_E). These correlations can range from −1.0 to +1.0. For example, genetic correlations of zero, 0.50, and 1.00 would indicate that the sets of genetic risk factors for the two disorders were, respectively, entirely unrelated, moderately related, and virtually identical. (See Sidebar 11.1 for details of this model.) This model should be familiar to readers, as it is very similar to the model introduced in the last chapter (Figure 10.2). Instead of examining one disorder measured at two occasions, we are now examining two disorders measured at one occasion.

Comorbidity of Major Depression and Generalized Anxiety

We begin with the simple case of two disorders, MD and GAD. We and others (Boyd et al., 1984) find that these two disorders have high rates of comorbidity in population surveys. That is, these disorders co-occur in the same individual far more commonly than would be expected by chance. Twin studies can tell us how much of the covariance in risk for these two disorders is due to overlap of genetic risk factors, shared environmental risk factors, and individual-specific risk factors.

We have fit bivariate (two-variable) twin models to MD and GAD using data from several different interviews. Figure 11.2 displays the results from one of these efforts using the first wave of interview data from our FF sample (Kendler, Neale, Kessler, Heath, & Eaves, 1992e). Several findings are noteworthy. First, shared environmental factors do not contribute to the observed MD–GAD comorbidity. This finding is consistent with prior results (Chapter 4) in suggesting that these factors do not contribute to liability to these disorders when considered separately.

SIDEBAR 11.1. Understanding Models for Comorbidity

The source of information needed to estimate a bivariate twin model can be described without the need for complex algebraic formulas. Assume that we have two disorders, A and B, and further assume, for simplicity, that shared environment does not impact on the resemblance for disorders A and B. For a twin study, we then focus on two correlations in liability between A and B: (1) the correlation obtained within individuals and (2) the cross-twin correlation in MZ pairs (that is, risk of A in twin 1 correlated with risk of B in twin 2 and vice versa). The within-individual correlation between disorders A and B could arise as a result of genes or unique environment. However, the cross-MZ twin correlation between disorders A and B could arise only as a result of genes. Therefore, the difference between these two correlations tells us directly about the contribution of the environment to the correlation in risk for the two disorders. If within-individual and cross-MZ twin correlations are approximately the same, then nearly all of the comorbidity observed between the two disorders is due to genetic factors. Cross-twin DZ twin correlations also contribute to these analyses because they allow us to distinguish the effects of genetic versus shared environmental contributions to comorbidity.

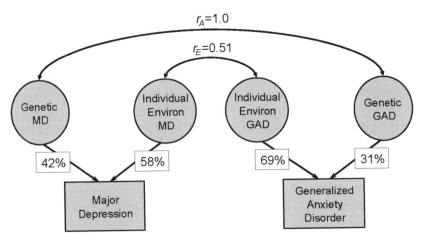

FIGURE 11.2. Results from best-fitting twin model for overlapping liability to major depression (MD) and generalized anxiety disorder (GAD) in women. Adapted from Kendler, Neale, Kessler, Heath, and Eaves (1992e, Figure 2). Copyright 1992 by the American Medical Association. Adapted by permission.

A second result is that the individual-specific environmental correlation (r_E) is 0.51, indicating that the environmental risk factors that influence MD and GAD are moderately correlated. This is of interest given our study of the effects of SLEs on MD and GAD syndromes (Chapter 8). In those analyses, some SLEs had relatively specific effects: They increased the risk for MD more than for GAD-like syndromes (or vice versa). However, most events were rather nonspecific in their effects. Thus these two very different analytic approaches to the same question produced similar results.

Third, and perhaps most interesting, the genetic correlation (r_A) is estimated to be unity. We do not have the statistical power to discriminate an estimate of 0.90 or even 0.80 from unity; but in any case, this estimate indicates a very strong relationship between the genetic risk factors for MD and GAD. These results suggest that from a genetic perspective, GAD and MD can be considered to be virtually the same disorder. We are confident of this result because we have replicated it using data from subsequent interviews with our FF sample (Kendler, 1996a) and in two samples of Swedish twins (Kendler, Gardner, Gatz, & Pedersen, manuscript in preparation; Roy, Neale, Pedersen, Mathe, & Kendler, 1995).

Comorbidity of Major Depression and Social Phobia

Let's now examine a bivariate analysis with quite a different outcome. This time, in our FF sample, we examined the sources of covariance in risk between lifetime MD and lifetime social phobia. The results of the best-fit model are shown in Figure 11.3 (Kendler, Neale, Kessler, Heath, & Eaves,

1993f). Although our earlier examination of social phobia alone in Chapter 4 detected evidence for a modest shared environmental effect, in these analyses with MD, this effect was not statistically detectable. In contrast to the MD–GAD results presented earlier, here our estimate of r_E is small (0.18), suggesting that the environmental risk factors for MD and for social phobia are largely independent of one another. This is the pattern we would expect if environmental experiences that increase risk for social phobia have little impact on risk for MD and vice versa. Finally, the estimate of r_A is only a bit higher, at 0.30. This result suggests that genetic risk factors for MD and social phobia are only modestly correlated.

Mechanisms for Comorbidity: Alcoholism and Major Depression

In addition to addressing the question of how much genetic overlap there is between disorders, information from twins (or other pairs of relatives) can be used to help us understand how comorbidity arises. In this section we describe the results of our study of the mechanisms underlying the comorbidity of alcoholism and MD.

It has long been observed that alcoholism and depression tend to co-occur within individuals. More recent evidence suggests that these two disorders also tend to co-occur within families (Merikangas & Gelernter, 1990). Three possible mechanisms for the comorbidity between depression and alcoholism are shown in Figure 11.4.[1] All three predict the same pattern of findings within individuals (that is, risk for alcoholism and risk for depression are correlated), but the models can be distinguished by observing the patterns of

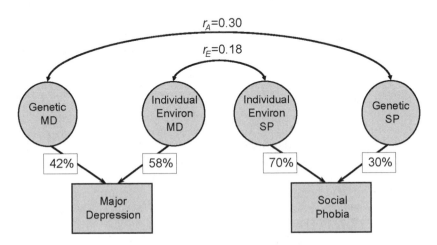

FIGURE 11.3. Results from best-fitting twin model for overlapping liability to major depression (MD) and social phobia (SP) in women. Adapted from Kendler, Neale, Kessler, Heath, and Eaves (1993f, Figure 4). Copyright 1993 by Cambridge University Press. Adapted by permission.

risk among pairs of relatives, such as twin pairs. Figure 11.4a shows a model for *phenotypic causation,* in which having depression directly increases the risk for developing alcoholism. This model predicts that if relative 1 has depression, risk for alcoholism in relative 2 is increased only if relative 2 also has depression. We could also test the opposite model, that having alcoholism directly increases risk for developing depression.

Figure 11.4b shows a *correlated liability* model, in which, within a person, the factors predisposing to alcoholism and depression are correlated. This is the same model as the one used to estimate the sources of overlap of MD with GAD and MD with social phobia. The liability to depression is correlated across relatives, as is the liability to alcoholism. Thus relatives will be *indirectly* correlated for their liability across disorders. For example, if relative 1 has depression, risk for relative 2 is increased for depression and to a lesser extent for alcoholism, and this occurs regardless of whether relative 2 has depression.

The third model, shown in Figure 11.4c, is the *alternate forms* model. Here the familial liability for alcoholism and depression are the same, but the development of one or the other disorder (or both) is influenced by individual-specific factors. According to this model, if relative 1 has depression, risk for relative 2 is increased equally (relative to population rates) for depression and alcoholism.

Figure 11.4d shows a variant of the alternate forms model, sex-dependent expression. As we discussed in Chapter 9, there are genes whose expression can be different in males and females. The observation that there is an elevated frequency of alcoholism among male relatives of individuals with depression led Winokur and colleagues to formulate the *depression-spectrum* hypothesis (Winokur, Cadoret, Dorzab, & Baker, 1971). This hypothesis proposes the existence of one set of familial risk factors that are preferentially expressed as alcoholism in males and as depression in females. This model is appealing because it helps account for the greater population prevalences of depression in women and alcoholism in men.

We compared how well these three models accounted for the twin-pair resemblance information for lifetime DSM-IV diagnoses of alcohol dependence (AD) and MD (Prescott, Aggen, & Kendler, 2000).[2] Figure 11.5 summarizes the twin-pair correlations for these disorders among males. (The results for females were similar.) For males from MZ and DZ pairs, risk for AD correlated 0.31 with that for MD. As was shown in Chapters 4 and 5, the MZ pair correlations for each disorder are about twice as great as those of DZ pairs (0.49 vs. 0.26 for AD, 0.31 vs. 0.11 for MD). The information relevant to understanding the sources of comorbidity comes from the cross-twin, cross-disorder correlations. For example, the correlation between MD in one twin and AD in the other is 0.20 in MZ pairs compared with 0.09 in DZs.

We applied our twin models to these data and obtained three major results. First, our findings were not consistent with the phenotypic causation model (Figure 11.4a). In general, it does not appear that alcoholism and

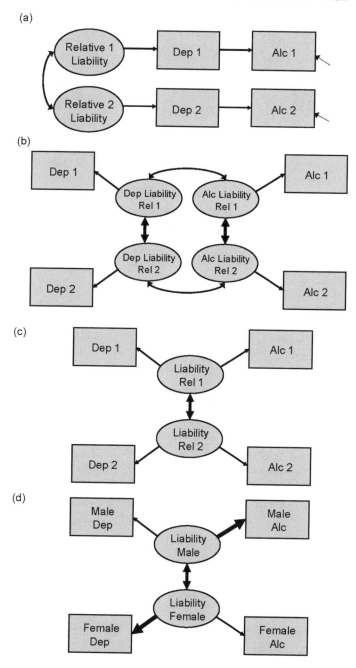

FIGURE 11.4. Predictions of alternative explanations for resemblance between relatives for alcoholism (alc) and depression (dep). (a) Phenotypic causation; (b) correlated liability; (c) alternate forms; (d) alternate forms—sex-dependent expression.

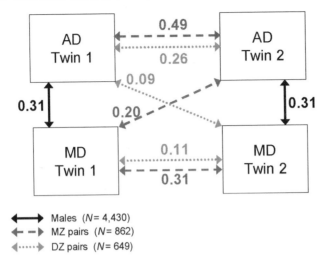

FIGURE 11.5. Twin-pair correlations for liability to alcohol dependence (AD) and major depression (MD) among male twin pairs. MZ = monozygotic; DZ = dyzygotic. Estimates are model based, so the cross-twin cross-disorder correlations are symmetric. For example, the MZ AD twin 1–MD twin 2 correlation is not shown but is also 0.20; the DZ MD twin 1–AD twin 2 correlation is also 0.09. Data from Prescott, Aggen, and Kendler (2000, Table 2).

depression co-occur largely because having one causes the other. Our second result was the finding that we could reject the alternate forms model (Figure 11.4c). Some of the familial liability to develop these disorders appears to be disorder specific.[3] By elimination, the most plausible model of those we tested was the correlated liability model (Figure 11.4b). The estimates indicate that all the familial liability is due to genetic factors. The genetic correlations for MD and AD were 0.52 for males and 0.39 for females. The individual-specific environment MD–AD correlations were 0.19 for males and 0.37 for females. This suggests that for females about half the risk for MD–AD comorbidity is due to genetic factors and about half to individual-specific factors. In contrast, for males the overlap between MD and AD is of about the same magnitude but due largely to genetic factors.

Our third major result was the finding that we could reject the hypothesis of sex-dependent expression. Liability to depression in females was not correlated with liability to alcoholism in males. Figure 11.6 portrays the correlations in opposite-sex twin pairs. The cross-sex MD–AD correlations did not differ from zero, providing no evidence for the depression-spectrum hypothesis. These results stand in clear contradiction to a common clinical dictum that a particular set of genetic and personality vulnerabilities, when occurring in a woman, will predispose to depression, whereas the same set of risk factors in a man will predispose to alcoholism. It is an appealing model—but probably wrong.

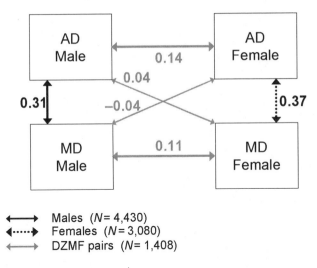

FIGURE 11.6. Twin-pair correlations for liability to alcohol dependence (AD) and major depression (MD) in opposite-sex twin pairs. Data from Prescott, Aggen, and Kendler (2000, Table 2).

Our results differ from some prior family studies of alcoholism and depression that have concluded in favor of the phenotypic causation model—that having depression causes alcoholism (Coryell, Winokur, Keller, Scheftner, & Endicott, 1992). There are several possible explanations for the differences among studies. One is the method of sample selection. Most of the studies producing these results have begun with depressed probands in treatment. As we discussed earlier, correlations between relatives can be biased if they are based on treatment rather than population samples. Another possibility is that different explanations may be correct in different families. It is plausible that there may be some families in which phenotypic causation is occurring, other families in which the shared liability model is correct, and still others in which the alternate forms model is acting. By chance or sampling, different studies reach different conclusions. Our statistical models and sample sizes do not allow us to detect such heterogeneity.

COMMON AND SPECIFIC RISK FACTORS FOR MULTIPLE DISORDERS

Now, let us take a large step up in complexity. When three or more disorders are examined, the modeling possibilities increase substantially. These *multivariate twin models* (*multi* meaning more than two) distinguish genetic and environmental risk factors that contribute to several disorders (i.e., common factors) from risk factors that contribute to one disorder only. These models, in essence, combine the power of the statistical technique of factor analysis with that of the twin design. Here we focus on one of the several plausible multivariate models, termed the *independent pathway model* (Kendler, Heath, Martin, & Eaves, 1987).

Common and Specific Influences on Phobia Subtypes

In Chapter 4, we examined the results of twin modeling for each of five phobia subtypes. As with most of the disorders we examined, our results suggested that the individual phobias were moderately influenced by genetic factors and that, except for social phobia, shared environment seemed to play only a small role. However, these analyses do not come close to exhausting the questions we can ask about the etiology of phobias. We can also examine how genetic and environmental factors contribute to the similarities and differences in risk for the individual phobia subtypes. The phobias are a set of syndromes all of which share a critical feature—an irrational, fearful avoidance of objects or situations that is inconsistent with the threat they truly pose. We might expect that the predisposition to develop a phobia is genetic but that the type of phobia one develops depends on one's individual-specific experiences. Thus cotwins might share a general predisposition to the development of phobias that is not specific to any particular subtype of phobia.

However, the phobia types differ in important ways. For situational, animal, and blood–injury phobias, the phobic stimulus is quite specific, whereas for social phobia and particularly agoraphobia the phobic stimuli are diffuse. Perhaps the three circumscribed phobias would share risk factors more closely among themselves than with the more diffuse phobia subtypes.

A second dimension that distinguishes phobia subtypes is physiological response. With typical phobias, exposure to the phobic stimuli produces increased sympathetic nervous system activity, manifested by symptoms such as rapid heartbeat, sweating, and flushing (Marks, 1988). By contrast, when individuals with blood–injury phobia are exposed to phobic stimuli (such as needles or the sight of blood), they usually experience increased parasympathetic nervous system activity, characterized by decreased pulse rate, lowered blood pressure, pallor, and sometimes fainting. Given these differences, we might expect the genetic and environmental risk factors for blood–injury phobia to be distinct from those of the other phobia subtypes.

We started by examining a model that included agoraphobia and social, animal, situational, and blood–injury phobias (see Sidebar 4.5). We used a three-level variable for each phobia type, consisting of *no fear, irrational fear*, and *fear with impairment*. Because we wanted to determine the degree to which these phobias share genetic and environmental risk factors, our model contained one set of common factors (for genes, shared environment, and individual-unique environment), as well as disorder-specific genetic and environmental factors. The first question we addressed was whether the pattern of phobia subtype overlap differs significantly in males and females. It did not, so we present results of the common factor model based on combining the male and female information. Figure 11.7 shows the variance percentages in each phobia attributable to each of the sources. For example, the common additive genetic factor (the A_c at the top of the figure) contributes to all of the phobias, but the proportions are largest for animal phobia (21%) and blood–injury phobia (22%) and weakest for agoraphobia (11%) and social phobia (5%).

The disorder-specific genetic factors (the A components in the lower part of the figure) account for 7–15% of the remaining variance in risk. This tells us that although the phobias are genetically related (they share the common A factor), they do not share all of their genetic risk. By comparing the proportions attributable to the common versus the disorder-specific genetic factors, we can determine the proportion of genetic risk shared with all other phobias versus that which is specific to a particular phobia type. For example, for situational phobia, the total heritability is 30%, half of which comes from genetic factors shared with all other phobias and half of which is unique to situational phobia. Blood–injury phobia has the highest proportion of genetic risk shared with other phobias (22% of the 29% heritability), and social phobia has the lowest (5% of the 17% heritability).

Overall, as we observed in the univariate analyses of phobias (Chapter 4), environmental experiences shared by siblings do not account for much of the

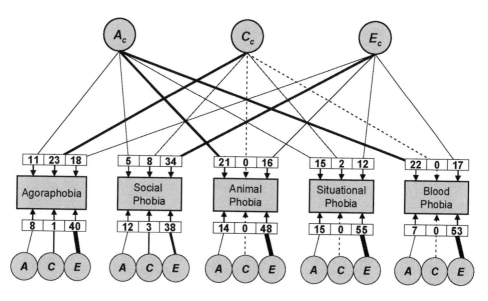

FIGURE 11.7. Estimated proportions of variance for phobia types from common and specific genetic and environmental factors. Estimates are variance %, model combined across MM and FF pairs. Values may not sum to 100 because of rounding; < 0.20 →; 0.20–0.39 →; 0.40+ ➡.

variation in risk for phobias. For three phobia subtypes (animal, situational, and blood–injury), the shared environmental variance is 2% or less. This means that the common shared environmental factor (Cc) is defined by agoraphobia and social phobia. It accounts for virtually all of the shared environmental variation in agoraphobia (23% of the total 24%) and most of that for social phobia (8% of the total 11%).

Finally, the common individual-specific environmental factor (Ec) contributes to all of the phobia types, with the highest proportion for social phobia (34%) and the lowest for situational phobia (12%). These results suggest the existence of a set of environmental experiences that are not shared with cotwins and that are nonspecifically "phobia-genic," affecting risk for all phobias. The disorder-specific individual-specific environmental effects are the largest in the model, ranging from 38 to 55%. These reflect environmental experiences that uniquely impact on risk for one phobia subtype only, as well as errors of measurement.

Stepping back from the welter of details, what are the broad take-home messages from this analysis? We suggest that there are four. First, individual phobias are caused by genetic and environmental risk factors shared with other phobia types, as well as risk factors unique to each type. So the results provide support both for the "lumpers" (those who consider the individual phobias to be just subtypes of one underlying disorder) and the "splitters" (those who view the individual phobias as largely independent disorders).

Second, social phobia and agoraphobia are somewhat different from the other, more "typical" phobias. They are less influenced by the genetic factor common to all subtypes and more influenced by the common environmental factors. To some extent, these results mirror the clinical differences between phobias with highly discrete versus more diffuse phobic stimuli.

Third, our results answer very clearly the question of whether blood–injury phobia is etiologically distinct from the other phobias. The answer is absolutely not! Indeed, blood–injury phobia has the *highest* loading on the common genetic factor. At least with respect to genetic risk, it is the most "typical" of the phobias.

Fourth, the multivariate analyses provided stronger evidence than did our univariate results in Chapter 4 that shared environment is really of importance (at least for social phobia and agoraphobia). In this respect, our results for phobias differ from those found for the other internalizing disorders of MD, GAD, and panic disorder.

What do prior studies tell us about the relationship between the genetic and environmental risk factors for the different subtypes of phobias? Age at onset (Marks, 1987; Ost, 1987) and patterns of comorbidity (Boyd et al., 1984; Schapira, Kerr, & Roth, 1970) suggest that there are meaningful differences among phobic subtypes. Family studies of phobia have found some evidence for the specificity of familial factors for individual phobic subtypes (Fyer et al., 1990; Noyes et al., 1986). In the only study to date that used multivariate genetic analysis, Phillips and colleagues (1987), in a twin-family design, examined seven categories of fears as assessed by self-report. Like ours, this study found evidence for a single genetic factor common to all categories of fears plus genetic factors specific to each fear.

Our results can be usefully compared with a recent study from Norway that examined responses to an extensive questionnaire about irrational fears given to nearly 800 twins and their families (Sundet, Skre, Okkenhaug, & Tambs, 2003). In examining the individual fears, the authors were able to extract four dimensions, which could be easily identified as situational, social/agoraphobia, animal, and illness–injury. Standard univariate analyses showed heritability estimates for these four dimensions of irrational fear that ranged from 22 to 47%, results broadly similar to our own findings. No evidence was found for an effect of shared environmental factors, however, a result that differs from that found in VATSPSUD. The authors then proceeded to fit a multivariate model and, again broadly consistent with our own results, found evidence for a broad genetic liability to all irrational fears, as well as evidence that genetic factors impact on each of the specific dimensions.

Common and Specific Influences on Substance Use Disorders

In the second set of multivariate analyses we present here, we examined a critical question in the etiology of substance use disorders: the extent to which genetic and environmental risk factors are substance-specific versus nonspecific in their effects. We included only the MM twin pairs in these analyses[4] and considered whether the twins had experienced abuse of and/or dependence on six classes of illicit psychoactive substances: cannabis, sedatives, stimulants, cocaine, opiates, and hallucinogens (Kendler, Jacobson, Prescott, & Neale, 2003d). The results of the best-fit model are shown in Figure 11.8. We focus here on the pattern of genetic risk factors. Consistent with the univariate results presented in Chapter 5, abuse of/dependence on all of the classes of illicit substances (with one exception) is highly heritable, with the estimates of heritability from the multivariate model ranging from 52% for sedatives to 74% for cannabis. The exception to this pattern is opiate abuse/dependence, for which heritability was estimated at 23%. Most notably, we found *no evidence* for substance-specific genetic effects. Rather, all of the genetic risk for the abuse of/dependence on these substances was due to one set of common genetic risk factors.

If true, these results tell us something important about the nature of the genetic vulnerability to illicit psychoactive substance abuse (Uhl, Liu, Walther, Hess, & Naiman, 2001). Interindividual differences in this vulnerability appear to be due to genetic factors, which increase or decrease risk for the abuse of *all* classes of illicit substances. Genetic variation in biological systems

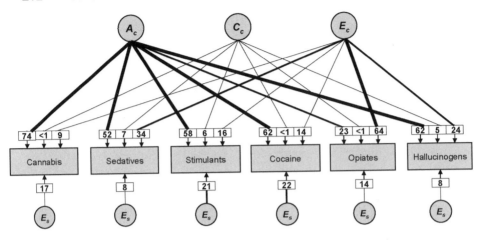

FIGURE 11.8. Estimated proportions of variance for illicit substance use disorders from common and specific genetic and environmental factors indicated, respectively, by the subscripts *c* and *s*. Estimates are variance % based on MM pairs. Values may not sum to 100 because of rounding; < 0.20→; 0.20–0.39 →; 0.40+ ➤. Adapted from Kendler, Jacobson, Prescott, and Neale (2003d, Figure 1). Copyright 2003 by the American Psychiatric Association. Adapted by permission.

that affects the action of only one or a small number of substance classes (e.g., specific variation in the receptor sites for individual drugs such as cannabis, cocaine, or sedatives) does not appear to be an important source of individual variation in vulnerability.

How do these results compare with those from other studies? Two twin studies and two large family studies have examined the specificity of familial/ genetic risk factors for drug abuse. Both twin studies (Karkowski, Prescott, & Kendler, 2000; Tsuang et al., 1998) and one of the two family studies (Merikangas et al., 1998), but not the other (Bierut et al., 1998), have produced results broadly congruent with our findings.

Where might these nonspecific genetic effects operate? We tentatively suggest two mechanisms, which are not mutually exclusive. First is a process that might be mediated through psychological traits. As we see later in this chapter, genetic variation in personality or in the liability to externalizing disorders may influence risk for the use and abuse of psychoactive compounds (Loeber, 1988; Zuckerman, 1972). Given this vulnerability, which class of substance is abused might be determined by opportunity or by chance. The second mechanism has a more direct physiological basis. There is substantial evidence that the pleasurable effects of most or all drugs of abuse (as well as other enjoyable experiences, such as eating and sex) are mediated by a common biological mechanism (Koob & Le Moal, 1997). Perhaps variation in those "hedonic" systems underlies the liability to abuse psychoactive substances.[5]

Multivariate Analyses of Psychiatric and Substance Use Disorders

In the final set of multivariate analyses that we present in this chapter, we sought to clarify the underlying structure of genetic and environmental risk factors for the common psychiatric and substance use disorders in men and in women (Kendler, Prescott, Myers, & Neale, 2003e). Because of practical limitations associated with analyzing many disorders simultaneously, we selected seven disorders: MD, GAD, any phobia, AD, drug abuse/dependence, AASB, and CD. These represent a broad range of conditions that are approximately balanced between *internalizing* and *externalizing* disorders.[6] We used information from more than 5,600 individuals from MM and FF twin pairs.

The first question we asked was whether the pattern of the resemblance within and between these disorders was the same in men and women. Men have higher rates of externalizing disorders and women higher rates of internalizing conditions, but the patterns of comorbidity were essentially the same in the two sexes. The rest of the results are based on combining the information from males and females.

Figure 11.9 shows the result of the "full" or unsimplified model, which we set up to have two genetic common risk factors, two shared environmental common factors, and two unique environmental common factors, as well as genetic and environmental factors specific to each disorder.[7] The structure of the genetic risk factors for these seven disorders is especially interesting. One genetic common factor (shown on the left side of Figure 11.9a) had high loadings on all three internalizing disorders. By contrast, a second genetic common factor (shown on the right side of Figure 11.9a) had high loadings on all four externalizing disorders. In addition, the two substance use disorders—AD and drug abuse/dependence—had substantial disorder-specific genetic loadings.

As shown in Figure 11.9b, the first shared environmental common factor had quite modest loadings on phobia and CD. The second shared environmental common factor had a substantial loading only on CD and a modest loading on AASB. All the shared environmental disorder-specific loadings were quite small.

The first common individual-specific factor had substantial loadings on MD, GAD, and AD, whereas the second factor had substantial loadings on only AASB and CD (Figure 11.9c). All of the disorder-specific unique environmental proportions, which include measurement error, were substantial.

What does all of this mean? These results suggest the existence of four major groups of genetic risk factors for these common psychiatric and substance use disorders. The first is a set of genes that predispose strongly to *all* externalizing disorders (and have little impact on risk for internalizing disorders). The second is a set of genes that predispose to *all* internalizing disorders (and influence only slightly the risk for externalizing disorders). The third and fourth sets of genes are more specific in their effect and have impact solely on the risk for AD and drug abuse/dependence, respectively. It is tempting to

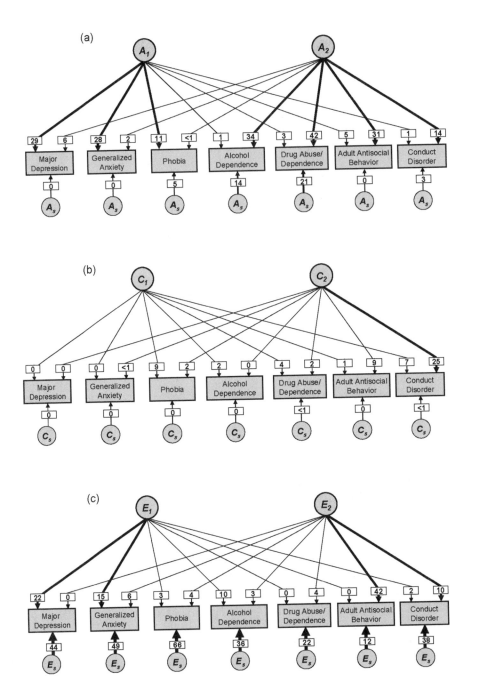

FIGURE 11.9. Estimated proportions of common and specific variance for psychiatric and substance use disorders. (a) Genetic sources of variance; estimates are variance %, model combined across MM and FF pairs; (b) sources of shared environmental variance; (c) sources of individual-specific environmental variance. Values may not sum to 100 because of rounding. Bold lines indicate > 10%. Data from Kendler, Prescott, Myers, and Neale (2003e, Table 2).

speculate that at least some of these disorder-specific genetic factors reflect genetic differences in the metabolism, end-organ responsiveness, and liability to the pleasurable versus noxious effects of psychoactive substances (e.g., Lyons et al., 1997; Thomasson et al., 1991).

Within the power of these methods, we were unable to find genetic factors that specifically influence the risk for MD, GAD, phobias, CD, or AASB. From a genetic perspective, these results permit us to reject two plausible hypotheses about the way in which psychiatric diagnostic categories "map" onto genetic risk factors. We can reject the "high specificity" hypothesis, which suggests that "DSM-IV got it right" in that each major disorder has specific genetic risk factors. We can also reject the "complete nonspecificity" hypothesis, which predicts only one global set of genetic risk factors for all disorders. Thus our findings are inconsistent with unitary etiological models for psychiatric disorders (Menninger, Ellenberger, Pruyser, & Mayman, 1958) and with viewpoints suggesting that psychiatric diagnoses are entirely arbitrary, man-made categories imposed on a single dimension of psychiatric or psychological dysfunction.

Our more textured results suggest that there are at least two broad dimensions of genetic risk factors for these common conditions, with the addition of specific sets of genes that predispose to alcohol and substance use disorders.

Consistent with the results from the univariate analyses described in Chapter 5, shared environment was not a potent contributor to risk for any of the externalizing disorders with the notable exception of CD. Clearly, some aspects of experiences shared by twins, such as the home environment or peer and community influences, are etiologically important for CD.

Interestingly, two meaningful unique environmental common factors were seen. However, the structure of these factors differed from the genetic risk factors in two important ways. First, AD loaded with MD and GAD, not with the other externalizing disorders. Second, CD and AASB loaded together without the substance use disorders.

These results demonstrate what we suspect is an important general principle for psychiatric disorders: *the patterns of comorbidity due to the effects of genetic and the effects of environmental risk factors often differ.* This means that the "phenotypic" patterns of comorbidity that we observe in clinical or epidemiological samples are really a sum of distinct patterns of comorbidity caused by both genetic and environmental risk factors. These findings have one final important implication. The overall tendency of common psychiatric disorders to sort themselves into two broad groups of internalizing and externalizing disorders (as has been seen in a number of recent analyses; see Krueger, 1999; Krueger, Caspi, Moffitt, & Silva, 1998) *is due to the effects of genetic and not environmental risk factors.*

In follow-up analyses, we explored the structure of genetic and environmental risk factors for the internalizing disorders. These results—consistent with results from epidemiological samples (Krueger, 1999)—suggest that the genetic risk factors for internalizing disorders can be further divided into those that predispose to chronic dysphoric conditions (e.g., "misery") and those that predispose to more acute anxiety disorders (e.g., "fear").

It is important to recognize that these results do not apply to all psychiatric conditions. Other studies suggest that genetic risk factors for schizophrenic illness are independent of the genetic factors identified here. We have not considered a host of other, less common, psychiatric disorders, including anorexia nervosa, obsessive–compulsive disorder, autism, and other developmental disorders.

RISK INDICATORS

Another way in which we apply data from twins to help us understand how genetic factors influence risk is by studying *risk indicators*. Risk indicators are quantitative traits that reflect the vulnerability to psychiatric and substance use disorders. Such traits are useful because they allow risk to be measured on a continuous scale (rather than the yes/no measurement of clinical diagnosis). They can also indicate vulnerability to a disorder in people even before the onset of illness or in those who may never develop the disorder.

In the rest of this chapter we examine three variables that have been proposed as risk indicators for different forms of psychopathology. These are: the personality trait of novelty seeking and cannabis use/abuse, drinking motives and alcoholism, and neuroticism and MD. Each example employs a somewhat different approach to studying risk.

Figure 11.10 displays a bivariate twin model that can be used to study risk indicators. This is similar (in fact, mathematically identical) to the bivariate model described previously (Figure 11.1). But here, rather than estimating two sets of paths and the correlations between the genetic and environmental factors, we estimate three sets of paths. The genetic and environ-

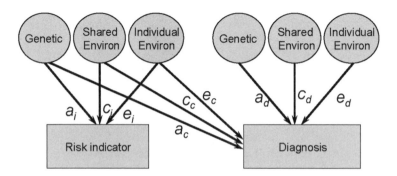

FIGURE 11.10. Twin model for correlated risk. Subscript i indicates factors influencing the indicator; d indicates influences on diagnosis from the diagnosis-specific factors; c indicates influences on the covariance between diagnosis and the risk indicator.

mental factors on the left side of the figure influence both the risk indicator and the outcome (e.g., clinical diagnosis). The second set of A, C, and E factors influence only diagnosis. By summing the two genetic contributions to diagnosis, we obtain the estimated heritability. But, more important, we can estimate what portion of the variation in liability to diagnosis is shared with the risk indicator and whether that variation is due to genetic or environmental sources. We illustrate the usefulness of this approach with an example.

Novelty Seeking as an Indicator of Risk for Cannabis Use and Abuse

We noted earlier that one possible explanation for the pattern of findings with illicit psychoactive drugs (that genetic factors are of substantial etiological importance but appear nonspecific in their effects) is that genes might act on substance use and abuse through genetic influences on personality traits. We used the risk indicator model to study the relationship between personality and the use and abuse of several drug classes in males and females (Agrawal, Jacobson, Prescott, & Kendler, 2004).

Here we present the results for males and cannabis, by far the most commonly used illicit drug. The personality trait we investigated was *novelty seeking* (see Sidebar 11.2). A substantial body of prior research suggests that individuals who score high on this trait (Fergusson & Horwood, 2000) or the closely related trait of *sensation seeking* (Zuckerman, 1972) are at increased risk for problem use of substances.

Figure 11.11a shows the results for cannabis use in males. The genetic factor contributing to novelty seeking and cannabis use accounts for 17% of the variance in novelty seeking and 18% of the variance in cannabis use. In contrast, the genetic factor specific to cannabis use contributes only 5% of the variance.[8] What is interesting about these results is that the shared genetic path to cannabis use is much larger than the specific genetic path. Over 70% (18/23) of the genetic liability for cannabis use is shared with novelty seeking. Shared and unique environmental factors account for little of the overlap between novelty seeking and cannabis use. These results suggest that the level of novelty seeking is a good index of the genetic risk for cannabis use among males.

The pattern of genetic results for cannabis abuse/dependence is different (Figure 11.11b). Here the path from the unique genetic factor is larger than that from the shared genetic factor. Of the total genetic effect on cannabis abuse/dependence in males, only about 26% (20/76) is shared with novelty seeking. Novelty seeking is not nearly as good at predicting genetic risk for developing problems with cannabis as it is at predicting genetic risk for cannabis use.

Interestingly, our analyses based on female twins indicate that novelty seeking is not nearly so good at indexing genetic risk for cannabis use in females as it is in males. Nor was it good at indexing genetic risk for the use of sedatives or hallucinogens.

SIDEBAR 11.2. Personality

Personality is typically defined as the totality of an individual's attitudes, behavioral patterns, and emotional responses that are generally stable over long periods of time. A huge amount of research has gone into defining and studying the major dimensions of personality. Many studies have also tried to understand the nature of the relationship between personality and risk for psychiatric and substance use disorders. In the VATSPSUD, we assessed three major dimensions of personality, two of which we examine in this book: novelty seeking and neuroticism. (The third is extroversion, which turned out not to be substantially associated with most forms of psychopathology in our sample.)

Novelty seeking (NS) assesses an individual's tendency to be impulsive and to seek out thrills and excitement. The 23 items that we used come from an early version of the Temperament and Character Inventory developed by the psychiatrist Robert Cloninger (Cloninger, Przybeck, Svrakic, & Wetzel, 1994). Some sample items used in our study include:

"Are you the type of person . . .
    who likes to think about things for a long time before you make a decision?
    who, when nothing new is happening, usually starts looking for something that is thrilling and exciting?
    who likes to stay at home better than to travel or explore new places?
    who often tries new things just for the fun or thrills, even if most people think it is a waste of time?"

As the reader might gather, in computing a score for NS, the answers to the first and third questions would be counted negatively, whereas the answers to the second and fourth questions would be counted positively. The personality dimension of novelty seeking is closely related to the trait of sensation seeking as articulated by the well-known psychologist Marvin Zuckerman (1994).

Neuroticism (N) is a personality dimension first conceptualized by the famous English psychologist Hans Eysenck (Eysenck & Eysenck, 1975). The term is now a bit dated, as "neurosis" is no longer commonly used in the mental health field. A more accurate term would be "emotional instability." What this dimension of personality assesses is a tendency to experience negative affect—mostly anxiety, sadness, or irritability. Here are some sample items used in our study:

"Are you the type of person . . .
    whose mood often goes up and down?
    who is irritable?
    whose feelings are easily hurt?
    who is a worrier?

Individuals who score low on neuroticism tend to be even-tempered, emotionally stable, and hard to upset. We assessed neuroticism by using the 12 yes/no items taken from the short form of the revised version of the Eysenck Personality Questionnaire (EPQ; Eysenck, Eysenck, & Barrett, 1985).

Recent years have seen much interest in the five-factor model for human personality (John, 1990). Neuroticism or a closely related trait appears in virtually all of the major five-factor models of human personality. A factor such as NS is also included in most of these models, although frequently the scale is named for the inverse of NS, for example, "conscientiousness."

218

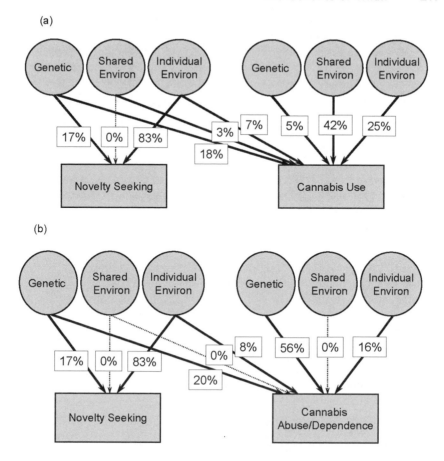

FIGURE 11.11. Results from bivariate twin model for overlap of novelty seeking and cannabis involvement among males. (a) Cannabis use; (b) cannabis abuse/dependence. Data from Agrawal, Jacobson, Prescott, and Kendler (2004, Table 1).

Mediators of Risk

A special case of risk indicators is *mediators*. These variables index risk because they sit in the causal pathway between basic genetic and environmental risk factors and the disorder. For example, excessive weight is a risk indicator for coronary artery disease. It is probably not a direct cause, but it indexes other causal variables (e.g., high-fat diet, lack of exercise, and hypertension). In contrast, high cholesterol levels could be considered a mediator of coronary artery disease because cholesterol is directly involved in the etiological pathway leading to blockages (technically atherosclerosis) in arteries in the body.

In cross-sectional observational studies of individuals, it is not possible to identify which risk indicators function as mediators. Doing so usually requires longitudinal or experimental studies. However, data from twins can help us

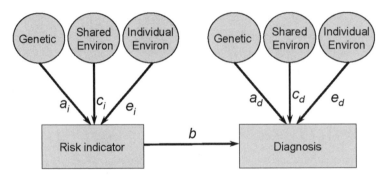

FIGURE 11.12. Twin model for mediated risk. The subscripts *i* and *d* stand for, respectively, indicator and diagnosis.

address this important issue. Figure 11.12 shows our twin model for studying mediators. Here the model, the association between the risk indicator and the outcome, is conceptualized as occurring *through* (or mediated by) the risk indicator (via path *b*). Mathematically this means that the genetic and environmental covariances (a_c, c_c, and e_c in Figure 11.10) are in the same proportions as the genetic and environmental influences on the risk indicator (a_i, c_i, and e_i).[9] If this is not consistent with the data, we can conclude that the variable is not a mediator. The results of the previous example are not consistent with novelty seeking being a mediator of risk for cannabis use. The proportions of the genetic and environmental covariance (18:3:7) are very different from the relative proportions for the variation in novelty seeking (17:0:83).

The difference between the basic risk indicator model (Figure 11.10) and the mediator model reflects another form of the old correlation versus causation question. Risk indicators are correlated with but do not appear to be a direct cause of the disorder. Mediators, by contrast, provide more evidence about causal relationships. Although the mediation model cannot prove causality, if it fits the observed data, then it is consistent with a causal relationship. If we can reject the mediation model, this suggests that the genetic and environmental causes of the index and outcomes are correlated but probably not causal.

Drinking Motivations as Mediators versus Indicators of Risk for Alcoholism

One proposed mediator variable for alcoholism is motivation for drinking. Some people use alcohol to help them deal with feelings of depression, anxiety, or stress, whereas others drink to enhance their comfort with and enjoyment of social situations. Longitudinal studies have found that people who have positive expectations about the effects of alcohol are more prone to develop drinking problems (Christiansen, Smith, Roehling, & Goldman,

1989). Not surprisingly, people who expect negative consequences from drinking, such as feeling sick, dizzy, or tired, are less likely to have problems with drinking. Thus the reasons people do or do not drink may have a direct impact on (or mediate) their risk for developing alcoholism.

Initially we might think that drinking motives should arise from individual-specific experiences with drinking. However, there is evidence that alcohol expectations run in families. Several studies have found that adolescents with an alcoholic parent tend to have more positive expectations about alcohol than adolescents whose parents do not have drinking problems. Two studies found that twins were correlated for their drinking expectations, although the studies differed on whether this was attributed to genetic or shared environmental factors (Slutske et al., 2002a; Viken, Johnson, Kaprio, & Rose, 2002).

We put these different pieces together in one analysis to test a mediational model for drinking motivations. We wanted to see whether motives for drinking provide a partial explanation of how risk for alcoholism is transmitted in families (Prescott, Cross, Kuhn, Horn, & Kendler, 2004). This transmission could come through genetic mechanisms (e.g., physiological differences among individuals in the degree to which they experience alcohol as pleasurable) or environmental paths (e.g., young adults modeling the drinking behavior of their parents).

As part of our MF2 and FF4 studies, we included scales from the Alcohol Use Inventory (AUI; Horn, Wanberg, & Foster, 1987; see Sidebar 11.3) to assess four motives for drinking: to manage mood (abbreviated below as

---

SIDEBAR 11.3. Assessment of Drinking Motives

As part of the questionnaires associated with our MF2 and FF4 studies, we included four scales from the Alcohol Use Inventory (AUI; Horn, Wanberg, & Foster, 1987). The AUI is a set of 16 factor analytically derived self-report scales developed in alcoholism treatment settings to characterize drinking styles. We selected four scales that seemed relevant to a general population sample. The Mood Management scale (MOOD) includes 7 items assessing drinking to unwind, to forget, to relieve tension, or to overcome depression. The Social Interaction/Gregarious scale (GREGAR) includes 9 items on whether a respondent's social life requires drinking, peer drinking, and drinking with others. The Social Anxiety scale (SOCANX) includes 9 items assessing drinking to feel more important, to overcome shyness, to make friends, or to meet people. The Mental scale (MENT) includes 5 items on drinking to be more mentally alert, to have better ideas, or to reach higher goals.

Scale scores were calculated by summing the number of yes responses and dividing by the number of items. This produced an average score in a metric that is comparable across scales. Test–retest correlations, based on 256 participants who were randomly selected for a reliability interview and who completed the AUI twice within 10 weeks, were: MOOD, $r = 0.85$; SOCANX, $r = 0.73$; GREGAR, $r = 0.77$; and MENT, $r = 0.69$. The scales were not administered to individuals who reported being lifetime abstainers because the items assume drinking experience.

Mood), to relieve social anxiety (SocAnx), to enhance social interaction and gregariousness (Gregar), and to improve mental functioning (Ment). These scales were completed by 2,545 female and 3,729 male drinkers, including 2,240 complete twin pairs. The first part of our analysis was to see if these drinking motives were associated with alcoholism in our sample. As shown in Figure 11.13, men and women who met criteria for a lifetime diagnosis of DSM-IV alcohol abuse or dependence (AAD) tended to have higher scores on each of the four drinking motives than did drinkers without AAD.

We tested both the risk indicator (Figure 11.10) and mediation (Figure 11.12) models as alternative explanations for the association between drinking motives and alcoholism. We found that the motives most strongly associated with alcoholism were drinking to manage mood and drinking to relieve social anxiety (Figure 11.13). However, the results from the twin models suggest that quite different processes underlie the associations of these two motives with alcoholism.

For SocAnx, the mediational model fit best. As shown in Figure 11.14a, 29% of the variation in AAD among females was shared with SocAnx, and about half of this was due to genetic factors. For males, about 21% of the variation in AAD was shared with SocAnx, including 6% attributed to genetic factors (Figure 11.14b).

In contrast, the mediational model was rejected for the Mood scale in favor of the risk indicator model. Mood was strongly associated with AAD but did not appear to be mediating alcoholism risk. The proportion of AAD risk shared with Mood was 31% for females and 35% for males, and the

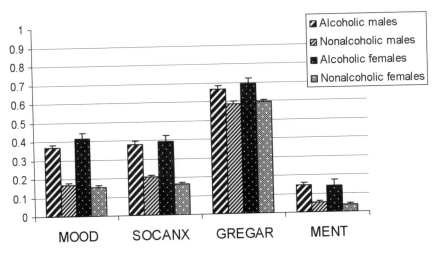

FIGURE 11.13. Association between drinking motives and lifetime diagnosis of alcohol abuse/dependence. See Sidebar 11.3 for an explanation of drinking motive scales. Adapted from Prescott, Cross, Kuhn, Horn, and Kendler (2004, Figure 3). Copyright 2004 by the Research Society on Alcoholism. Adapted by permission.

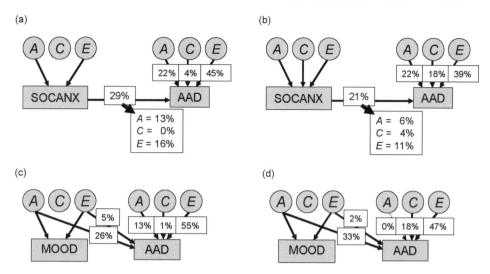

FIGURE 11.14. Results from twin models for drinking motives and alcoholism. (a) AUI SOCANX for females; (b) AUI SOCANX for males; (c) AUI MOOD for females; (d) AUI MOOD for males. See Sidebar 11.3 for an explanation of drinking motive scales. Adapted from Prescott, Cross, Kuhn, Horn, and Kendler (2004, Figure 4). Copyright 2004 by the Research Society on Alcoholism. Adapted by permission.

large majority of this was attributed to genetic factors contributing to both Mood and AAD (Figures 11.14c and 11.14d). These results suggest that there may be other factors, which are strongly genetically influenced, that contribute both to risk for alcoholism and to the need to manage dysphoric mood.

These results are provocative, but we should mention some limitations of this study. The analyses were cross-sectional (we measured motives at the same time as or after we assessed drinking problems), and we included individuals with a range of drinking experiences. Ideally, we would like to measure motives longitudinally to see whether they change in response to drinking experience. A study of drinking motives among adolescent twins suggests that MZ and DZ pairs are about equally similar in their expectations about the positive effects of alcohol before they begin drinking but that after they have had experience with alcohol, DZ pairs become less similar (Slutske et al., 2002b). That is, before adolescents use alcohol, their expectations about its effects are based on learning (e.g., from parents, peers, the media). Thus MZ and DZ pairs are expected to be correlated for drinking expectancies to a similar degree. But after the experience of drinking, genetic differences in alcohol response are expressed and influence subsequent expectations about the effects of alcohol.

If the results of our study are replicated, particularly by longitudinal studies of twins, they have implications for the prevention of problem drinking.

Although drinking to manage mood does not seem to be causally associated with risk for alcoholism, a high score on this scale is a good risk indicator for alcohol problems. Drinking to alleviate social anxiety appears to be a partial mediator of alcoholism risk. High scores on this measure could be used to identify at-risk individuals and to provide them with other strategies for coping with their social fears before they develop drinking problems.

Neuroticism as an Indicator or Mediator of Risk for Depression

Our third example again looks at personality and psychopathology, but this time we studied the relationship between the personality dimension of neuroticism and MD. Neuroticism measures the predisposition to negative emotions such as worry, anxiety, and depression (Eysenck & Eysenck, 1964; see Sidebar 11.2). A large literature (see Fanous, Gardner, Prescott, Cancro, & Kendler, 2002; Kendler et al., 1993b) suggests that: (1) individuals with MD tend to have higher levels of neuroticism than those without MD; (2) individuals with a history of MD but who are not currently depressed also tend to have higher levels of neuroticism (although not generally as high as those who are currently depressed); (3) individuals with a history of MD tend to have higher levels of neuroticism when in an episode of MD than when in remission; and (4) among individuals without prior MD, higher neuroticism strongly predicts future risk for MD.

As with the analyses of novelty seeking and cannabis use and abuse, we wanted to know how much of the genetic contribution to MD was shared with neuroticism and how much was specific to MD. However, our repeated measurements of MD and neuroticism allowed us to ask some additional questions about the nature of the relationship between them. First, does neuroticism mediate the impact of genetic and environmental factors on risk for MD, or is neuroticism better understood as an index of one or more of these risk factors? Second, to what extent is neuroticism a risk factor or mediator for MD versus just an indicator of a recent depressive episode? That is, are elevated levels of neuroticism associated with MD because neuroticism reflects an enduring trait that is associated with vulnerability to depressive episodes, or could neuroticism be associated with MD because being in (or just having recovered from) an episode of depression causes a transient elevation in neuroticism?

These analyses were based on female twin pairs who participated in the wave 1 interview. The model we used for these analyses is depicted in Figure 11.15a. It includes neuroticism assessed at time 1 and time 2 (the original questionnaire and the wave 1 interview) and past-year episodes of MD (i.e., occurring between these two times of measurement). As with the model in Figure 11.10, there are genetic and environmental factors that are shared among all the outcomes and factors that are specific to each outcome.[10] The contributions from the common factors are set to be equal for time 1 and time 2 neu-

(a)

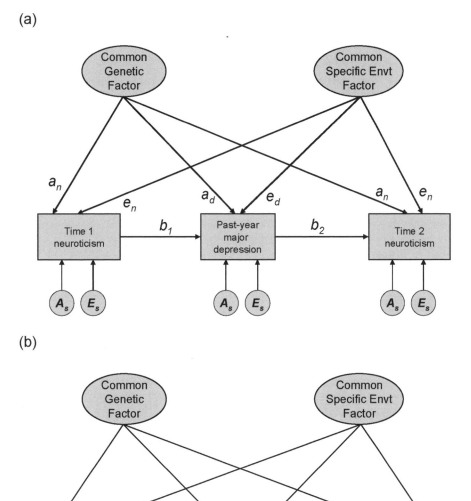

(b)

FIGURE 11.15. Model for the association between neuroticism and major depression over time (one twin shown). (a) Full model; (b) results from best-fitting model. Adapted from Kendler, Neale, Kessler, Heath, and Eaves (1993b, Figure 2). Copyright 1993 by the American Medical Association. Adapted by permission.

roticism. A new feature of this model is the inclusion of paths between neurot-icism and MD. This version of the mediation model differs somewhat from the one used in the drinking motivations example (Figure 11.12). Here the b_1 path includes the proportion of the covariance between neuroticism and MD that could be considered mediated. This more complex version of the model is possible because we have multiple assessments of neuroticism. A significant estimate of b_1 would be consistent with the hypothesis that genetic and envi-ronmental risk for depressive episodes is mediated in part by neuroticism. The b_2 path tests whether risk for a recent episode of MD is more closely associ-ated with future neuroticism (as measured at time 2) than with neuroticism measured earlier. A significant b_2 path would be consistent with the hypothe-sis that experiencing MD alters neuroticism (rather than the reverse).

The results from the best-fitting model are depicted in Figure 11.15b. There are three important results. First, the major reason that neuroticism is closely related to liability to MD is that a set of genetic risk factors influences both traits. Of the total variation in past-year MD shared with neuroticism (29%), the large majority (26/29) is due to overlapping genetic factors. Put another way, of the total genetic influence on past-year MD (46%), over half arises from the genetic factor that also contributes to neuroticism.

The second result is that, in contrast to the genetic results, the environ-mental influences on neuroticism and past-year MD are only slightly related. Of the total environmental contribution to the liability to MD (54%), approx-imately 95% (51/54) is unique to MD and only 5% is shared with neuroti-cism.

Perhaps most interesting are the results concerning the b paths. The b_1 path was not significantly different from zero. This is inconsistent with the mediational model. That is, a genetic factor influences both neuroticism and MD, but the genetic risk for MD does not "run through" neuroticism itself. Thus neuroticism is a risk indicator for MD, not a mediator. Also of note, the estimate for the b_2 path was small but significant, accounting for 4% of the variation in time 2 neuroticism. This suggests that neuroticism is influenced to a small extent by the recent occurrence of an MD episode.

SUMMARY

In the first part of this chapter, we examined a range of multivariate twin models. Starting with two disorders at a time, we showed how such studies could partition the sources of comorbidity between two disorders into the portions due to genetic, shared environmental, and unique environmental influences. We found that MD and GAD shared nearly all of their genetic risk factors, whereas the genetic relationship between MD and social phobia was quite modest. We found that MD and alcoholism shared a moderate propor-tion of their genetic risk factors, and we were able to reject a model of phenotypic causation in which the comorbidity arose from MD directly leading to alcoholism. Contrary to clinical wisdom, we also found no evidence that our alternate forms model explained the pattern of family resemblance for depression and alcoholism in men and women.

By analyzing multiple disorders at a time, we were able to study the common and specific genetic and environmental influences across disorders. We examined the pattern of genetic and environmental contributions to the subtypes of phobias, to abuse of/dependence on different illicit substances, and to seven common psychiatric and substance use disorders. The findings were diverse. For example, for the six classes of psychoactive substances, genetic factors appeared to be entirely nonspecific in their effect. By contrast, for phobia subtypes, we found a mixture of nonspecific and specific genetic effects.

Finally, we examined models that included risk indicators, variables more "basic" than the disorders themselves. These could function either as indicators of genetic or environmental risk for the disorder or as variables that mediate genetic or environmental influences. We showed that the personality trait of novelty seeking is a good risk indicator for genetic liability to cannabis use in males. The relationship between drinking motives and alcoholism appears to be complex. A risk-indicator model fit best for drinking to manage moods, whereas a mediational model provided the best explanation for drinking to relieve social anxiety. Neuroticism is a good index of genetic risk for MD in females but does not appear to directly mediate genetic risk.

We hope this chapter illustrates the richness of this more complex twin modeling. The use of these approaches allows us to ask questions of real clinical importance in a conceptually (and statistically) rigorous manner. These models are more difficult but ultimately more useful and informative about the nature of psychiatric and substance use disorders than are the simpler twin models that merely estimate genetic and environmental proportions of variance.

NOTES

1. Many other models for comorbidity are possible (see Neale & Kendler, 1995).

2. The results are based on 4,430 males and 3,080 females who participated in the fourth wave of interviews with FF twin pairs or first wave of interviews with MM and MF pairs. We used several definitions of alcoholism and depression, and all the results were similar to those reported here. This work appeared originally in Prescott et al. (2000).

3. This is indicated by the fact that the MZ pair correlations within disorders (0.49 and 0.31) are greater than the correlation across disorders (0.20).

4. The prevalences of several forms of substance abuse/dependence in the females, particularly opiates, were too low to permit analysis of these substances.

5. We do not mean to imply that all psychoactive substances share a common set of genetic risk factors. Indeed, our previous multivariate analysis suggested that alcohol and illicit drugs in part have independent genetic risk factors. Other pre-

liminary results we have obtained suggest that the genetic liability to become dependent on nicotine or caffeine (the two other legal forms of psychoactive substances) is also at least partly independent of the genetic risk factors for illicit substance abuse.

6. See Chapters 4 and 5 for descriptions of diagnostic definitions of these disorders.

7. Usually we report results of the "best-fitting" model. However, in this case, the modeling process was quite complex because the number of alternative models was so large and because the best-fit model did not provide more insight into the underlying processes than the full model. We selected a model with two common factors for each of the three components because with only seven disorders we could not reliably estimate models with more complex structure.

8. The total genetic effect on novelty seeking in our sample is rather modest and smaller than is typically seen for novelty seeking and other personality traits, in which heritabilities are usually in the range of 30–45% (Loehlin, 1992). We suspect that this is just a result of sampling fluctuation. In any event, our focus here is on sources of variance in drug use and abuse/dependence: the one shared with novelty seeking and the other independent of novelty seeking.

9. The covariance is assumed to be measured without error. We separated individual-specific covariance from Alcohol Use Inventory (AUI) scale measurement error by using an estimate of error based on short-term test–retest reliability.

10. For simplicity of presentation, we have omitted the shared environmental factors from the figures. They did not contribute either to neuroticism or MD risk.

CHAPTER TWELVE

Three Extensions of the Twin Model

In this chapter we present three extensions of the twin model that address some limitations of standard analyses of data from twin pairs. These extensions include studying multistage conditional processes (in which individuals must develop one trait to become susceptible to another), understanding the transmission of disease risk between parents and offspring, and allowing for unreliability or error in our assessment of disorders.

GENETIC INFLUENCES ON CONDITIONAL PROCESSES

Our initial approach to studying genetic and environmental influences on substance use disorders, presented in Chapter 5, was to treat these conditions just as we treat psychiatric disorders such as MD and phobias. That is, we divided the population into two categories: those who have had the disorder and those who have not. However, as we noted, substance use disorders differ from psychiatric disorders in a simple but fundamental way: *to develop drug abuse, you first need to use drugs.*

Therefore, for substance use disorders we needed to consider the following three categories: (1) those who have never used (or, more technically, "initiated") the substance, (2) those who initiated use but did not develop a disorder, and (3) those who initiated use and subsequently developed a substance use disorder. The standard method for analyzing substance use disorders as presented in Chapter 5 has the limitation of combining categories 1 and 2 into one group, which we called "unaffected." Although we were right to conclude that the average liability to drug abuse for an individual in category 2 is low, the liability to drug abuse for individuals in category 1 is really unknown. It could be low. It could be high.

How can we best study this kind of situation? First, there is a *contingent* element that cannot be ignored: One must try a drug in order to abuse it. Second, we must consider the relationship between the genetic and environmental factors that contribute to drug initiation and those that influence the progression to abuse. Finally, at a more technical level, we have to deal with what differentiates this problem from more standard bivariate twin analyses that consider the relationship between the genetic and environmental risk factors for two disorders (such as that between MD and GAD, which we examined in Chapter 11). We are missing a key piece of data. We cannot estimate liability to drug abuse for individuals who have never used drugs.

Taking these factors into account, Neale and Kendler developed what we think is a particularly helpful and elegant solution to this problem, illustrated in Figure 12.1.[1] Our term for this model is the *causal, contingent, common pathway*, or CCC, model (Kendler et al., 1999d). The model is *causal* because it assumes a direct path (*b*) from the liability to substance initiation to the liability to substance misuse; it is *contingent* because misuse can be assessed only in those who have initiated substance use; and it posits a *common pathway* in that genetic and environmental effects on initiation can affect misuse only by flowing through the phenotype of initiation. This model suggests that risk factors exist for initiating drug use that are divided into the usual categories of additive genetic (A_i), shared environmental (C_i), and individual-specific environmental components (E_i), where the subscript $_i$ indicates that they are specific for *initiation*. Individuals with high liability on this dimension initiate drug use, thereby creating the possibility that they will progress to drug abuse.

The key to understanding this model is the way in which it handles risk factors for drug abuse.[2] One set of risk factors for abuse is shared with initiation and flows into abuse through path *b*. For example, as noted in Chapter 11, novelty seeking is a personality trait that predisposes individuals to initiate drug use and, somewhat less powerfully, to develop drug abuse given initiation. Thus, in our model, the genetic and environmental risk factors for nov-

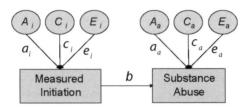

FIGURE 12.1. Model for estimating genetic and environmental influences on substance abuse conditional upon initiation (shown for one twin).

elty seeking would be expressed in two ways: first, through the factors A_i, C_i, and E_i, which would influence liability to initiation, and then through initiation, which would influence the risk for subsequent abuse. Second, however—and this is critical—the model also contains a set of risk factors for drug abuse that are *independent* of the risk factors for initiation. We label these additive genetic (A_a), shared environmental (C_a), and individual-specific environmental components (E_a), where the subscript $_a$ indicates specificity for *abuse*.[3]

An example of the A_a component would be genetic factors that influence an individual's subjective response to drug taking. When first exposed to a drug, individuals experience a wide variety of both positive and negative effects. Not surprisingly, individuals who experience predominantly pleasurable effects will be more likely to continue to use that drug (and hence put themselves at further risk for developing problems) than will those who have more negative experiences (Eissenberg & Balster, 2000; Fergusson, Horwood, Lynskey, & Madden, 2003). Genetic factors probably influence the intensity of both the pleasurable and aversive effects of psychoactive drugs, in part through the brain dopamine pathways (Koob & Le Moal, 1997). However, it is rather unlikely that these genetic factors directly influence the decision to use a drug in the first place. These factors would thus be specific to the risk for abuse, given use, and would be reflected in the latent variable A_a.

Turning to the key path b, if *all* of the risk factors for drug abuse were also risk factors for drug initiation, then the value of b would approach 1 and the values of a_a, c_a, and e_a would approach 0. That is, there would be no genetic or environmental risk factors specific for abuse, as they all would be shared with initiation. If risk factors for initiation and abuse were, by contrast, entirely unrelated, b would approach zero, and the risk for abuse would be due only to the effects of a_a, c_a, and e_a. If risk factors for initiation and abuse are related, but not identical, then b would be between zero and unity, and abuse would be caused *both* by genetic and environmental risk factors common to initiation and unique to abuse.

Now we present the results we obtained when fitting this model to our twin data on any illicit psychoactive substance use and the combined category of abuse/dependence.[4] We focus on the "any drug" category because it provides us with the greatest statistical power. We first fit the model depicted in Figure 12.1 separately for males and females and then asked whether the model would still fit if we required the estimates to be equal in the two sexes.[5] We did this for any illicit substance and also for four of the specific substances that we examined (those with sufficient prevalence: cannabis, cocaine, stimulants, and sedatives). Although men and women vary in their rate of drug use and especially their rates of abuse/dependence, the pattern and magnitude of effect of genetic and environmental risk factors appear to be the same across sexes.

Figure 12.2 depicts the results of our CCC model fitted to use and abuse/dependence of *any illicit substance* (Agrawal, Neale, Jacobson, Prescott, & Kendler, 2005). We want to emphasize four aspects of the results. First, initia-

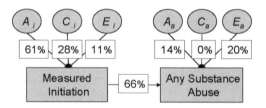

FIGURE 12.2. Results from conditional twin model for initiation and abuse of any illicit substance, combined across sex (shown for one twin). Data from Agrawal, Neale, Jacobson, Prescott, and Kendler (2005, Table 1).

tion is strongly influenced by genetic factors (the heritability is 61%; 95% CI = 49, 80). Of substantial interest, however, is that shared environment is also of importance, accounting for 28% of the variance in liability (95% CI = 25, 74).

Second, there is substantial continuity between the risk factors for initiation of drug use and the progression from use to abuse. Our estimate of b indicates that 66% of the variance in substance abuse/dependence is shared with substance initiation. This means that about two-thirds of the variance in risk for developing abuse of or dependence on any illicit substance results from the same factors that influence use in the first place. However, one-third of the risk factors are new—specific to the stage of abuse.

A third important result is that we can quantify the sources of the liability that are *specific* to abuse. In particular, we found no evidence that shared environmental factors affect risk for abuse given use. These results are one of the clearest examples of the dictum that *genetic designs can often inform us in critical ways about the actions of environmental risk factors.* Our results present compelling evidence that shared environmental factors (which probably include peer influences, parental attitudes, and family and community religious beliefs) influence the decision to first use a substance. However, we also find that after initiation there are no "new" shared environmental factors that affect the chances of developing abuse or dependence.

The pattern is quite different for genetic factors. Fully 40% (i.e., 14/34) of the liability that is specific to abuse is due to genetic factors. Critically, these are genetic factors that are entirely independent of those factors that influenced the initiation of illicit drugs. The remaining 60% of the liability to abuse/dependence given use is a result of individual-specific environmental factors.

A fourth result is that this model can be used to separate the sources of risk for abuse into those that are "shared" with use and those that are "unique" to the development of abuse. As noted earlier, all the shared environmental influences on abuse are shared with use. The story with genetic factors is different. With a bit of elementary algebra, we can calculate that genetic risk factors account for ~54% of the total variance in liability to abuse of any illicit drug. Of this amount, three-fourths is shared with factors that also influence drug use, and one-fourth is unique to the stage of abuse/dependence. Some will likely find this result surprising. Although there clearly are genes whose only action is to alter the risk for progressing to abuse or dependence after first trying a drug, the bulk of the genetic risk factors act at both stages. Such risk factors affect both the chances that individuals will try the drug *and* the risk that they will develop drug-related problems.

We then went on to examine the results of this model when applied to specific classes of psychoactive substances, including cannabis, cocaine, stimulants, and sedatives. The results were quite similar to those seen for any illicit substance.[6] We also examined the progression from smoking initiation to nicotine dependence (ND; defined by the FTQ; Fagerstrom & Schneider, 1989; see Sidebar 5.4) in our sample of female–female twin pairs (Kendler, Neale, et al., 1999d). The pattern of findings was also broadly comparable to what we found with illicit drugs. The best-fit model indicated that ND is highly heritable. Approximately 40% of the variance in liability to ND is due to factors specific to dependence, and the remaining 60% is shared with factors that affect smoking initiation. The estimated heritability of ND is high (72%). About two-thirds of these genetic risk factors are shared with smoking initiation, and one-third are unique to the stage of ND.

What can we learn from these examples of the genetics of conditional processes? At a practical level, it is much more satisfying to approach the analysis of drug involvement by conceptualizing it as a multistage process.[7] As might be predicted, the risk factors are neither entirely the same across the different stages nor entirely distinct. The largest difference we saw was for shared environment. These results might suggest something like the following:

> As a parent, teacher, or minister, your behavior is much more likely to influence the chances that a child will use drugs than that he will go on to abuse a drug once he tries it. Although family and community environments seem to influence the decision to use a drug, they do not appear to have much influence once one has experienced the drug's effects. Thus similarity among relatives for developing problem drug use (once use has started) seems to result largely or entirely from genetic factors.

These models could be applied to other multistage processes within psychopathology. For example, they could address the relationship between the risk factors that lead an individual to develop MD and those that influence level of impairment given that someone is depressed. Or they could be used to study how similar or different the genetic risk factors are for the development of irrational fears from those that make fears sufficiently disabling to produce a phobia. Answers to these and other such questions will have to be left for future studies.

CROSS-GENERATIONAL TRANSMISSION OF RISK

By this point in the book, it is probably clear to our readers that we are rather enamored of the power of the twin method to understand the sources of individual differences in risk for psychiatric disorders. However, the twin method does have some limitations. An important one—the focus of this section—results from the fact that twins are always members of the same generation. Therefore, twin studies cannot, on their own, tell us much about *how risk for disorders passes from one generation to another.*

However, when information from twins is combined with information from their parents or children—as part of what is called a *twin–family design*—this situation changes quite dramatically. Indeed, given some reasonable assumptions, twin–family designs compare quite favorably with adoption studies (Heath, Kendler, Eaves, & Markell, 1985) for sorting out why children resemble their parents in risk for illness.

Children resemble their parents due to parent–offspring transmission of genes and what we might call environmental transmission. *Genetic transmission* occurs because parents pass one copy of each of their genes to their offspring. *Environmental transmission* (also called *cultural transmission*) occurs because parents influence their offspring directly (by teaching, by serving as models, and by otherwise cajoling the children in order to influence their behavior) and indirectly (by creating a certain kind of rearing environment according to their social class and their choices of neighborhood, schools, church, etc.).

How can we discriminate genetic from cultural transmission?[8] In adoption studies, it is quite easy. Given some assumptions, the resemblance between adoptive parents and their adopted children should be due solely to cultural transmission. The resemblance between biological parents and their adopted-away children should result only from genetic transmission.

When studying twins and their families, we can also discriminate these two mechanisms, but the reasoning is less direct. By studying MZ and DZ pairs, we can estimate the importance of genetic factors for a given trait, and based on this information we can predict the level of expected resemblance between parents and children that should result from genetic mechanisms. If cultural transmission is occurring, it will produce parent–offspring resemblance *greater* than that predicted by genes alone.[9]

We studied the sources of parent–offspring transmission in risk for alcoholism in our sample of female twin pairs (Kendler, Neale, Heath, Kessler, & Eaves, 1994a) whose parents had participated in personal interviews (see Chapter 2). As described in Chapter 5, there is substantial evidence that genetic factors contribute to the risk for alcoholism. It is less clear whether the liability to alcoholism is also transmitted from parent to child by nongenetic means. For example, children might model their approach to alcohol use on their parents by the process of imitation or social learning (Bandura, 1986). Alternatively, religious and social attitudes passed from parents to children (which usually include attitudes toward alcohol use) might contribute to parent–offspring resemblance for alcoholism. Results of empirical studies of the role of cultural transmission—most done in the setting of adoption designs—are mixed. Some studies suggest that being raised by parents with alcoholism increases the risk for alcohol problems above and beyond that expected from genetic effects alone (Beardslee, Son, & Vaillant, 1986; Cadoret, O'Gorman, Troughton, & Heywood, 1985; Cadoret et al., 1987), whereas other studies find no such effect (Cadoret, Cain, & Grove, 1980; Cloninger, Bohman, & Sigvardsson, 1981; Goodwin, Schulsinger, Hermansen, Guze, & Winokur, 1973).

The model that we applied to the twins and their parents is portrayed in Figure 12.3. It has several features that distinguish it from our standard twin models. In addition to our usual sources of resemblance among relatives (A and C), we have added cultural transmission, depicted here as path w, which goes from the phenotype of the parent to the shared environment of the twins. Cultural transmission is allowed to differ between fathers (w_f) and mothers (w_m). Furthermore, because social attitudes toward alcohol consumption have changed dramatically in this century, it is possible that the genetic factors that predispose to drinking problems may differ over generations. To capture this in our model, we include two latent variables representing the genotypes that are transmitted to the offspring (A_F' and A_M'). The paths from the parent's own genotype (A_F and A_M) to his or her transmitted genotype are estimated as

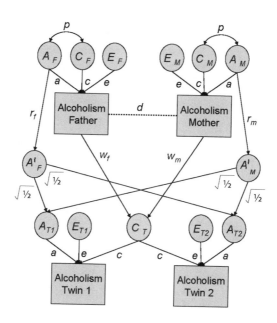

FIGURE 12.3. Parent–offspring model for alcoholism with phenotypic cultural transmission.

free parameters (r_f and r_m), which represent the genetic correlation between generations. Finally, the model assumes that spousal resemblance for the liability to alcoholism results from assortative mating (path d), in which spouses select one another (in part) on the basis of their predisposition to alcoholism.[10]

The results from the best-fitting model for our narrow definition of alcoholism are shown in Figure 12.4.[11] The results could not have been simpler. We found no significant evidence for spousal resemblance for this definition of alcoholism, nor could we find evidence for cultural transmission. Finally, the genetic risk factors that influence alcoholism are the same in the parent and twin generations. The results indicate that all family resemblance for liability to alcoholism is a result of genetic factors. Being raised by an individual with alcoholism produced no additional risk for illness beyond that due to genetic transmission. The key result of this analysis—the absence of evidence for cultural transmission—was also seen when we examined a broader definition of alcoholism.

Our main goal in this section was to illustrate one important extension of the twin model—examining twins along with their families. In so doing, we can expand considerably the breadth of research questions that can be addressed. In particular, we can better understand how the vulnerability to psychiatric and substance use disorders is passed from parents to their offspring.

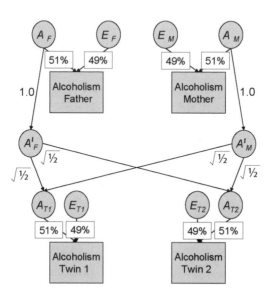

FIGURE 12.4. Estimates from best-fitting model for parent–offspring transmission of alcoholism. Adapted from Kendler, Neale, Heath, Kessler, and Eaves (1994a, Figure 2). Copyright by the American Psychiatric Association. Adapted by permission.

DEALING WITH UNRELIABILITY

In our description of the twin method (Chapter 3), we noted that the set of risk factors we call *unique* or *individual-specific environment* (E or e^2) is, in most instances, entirely confounded with errors of measurement. This point can be most clearly illustrated by an example. Assume that we have members of a pair of reared-together MZ twins, who of necessity have all their genetic (A) and all their shared environmental (C) risk factors in common. We personally interview these two individuals, and twin 1 reports a lifetime history of disorder X, whereas twin 2 denies such a history. If we knew that a lifetime history of illness is always reported with complete accuracy, we could conclude that this pair is truly discordant. We would then know that this discordance must be due to environmental experiences not shared by the twins, which either precipitated the disorder in twin 1 and/or protected twin 2 from developing the disorder. However, individuals are far from completely accurate in reporting their lifetime history of illness. Given this unreliability, we cannot with certainty distinguish among three alternatives: (1) the twin pair is truly discordant; (2) the twin pair is truly concordant for not having the disorder and twin 1's report is a false positive (i.e., twin 1 exaggerated his symptoms and did not really meet criteria for the disorder); or (3) the twin pair is truly concordant for having the disorder and twin 2's report is a false negative (i.e., twin 2 forgot about a prior episode of illness).[12]

There is a large literature on the reliability of psychiatric diagnoses obtained by structured interview.[13] The design of most such studies is straightforward. A reasonably-sized sample of patients or community respondents is given the same structured interview on two separate occasions, and the similarity of their responses is compared. In most studies, the test–retest reliability of most diagnoses is in the "moderate" range (i.e., a κ of 0.40 to 0.60; see Chapter 2, p. 32). Generally, reliability is higher when assessed in clinical rather than community samples, perhaps because the disorders are more severe and hence more "memorable." Reliability is typically higher for drug use than for standard psychiatric disorders, probably because drug use and many of the drug-related criteria are more objective than most of the criteria for psychiatric disorders.

Unreliability is an enemy to research in genetic epidemiology. Such "errors of measurement" cause the true effect of genetic or shared environmental risk factors to be underestimated. If, for example, the estimated heritability of a disorder is modest, the reason may be that either true environmental effects are quite important for the disorder or assessment of the disorder is unreliable. It would be helpful to distinguish between these two possibilities.

In this section we describe the use of two methods to correct for unreliability of measurement. The first involves measuring the same thing (e.g., lifetime diagnosis of MD) on two occasions; the second involves obtaining information on the same diagnosis (e.g., lifetime MD) from two different informants.

Twin Measurement Model

We applied the first model—which we have called the *twin measurement model*—to a lifetime diagnosis of MD in 847 female–female twin pairs in which both members completed both the first and third waves of personal interviews (Foley, Neale, & Kendler, 1998). For the sake of simplicity, we refer to these assessments as time 1 and time 2. This model differs from that presented in Chapter 10. There we studied past-year depression as reported for two nonoverlapping periods. Here we study lifetime depression as reported on two different occasions.

The basic model that we used is illustrated in Figure 12.5. The model assumes that each twin has a "true" but unobserved (or "latent") liability to MD. Our two assessments of the lifetime history of MD in these twins partly reflect their true liability to MD and partly reflect error. The paths l_1 and l_2 represent the degree to which the assessments of the lifetime history of MD obtained at time 1 and time 2, respectively, reflect true liability. The other paths to the assessment of MD at each point (u_1 and u_2, respectively) represent error in the individual assessments.[14]

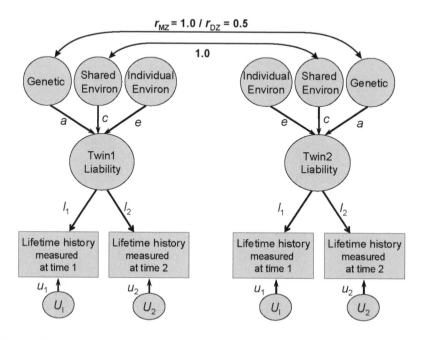

FIGURE 12.5. Longitudinal twin model to correct for unreliability of measurement.

There are two critical differences between this model and the standard twin model. First, this model *separates* error of measurement (*u*) from true individual-specific environment (*e*) that contributes to the true liability to MD. Second, it provides a direct estimate of the degree to which the individual assessments of lifetime history of MD reflect the latent liability (*l*).

We fitted a series of different models to these data, the best-fitting model of which is shown in Figure 12.6. This model has a number of interesting features. The l_1 and l_2 paths could be set equal. This means that the degree to which the assessed history of MD reflects the true liability to MD is the same at the two interviews. The best-fitting model estimated that about 66% of the variance in liability assessed at personal interview is "reliable" and is thus assumed to reflect "true" disease liability. The remaining variance (34%) in liability to MD, as assessed at either our first or second interview, is unreliable and probably reflects measurement error.

What we called measurement error probably reflects a number of distinct processes. For example, there is evidence that current mood influences one's tendency to recall prior experiences of depression (Bower, 1987). So imagine that we had a pair of twins who were truly concordant for lifetime MD but

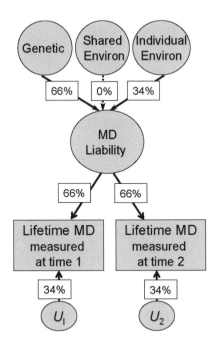

FIGURE 12.6. Results from twin analyses to correct for unreliability of measurement in risk for lifetime major depression (MD) (shown for one twin). Adapted from Foley, Neale, and Kendler (1998, Figure 1). Copyright 1998 by Cambridge University Press. Adapted by permission.

whose episodes were relatively mild and occurred a long time ago. One of them has a particularly bad day before her interview and remembers her prior depression. The other is in a very good mood during the interview and does not recall her prior depression. This measurement error would result in the twins' appearing to be discordant for MD.

We also know that in interview situations the behavior and attitude of the interviewer can influence the degree to which respondents will reveal information about themselves. Despite the fact that all of our interviewers went through the same rigorous training, it is certainly possible that some of them were better than others at providing an interview environment that encouraged the twins to report about their prior psychiatric problems. Such effects would also come out as measurement error in our study.

What is most important about this model is that it allows us to "subtract" the effects of error from the estimates of the etiological role of genetic and environmental risk factors in MD. If we analyzed the data from time 1 on its own in a standard twin model (such as the ones we used in Chapters 4 and 5), we would estimate that the heritability of MD is 43%, with the remaining 57% of variance in risk due to individual-specific environment. This is very close to the results we report in Chapter 4 based on all-female pairs interviewed at least once. However, those estimates include the effect of error. Corrected for unreliability, the heritability of liability to MD is now estimated at 66%, with 34% of risk due to "true" individual-specific environment. These changes are substantial. Estimated heritability increases from 43 to 66%. It is also important to note that, had we detected evidence for shared environment (c^2) for MD, this estimate would also increase after correcting for unreliability. Thus this method reveals that a substantial proportion of what our standard twin models estimate as individual-specific environment actually represents error of measurement.[15]

We also applied this measurement model to our diagnoses of phobia using information obtained from our female–female twin pairs at the first and fourth interview waves (Kendler, Karkowski, & Prescott, 1999c). The long-term stability of a lifetime diagnosis of phobias was among the lowest we found in our study. When we corrected for that unreliability of measurement, the heritability increased substantially, with results for most phobia subtypes in the range of 50–60%. As with MD, our results suggest that a good deal of what we called individual-specific environment in our standard twin models for lifetime psychiatric disorders reflects unreliability of measurement.

Multiple-Rater Model

The second analytic approach we have taken to address the problem of measurement error also involves two reports of the presence or absence of a history of psychiatric illness in a twin. However, instead of asking the twin twice about his or her own history of MD, we used self-reports (twins reporting on their own history of MD) and cotwin reports (twins reporting on the

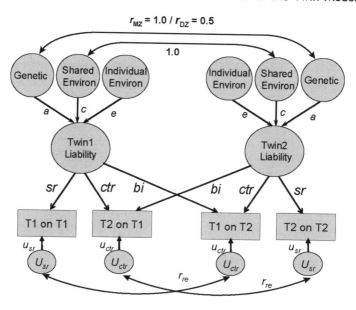

FIGURE 12.7. Twin model for multiple raters.

history of MD in their cotwins).[16] The *multiple-rater model* used to analyze these data is portrayed in Figure 12.7. This model depends on four kinds of diagnostic reports for each twin pair, including two self-report measures: "T1 on T1" (twin 1's report on twin 1) and "T2 on T2" (twin 2's report on twin 2), and two cotwin reports: "T2 on T1" (twin 2's report on twin 1) and "T1 on T2" (twin 1's report on twin 2).

As in our twin measurement model, we assume that there is a latent "true" liability to MD. As usual, this latent liability results from variation in A, C, and E. This latent liability is reflected primarily in two diagnostic measures. For twin 1's liability, these would be measured by self-report (T1 on T1) and cotwin report (T2 on T1). The latent liability to MD is connected to the self-report history through the path labeled *sr* (for self-report). The higher the value of this self-report path, the more closely related twin 1's self-report history is to the "true" latent phenotype. The latent liability to MD is also reflected in the cotwin report through a path labeled *ctr* (for cotwin report). The higher this cotwin report path is, the more closely related the cotwin report about a twin and the true liability of that twin are. One of the interesting results from this model is that we can quantify how well our twins have followed the old Greek maxim of "know thyself." By comparing the coefficients of these two paths, we can assess whether twins know themselves better than their cotwins know them.

What makes this model different from our measurement model is the need to account for potential biases in cotwin report. A large body of data indicates that the report about the history of illness obtained from one relative (typically called an *informant*) about another relative is influenced by characteristics of both the relative and the informant. In particular, the probability that an informant will report that a relative has a particular disorder is influenced by the informant's own history of that disorder (Breslau, Davis, & Prabucki, 1987; Chapman, Mannuzza, Klein, & Fyer, 1994; Heun, Maier, & Muller, 2000; Kendler et al., 1991b; Rice et al., 1995; Roy, Walsh, Prescott, & Kendler, 1994; Roy, Walsh, & Kendler, 1996). This potential bias was taken into account in our model in two ways. The first and most obvious way is to include a path by which the cotwin report is influenced by the latent liability of the cotwin. This is portrayed in Figure 12.7 by the path with the coefficient bi for "bias." A large estimate for the bias path means that a cotwin report is strongly influenced by the cotwin's own liability to illness. For example, if individuals with high liability to MD are more likely to observe and report MD in their relatives (perhaps because they are more sensitive to the symptoms), this would result in a positive estimate for the bias path. A negative bias is also possible.

The second method used to account for informant effects begins with a feature that this model shares with the measurement model. We included in both models an error term (U for unreliability), which reflects everything that might influence self-report or cotwin report of MD except the disease liability. The path coefficients u_1 and u_2 express the magnitude of the impact of these residual effects on the observations of self- and cotwin report, respectively. Some of these residual effects (such as impressions of the interviewer, a tendency to generally underreport or overreport symptoms) could affect the tendency of an individual to report on both him- or herself and his or her cotwin. This *correlation of residual errors* is reflected by the path r_{re}. Thus this model contains two different paths whereby "excess" resemblance[17] might arise between a twin's self-report (i.e., T1 on T1) and his report on his cotwin (i.e., T1 on T2). The first of these is via the bias path and the second is through correlated errors.

We fit this model to five disorders and regular tobacco use assessed in approximately 1,200 of our male–male pairs (Kendler, Prescott, Jacobson, Myers, & Neale, 2002b).[18] We review the results for two disorders that illustrate the range of findings, MD and AASB. The results from the best-fitting multiple-rater model for lifetime MD are summarized in Figure 12.8. Four results are particularly noteworthy. First, "true" liability to MD constituted an approximately equal combination of the *self-report* and *cotwin report* information (i.e., $sr = ctr$) . This means that these two different methods of obtaining a lifetime diagnosis of MD (asking twin 1 about his own history or asking twin 2 about twin 1's history) equally reflect twin 1's true liability to MD.

Second, there was substantial unreliability in both self- and cotwin report of lifetime MD. These measures are about equally the result of true liability to illness and of error.

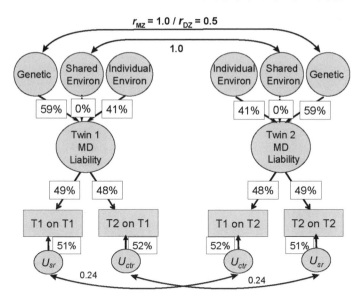

FIGURE 12.8. Results from multiple-rater model for lifetime major depression (MD). Adapted from Kendler, Prescott, Jacobson, Myers, and Neale (2002b, Figure 2b). Copyright 2002 by Cambridge University Press. Adapted by permission.

Third, the heritability of the true or latent liability to MD is 59%, substantially higher than was obtained from applying a standard twin analysis to self-report diagnoses (Chapter 4). These results are reassuringly similar to the estimate obtained earlier based on our measurement model. At least with respect to depression, errors of measurement can be estimated equally well by assessing the same twin twice or by asking twins to report on each other. The latter, we should note, generally demands much less effort.

Fourth, the best-fit model had a zero estimate of the *bias* path but did contain a substantial and positive correlation between the error terms. This result tells us that there is some "extra" resemblance between self- and cotwin report. Individuals who report that they themselves have a history of MD are more likely than would be predicted by other parts of the model to report that their cotwins have a history of MD.

The results for AASB are summarized in Figure 12.9. They differ substantially from those found for MD in several key ways. First, the cotwin report path is much larger than the self-report path. These results suggest that you would obtain more accurate information about twin 1's history of ASB by asking his cotwin than by asking twin 1 himself. This result probably rings true to readers who are clinicians. Individuals with antisocial traits are often remarkably good at justifying their own behavior so that it is seen in a favorable light (Cleckley, 1982). Usually, their relatives are not quite so sympathetic, perhaps because they are often the victims of the antisocial behavior.

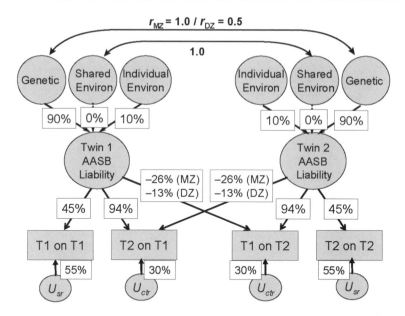

FIGURE 12.9. Results From multiple-rater model for adult antisocial behavior (AASB). Adapted from Kendler, Prescott, Jacobson, Myers, and Neale (2002b, Figure 2c). Copyright 2002 by Cambridge University Press. Adapted by permission.

A second difference between the results for MD and AASB is that there was evidence of a significant negative bias path for AASB.[19] This means that individuals with high levels of liability to ASB are *less* likely to report such behavior in their cotwins. Such individuals probably have a higher threshold for what they consider to be abnormal or deviant behavior than do individuals without AASB. This reminds us of the bad joke in which an alcoholic is defined as someone who drinks more than his doctor. Our view of what is deviant in the world is probably substantially influenced by the benchmark of our own behavior.

A third result is that the latent genetic liability to AASB when assessed by both self- and cotwin report is quite high, approximately 90%! This is considerably higher than that reported in Chapter 5. The explanation for this high estimate of heritability for the reliable liability to AASB is that prior studies of ASB have often relied largely or exclusively on self-report measures. As the model results show, these measures are quite unreliable. Although our result has substantial statistical precision (the 95% CI is 88%, 94%), we would caution against an overzealous interpretation of this finding and emphasize that replication is needed. However, other studies also suggest that the reliable portion of externalizing liability is quite high. For example, a study of adolescent male twins estimated the heritability of the latent liability to externalizing behavior to be about 80% (Hicks et al., 2004).

Conclusions about Unreliability

There are three main messages to take away from our analyses of unreliability. First, as has been shown previously by us and by other researchers, unreliability is substantial when psychiatric diagnoses are based on a single report of what people say about their lifetime history of psychiatric disorder.[20] Second, several powerful approaches are available in twin studies to assess and correct this unreliability. The extra effort they require is likely to be worthwhile. Third, correcting unreliability can increase estimates of heritability and decrease estimates of the importance of individual-specific environment. The typical twin study that is based on a single assessment is likely to underestimate heritability, perhaps substantially, and to overestimate the impact of unique environmental factors.

SUMMARY

In this chapter we have described three extensions of the traditional twin model used to address conditional multistage processes, transmission of risk across generations, and the unreliability of measurement. We examined these subjects for two reasons. First, we believe the substantive results are of considerable interest in clarifying important questions about how genes and environment influence the risk for psychiatric and substance use disorders. Second, these results show how it is possible, with some creative thinking and proper statistical methods, to develop ways to rigorously address important questions in the etiology of psychiatric illness that have too long been left to the realm of speculation or clinical intuition.

NOTES

1. We are not the first to approach this overall problem, although our solution may have some advantages over those proposed earlier (e.g. Heath & Martin, 1993; Madden et al., 1999).

2. Here we use the term *drug* to refer to any illicit psychoactive substance and the term *abuse* to refer to any form of misuse.

3. The model we fit also included a fixed estimate of the unreliability of initiation (based on test–retest reliability) so that the variation transmitted to substance abuse is from the reliable portion of initiation. For simplicity this is not shown in the figures.

4. We study abuse and dependence together to increase our statistical power. This is especially needed for the female twins, in whom dependence on some of the substances is quite rare. Even so, the sample sizes of individuals with abuse/dependence for opiates and hallucinogens were too small to permit useful analysis. When we examine results for dependence only versus the combined category of abuse and dependence, the pattern of findings is nearly always quite similar.

5. These analyses included only same-sex twin pairs. We included an unre-

liability component, U, in this model, which represents the unreliability in our assessment of initiation, although for simplicity, this is not shown in the figures. Our measure of drug initiation will never be perfectly reliable and will always contain some error of measurement. It distorts the model to expect that "error" in drug use would be passed, via the b path, downstream to influence risk for drug abuse.

6. Genetic risk factors specific to the stage of abuse were relatively more important for stimulants and less important for cocaine, at least in males. The degree of communality between risk factors for use and risk factors for abuse/dependence (i.e., the magnitude of the b path) was highest for cannabis and lowest for sedatives.

7. This need not be restricted to two stages; we have fit models for tobacco use that included initiation, regular use, and ND.

8. We use a broader definition of the term *cultural* than is employed in anthropology. This terminology has been a source of confusion when genetic epidemiologists and anthropologists talk about sources of family resemblance.

9. Another twin–parent design is possible—the study of twins and their children. Although the latter design has some advantages over the former, it was not used in the VATSPSUD and thus is not further discussed.

10. Parent–offspring models include several complex constraints. For estimating the parental correlation in liability, we selected the delta path method (see Fulker, 1988; van Eerdewegh, 1982). Models that contain both w (w_f and w_m) and r (r_f and r_m) are not identified in the usual twin–family design. We estimated them by testing a series of models with differing constraints (see Kendler, Neale, Heath, Kessler, & Eaves, 1994a, for details). Another feature of the parent–offspring model is that the correlation between the additive genetic and common environmental components can be estimated (path p), but this did not turn out to be significant in the current example.

11. The narrow definition used DSM-III-R criteria for AD, including the tolerance or dependence criteria. This study included 2,060 female twins, 853 mothers, and 615 fathers. Four family types were studied: twins only (n = 129 pairs), twin pairs and their fathers (n = 48), twin pairs and their mothers (n = 286), and pairs with both parents (n = 567).

12. We know from prior research that the third possibility is quite a bit more likely: People are more prone to forget about episodes of illness that did happen than to report episodes that did not happen.

13. Some of the more important recent references to consult on this issue include Aneshensel, Estrada, Hansell, and Clark, 1987; Bromet, Dunn, Connell, Dew, and Schulberg, 1986; Fendrich, Weissman, Warner, and Mufson, 1990; Prusoff, Merikangas, and Weissman, 1988.

14. By definition, $l^2 + u^2 = 1.0$. Further elaborations of this model are possible. In particular, the occasion-specific effects could be a result of factors other than just random error. For example, we tested whether there were genetic effects specific to the time 1 or the time 2 interview but found no evidence for any twin resemblance for the occasion-specific factors. Another assumption of the measurement model is that the lifetime assessments of two interviews cover the same risk period. Our interviews were designed so that at the time 2 interview we assessed lifetime history for MD up to the date of the time 1 interview.

15. The most instructive way to appreciate the results of this model is to partition the variance of the lifetime history of MD as assessed at one of the specific times. At the first level, this can be divided into 34% due to unreliability and 66% due to systematic effects. Now the systematic effects can be divided into genetic effects (equal to

44% of the variance in the lifetime history) and "true" individual-specific environment (equal to 22%). Thus, of the 56% of the variance in liability attributed to individual-specific environment in a standard twin model about 60% (34/56) comes from measurement error and about 40% (22/56) reflects "true" individual-specific environment.

16. We are by no means the first or only group to use multiple-rater models, although most prior uses of such models have been applied to data collected about children. See, for example, Neale and Stevenson, 1989; Simonoff et al., 1995; Vierikko, Pulkkinen, Kaprio, and Rose, 2004.

17. By excess resemblance, we mean beyond that expected from the correlations in the genetic and environmental risk factors on the latent phenotype.

18. FF pairs were not included because we never asked them about the history of psychiatric and substance use disorders of their cotwins.

19. The net effect of the bias path differs for MZ and DZ pairs because the path goes from one twin to the other and thus includes differences in the degree of genetic resemblance. The observant reader will note that the two positive paths to the "T2 on T1" and "T1 on T2" boxes sum to more than 100%—to 124% to be precise. This occurs because of the negative bias paths. When averaged across both MZ and DZ twins, the sum of the three paths to these boxes approximates 100%.

20. Studies that rely on medical records collected at the time of illness or other official records (such as registration for alcohol problems) do not have this problem of low test–retest reliability, but there are often other problems with the validity of such data, including incomplete identification of cases and inconsistent diagnostic procedures.

PART V

BRINGING IT ALL TOGETHER

CHAPTER THIRTEEN

The Genetics of the Environment

In Part II of this book, we took the perspective of the psychiatric geneticist, asking basic questions about the magnitude of the role of genetic factors in the etiology of psychiatric and substance use disorders. In Part III, we acted as psychiatric epidemiologists, trying to relate proximal and distal environmental risk factors to liability to illness. In Part IV, we tried to show the breadth and depth of the questions that the psychiatric geneticist can answer beyond the simple question of heritability. Although the environment played a role in these analyses, it was an unobserved component, the presence of which we inferred by patterns of correlations in twin pairs. In this final section of the book, we weave together the genetic and environmental risk factors, showing the complex and interesting ways in which they relate to one another in the etiology of psychiatric and substance use disorders.

Traditional models for the etiology of psychiatric disorders assume that genetic and environmental risk factors are independent and add together to produce low or high risk for a disorder. The environment is usually conceptualized as something "out there" that happens to us. In this chapter we show that neither of these assumptions is correct. We present evidence that *genetic risk factors influence the probability of exposure to environmental risk factors*, including stressful life events, low levels of social support, and poor parenting.

STRESSFUL LIFE EVENTS

We began Chapter 8 by showing that the occurrence of stressful life events (SLEs) strongly predicts the subsequent onset of episodes of major depression (MD) and generalized anxiety disorder (GAD). In this chapter, we ask a different question: What causes people to have SLEs?

Most studies of SLEs assume that their occurrence is random, that having a large number of SLEs is due to "bad luck." However, several lines of evidence suggest that a "bad luck" model of life events is implausible. First, the number of recent SLEs that individuals report is moderately stable over time; some individuals experience large numbers and others small numbers of life events (Andrews, 1981; Fergusson & Horwood, 1984). Second, the number of life events a person experiences can be predicted by personal characteristics, such as social class, self-esteem, social support, mood, and personality (Brett, Brief, Burke, George, & Webster, 1990). Third, research has shown consistent differences among people in how frequently they experience specific events, such as automobile accidents, industrial injuries, and criminal victimization (McFarland, 1957; Tillmann & Hobbs, 1949).

As we demonstrated in prior chapters, the twin design is a powerful technique for understanding the sources of individual differences in human populations. To begin to answer the question of the genetic control of exposure to the environment simply requires that we turn the twin method from the study of the causes of disorders and apply it to the study of environmental risk factors. We first consider twin resemblance for stressful life events.

Sources of Individual Differences in Reported Life Events: A Cross-Sectional Study

In the mailed questionnaire that represented our first contact with the female–female twins, we asked respondents whether they had experienced any of 44 SLEs during the preceding year. As with SLEs assessed by interview (see Figure 8.1), the frequency varied widely across different types of events. The most commonly reported events (by over 40% of women) were interpersonal difficulties and a crisis within their social networks. The events reported least commonly were being the victim of a crime (3.9%) and experiencing legal problems (2.6%). The average number of prior-year life events was three, with 18.4% of twins reporting no events (Kendler, Neale, Kessler, Heath, & Eaves, 1993g).

As shown in Figure 13.1, we found substantial twin-pair resemblance for the total number of SLEs experienced, with correlations of 0.43 among MZ pairs and 0.31 among DZ pairs. MZ correlations for each of the nine classes of life events consistently exceeded those for DZ pairs, although the difference was sometimes small.

Figure 13.2 depicts the genetic and environmental proportions of variance for predisposition to experience life events. Genetic factors were esti-

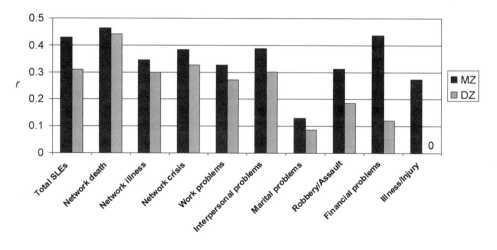

FIGURE 13.1. Twin-pair correlations for 1-year occurrence of stressful life events (SLEs). *r* = correlation; MZ = monozygotic; DZ = dizygotic. Data from Kendler, Neale, Kessler, Heath, and Eaves (1993g, Table 2).

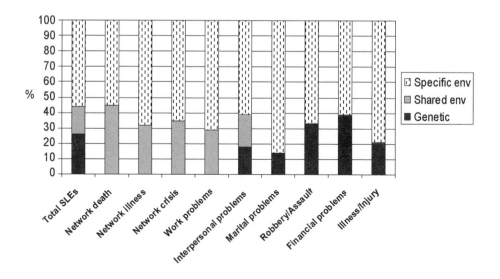

FIGURE 13.2. Estimated proportions of variance for 1-year occurrence of stressful life events (SLEs). Env = environment. Data from Kendler, Neale, Kessler, Heath, and Eaves (1993g, Table 3).

mated to account for 26% of the variance in total life events. Shared environmental factors contributed 18%, and the remaining 56% came from individual-specific environmental factors. The model-fitting results differ for different classes of life events. For all the network events (death, illness/injury, and crisis) and work difficulties, genetic factors appear to play little to no role; twin resemblance appears to result largely from shared environmental influences. This makes sense, as one would not expect an individual's genetically influenced behavior to affect the illnesses, crises, or deaths of her family and friends.

For interpersonal difficulties, twin-pair resemblance resulted from about equal proportions of shared environment and genetic factors. This also seems reasonable. As twins share all of the same family members and some of the same friends, they are also likely to share many interpersonal difficulties.

For the remaining four "personal" events and difficulties, nearly all twin resemblance was due to genetic factors. For illness, marital, and financial problems, this seems sensible. These kinds of events are influenced by an individual's health or personality—characteristics that are genetically influenced. For being robbed or assaulted, we note that most of the variation came from individual-specific environment—consistent with the "bad luck" model of SLEs. However, most of the modest twin resemblance appeared to be the result of genes. Perhaps these effects are mediated by genetically influenced temperamental traits such as risk taking or impulsivity.

We conducted a number of additional analyses to test for possible biases in our results. We were particularly concerned about violations of the equal environment assumption (EEA; see Chapter 6). Frequency of social contact between the twins as adults significantly predicted twin similarity for total life events. Because twins from MZ pairs have more contact with each other than do DZ pairs, it is possible that greater twin resemblance in MZ twins, which our model attributes to genetic influences, could have resulted from closer contact between the MZ twins. However, including measures of social contact did not change the results of our analyses to any substantial degree. This supports our interpretation that the evidence for genetic influences is not due to a contact bias.

We also conducted additional analyses to identify the sources of the shared environmental influences on life events. Because some SLEs tend to decrease with age (e.g., relationship difficulties) and others increase (e.g., health problems), we hypothesized that some of the shared environmental effect was due to twins in a pair being the same age. In fact, we found that age effects were not important. Another possibility is that some of the shared environmental effects were due to twins reporting the same event. This was true in part for network events; however, for personal events, shared environmental effects appear more likely to be the result of "enduring" factors shared by twins, such as might result from being reared in the same environment.

Sources of Individual Differences in Reported Life Events: A Longitudinal Study

Our initial analysis of SLEs had at least two methodological weaknesses. First, we used questionnaire-based measures. As we discussed in Chapter 8, this method of assessment is probably more influenced by personality and perceptual biases than are measures obtained by structured personal interviews. Second, our results were based on a single time of assessment. As we noted previously (see Chapter 3), cross-sectional studies cannot discriminate among enduring individual-specific environmental effects, occasion-specific effects, and errors of measurement. However, as we illustrated for MD in Chapter 10, when the same trait is measured on more than one occasion, we can make some distinctions among these forms of individual-specific factors.

We consider this issue to be of particular interest for SLEs because we would like to distinguish the portion of individual differences in SLEs that is truly "bad luck" from that which is an enduring characteristic of the person. This distinction is portrayed in Figure 13.3. On the left are enduring factors, which produce similarity over time in an individual's risk for experiencing SLEs. The genetic and shared environmental factors would produce resemblance between members of a twin pair. On the right are time-specific factors, including bad luck and measurement error, as well as temporary factors about a person, such as short-term fluctuations in mood, that might alter his or her risk. These time-specific factors act at the individual level and generally would not be correlated across twins in a pair (although bad luck could cause an SLE that both twins shared). The time-specific (or "transient") factors are shown in a single circle because they cannot be estimated separately using a longitudinal twin study such as we conducted.

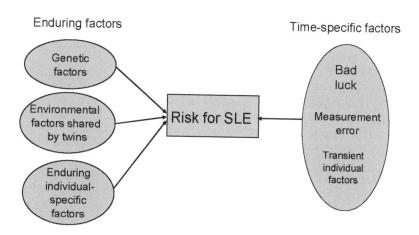

FIGURE 13.3. Causes of stressful life events (SLEs) estimated in a longitudinal study of twins.

To separate enduring and time-specific effects on SLEs, we analyzed data from 937 female–female twin pairs who completed the wave 1 and 2 personal interviews (Foley, Neale, & Kendler, 1996). The measures of SLEs were the same as those described in Chapter 8 (see Sidebar 8.1). The study, which was performed along with our colleague Debra Foley, examined each type of life event separately, but here we focus on the results for two broad categories: network events and personal events. Total personal SLEs correlated 0.43 across the two interview waves, confirming the idea that there are stable differences among individuals in the occurrence of SLEs. Occurrence of network events was somewhat less stable, correlating 0.24 across the two interviews. The twin-pair correlations for personal and network SLEs, though quite variable, were nearly always higher in MZ than in DZ pairs. The exception (as expected) was for reports of deaths of parents and siblings, for which MZ and DZ correlations were nearly identical, indicating very high reliability between twins for the recall of these salient events. The twin-pair correlations and results of model fitting for personal events and network events for each wave analyzed separately were similar to those obtained for the questionnaire-based study (shown in Figures 13.1 and 13.2).

The unique results from this study came when we analyzed the data from both waves together. Nearly half of the variability among people in the tendency to experience SLEs was due to factors that are *stable* across time. Stable effects (those on the left side of Figure 13.3) accounted for 45% of the variation in risk for personal life events, whereas the time-specific effects (shown on the right side of this figure) accounted for 55%. Of the 45% stable vulnerability to SLEs or "event-proneness," 29% was due to genetic effects and 16% to stable individual-specific environmental effects. The stable liability to SLEs is quite heritable—nearly two-thirds of differences between people in their tendency to experience small versus large numbers of personal SLEs is genetic. Another important result is that environments shared by siblings do not seem important (except when both siblings are experiencing the same event). Finally, as we expected, many SLEs seem to be caused by transient time-specific factors, which are probably largely bad luck.

Our findings of heritable influences on SLEs have been replicated in several other twin studies. Significant genetic effects have been found for specific SLEs, such as combat trauma and divorce, as well as for summary measures of SLEs (Lyons et al., 1993; McGue & Lykken, 1992; Plomin, Lichtenstein, Pedersen, McClearn, & Nesselroade, 1990; Thapar & McGuffin, 1996).

These results provide convincing evidence supporting one of the major themes of this book: The relationship between individuals and their environments is complicated. Certainly, life does sometimes deal us a bad hand. Sometimes we are stung by "the slings and arrows of outrageous fortune," as Shakespeare's Prince Hamlet said. But as we found in this study, the tendency to have high versus low levels of life stress is a somewhat stable trait. And, more interestingly, genetic factors play a strong role in that stability. To put it more succinctly, we are responsible, directly or indirectly, for a fair proportion of the stressful situations we experience. Part of what makes us prone to create stressful environments is earlier environmental experiences, but more of this tendency appears to come from genes that we have inherited. For example, people who, because of their genetically influenced temperament, are irritable and hot tempered or those with strong, domineering personalities will provoke hostility in others much more often than will their sunnier, more imperturbable counterparts and thus may experience more interpersonal difficulties.

SOCIAL SUPPORT

In Chapter 8, we introduced the concept of social support, which we defined broadly as the caring and sustenance an individual obtains from the social environment. In the thousands of studies that have examined social support, it has nearly always been conceptualized as an environmental variable—something the environment provides for the person. Three lines of evidence suggest that this unidirectional model—in which the social environment impinges on the individual but not vice versa—may be unrealistic.

First, level of social support is significantly correlated with personality, suggesting that personal characteristics influence the amount of social support an individual receives (Sarason et al., 1986; Monroe & Steiner, 1986). Extraverts tend to report higher levels of social support than introverts. Individuals who are highly neurotic tend to report lower quality of social support than those with easygoing personalities.

Second, positive social interactions result from active efforts that individuals make to develop and sustain supportive relationships (Antonucci & Jackson, 1990). Good social relationships do not just happen but are created.

Third, level of social support is moderately stable over time, even when there is substantial environmental change (Sarason et al., 1986). A particularly good demonstration is provided by a study of social support among Japanese high school exchange students who were placed with host families in other countries (Furukawa & Shibayama, 1997). A social support scale was administered before the students left Japan, after they had lived 6 months in an unfamiliar foreign community, and 6 months after they returned home. The correlations in level of social support across the three contexts were relatively high. To a substantial degree, individuals created social environments during their exchange similar to those they had experienced in their "home" environments.

In the VATSPSUD we wanted to understand the causes of such stability of social support. We applied the same longitudinal twin design to social support that we used with SLEs. During our first and third personal interviews with the female twin pairs, we assessed the dimensions of social support using a 16-item Social Interaction Scale (Schuster, Kessler, & Aseltine, 1990) developed at the Institute for Social Research. In these analyses we wanted to look more closely at the dimensions of social support and their stability over time. Rather than using a global measure (as in Chapter 8), we identified six aspects of social support based on factor analysis of our data (Kendler, 1997). *Relative Problems* and *Friend Problems* reflect the degree to which the twin reported relatives or friends as "making too many demands," "criticizing," and "creating tension or arguments." *Relative Support* reflects the frequency of contact with relatives and the degree to which relatives made the twins feel "they care about you" and expressed "interest in how you are doing." The *Confidant* factor reflects the access to a confidant and the number of available confidants. *Friend Support* indexes positive emotional relations with friends. *Social Integration* reflects the number of friends, the frequency of contact with them, and the frequency of club attendance.

The dimensions of social support were moderately stable over the 5-year interval between our two assessments of these measures. The time 1–time 2 correlations were: Relative Problems, 0.51; Friend Problems, 0.39; Relative Support, 0.42; Confidants, 0.42; Friend Support, 0.44; and Social Integration, 0.45.

The estimates from our twin analyses are summarized in Figure 13.4. The time-specific (transient) effects are substantial, ranging from 47 to 62% of the variance. As we discussed in the context of SLEs, these effects include short-term effects (e.g., a short-lived argument with a friend or relative a few days before the interview), as well as errors of measurement. After removing these short-term effects, the stable variation in all six dimensions of social support is substantially heritable. The results from our best-fit models indicate that 43–

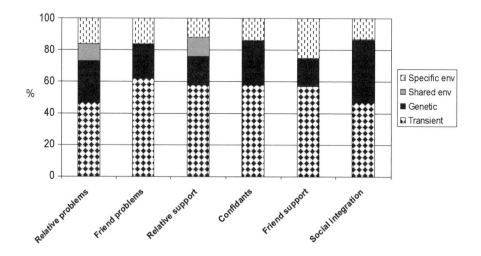

FIGURE 13.4. Proportions of variance for social support measured on two occasions. Env = environment. Data from Kendler (1997, Table 2).

75% of the variance in stable social support is due to genetic differences between individuals. Because an individual's genetically influenced temperament might influence the kinds of friends she selects, the degree to which she forms confiding relationships, and the extent to which she joins social organizations, it is reasonable that these dimensions of social support might be more heritable.

Shared family effects contributed to twin-pair resemblance for social support only for the two factors that involved relatives. These results suggest that the quality of social support from relatives may be related to the temperaments of the relatives, as well as to the temperaments of the twins. For example, if a mother is particularly critical and demanding, both of her twin daughters would have higher Relative Problem scores. This would be true both for MZ and for DZ twins, resulting in shared environmental variance. It is worth noting that genetic effects are present even for the measures of social support from relatives. This suggests that—given such a critical mother—twins from MZ pairs are, on average, more likely to develop a similar kind of relationship with her (for good or ill) than are DZ twins. As with stressful life events, the *environmental* risk factor of social support is relatively heritable.

An important issue in social support research is the distinction between objective and subjective measures. That is, have we measured how the world truly treats the twins or only how the twins see themselves as being treated? Our results are based on respondent report, so we cannot determine definitively whether we have found evidence for genetic factors that actually influence how individuals interact with their social environments or genetic factors that influence the ways twins perceive their social environments.

However, we can obtain some information by comparing the pattern of results for the four scales on which the twins reported about emotional aspects of their social relations (Relative Problems, Relative Support, Friend Problems, and Friend Support) with the results for the remaining two scales (Confidants and Social Integration), on which the twins report the more objective measures: number and frequency of their social contacts. If the observed heritability of social support was a reflection of a *plaintive set* that individuals bring to the world (e.g., as the childhood song goes, "nobody likes me, everybody hates me, guess I'll eat some worms"), we would predict *higher* heritability estimates for the four scales that reflect the emotional nature of social relations than for the two scales that measure social contact. However, the opposite is observed. The highest heritability estimates are for the two scales that report more objective phenomena: Confidants and Social Integration. These results suggest that we are assessing some features of the objective social reality.

We are aware of one other twin study that has examined social support across multiple occasions. This study was performed in Sweden and involved older twins, some of whom were reared together and others who were reared apart (Bergeman, Neiderhiser, Pedersen, & Plomin, 2001). Despite the age and cultural differences between this study and our own, the results are similar. The investigators reported moderate heritability for three factors of social support and evidence that the same set of genes influenced social support across time. So, as we saw with SLEs, it is far more correct to say of the relationship between individuals and their environments that each affects the other (person ↔ environment) than to say only that people are affected by their environments (person ← environment).

PARENTING

As we described in Chapter 7, the manner in which a child is reared by his or her parents has long been considered a crucial determinant of mental health. Many studies, including our own, suggest a relationship between parenting received and risk for psychopathology later in life. Nearly all studies of parenting consider it to be an "environmental" variable, but as we just saw for social support, this perspective is probably an oversimplification. Parenting is a complex, dyadic process that is influenced by many factors, including temperamental characteristics of the parent that influence *provision* of parenting and temperamental characteristics of the child that *elicit* the type of parenting received.

As with SLEs and social support, we set out to understand the sources of individual differences in parenting using a twin design. Our sample of female–female twins provided an opportunity to explore the role of genetic and environmental influences on parenting from two different perspectives: twins reporting on the parenting they received from their fathers and mothers and twins reporting on the parenting they provided to their own children. These two viewpoints make for a more complex but richer view of the phenomenon of parenting than we obtained for SLEs or social support. We can, in effect, study the genetics of parenting as seen from the perspectives of both parent and child. We used the same measures of parenting described previously (see Sidebar 7.1), using three factors derived from a brief version of the Parental Bonding Instrument (PBI; Parker, Tupling, & Brown, 1979). Here we focus solely on the dimension of parental *warmth*, because this was the dimension most strongly related to risk for psychiatric and substance use disorders (see Chapter 7).

Parenting Received

First, let's consider three simplified scenarios for influences on how parents treat their children and what these predict for the results of a twin study of parenting received. In the first scenario, each parent treats all of his or her children exactly the same, regardless of the genetic similarity of the children. In this case, twins from MZ and DZ pairs would be equally similar for parenting received and twin resemblance, for parenting received would be estimated as entirely due to shared environmental factors. In the second scenario, parents modify their parenting style in reaction to genetically influenced characteristics of their children. Now the similarity of parenting received by twins in a pair would be a direct result of the twin-pair genetic resemblance; that is, the level of similarity in parenting received by MZ pairs would be twice as great as that received by DZ pairs (because MZ twins are, on average, twice as genetically similar as DZ twins). In this case, a twin study would find that all similarity for parenting received would be due entirely to genetic factors. In our final scenario, parents treat their children differently from one another but in a way that is unrelated to the child's genetic constitution (perhaps engaging in unpredictable, erratic parenting). In this case the parenting experience of each child in a family would be uncorrelated, and a twin study would find that variability in parenting is due entirely to individual-specific factors.

We analyzed information from members of 547 MZ and 390 DZ twin pairs who provided ratings of the parenting provided to them by their mothers and fathers (Kendler, 1996b). The pair correlations for levels of paternal and maternal warmth were much higher for MZ pairs ($r = 0.71$ and 0.61, respectively) than for DZ pairs ($r = 0.48$ and 0.38, respectively). The estimates from twin model fitting, shown in Figure 13.5, suggest that genetic factors are a major influence on twin resemblance for parenting received. For paternal warmth, shared environment also played a significant role.

These results reflect genetic influences on *elicitation of parenting*. Presumably, the level of parental warmth shown by parents reflects genetically mediated characteristics of their offspring.

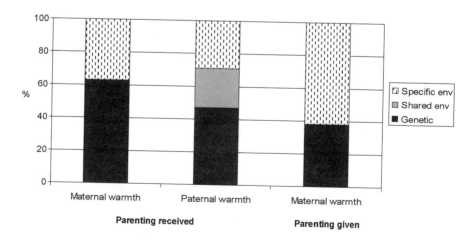

FIGURE 13.5. Proportions of variance for parental warmth as rated by the twin: Received and given. Env = environment. Data from Kendler (1996b, Table 2).

Parenting Given

Now let's consider what genetic and environmental influences mean when twins report on the parenting they provide to their own children. If the way a woman raises her children is entirely a result of attitudes and values obtained from her family of origin, then variation in parenting style would be entirely due to shared environment; the similarity of the parenting received in offspring of pairs of female–female MZ twins and DZ twins would be the same. If the way a woman raises her children is solely a result of her own genotype, then parenting given would be entirely genetically based; the similarity of parenting received from mothers who are twins would be twice as great for the offspring of MZ twin pairs as for the offspring of DZ pairs. If the way a woman raises her children is unrelated to her family background and to her genotype, then parenting would be entirely individual specific; the parenting experienced by offspring of MZ and DZ twin pairs would be uncorrelated.

We analyzed data from 145 MZ and 117 DZ pairs of female twins who reported on the parenting they provided to their own children (Kendler, 1996b).[1] We found moderate resemblance for the parenting reports of MZ pairs ($r = 0.44$) and no resemblance for DZ pairs ($r = -0.01$). As shown in Figure 13.5, the source of the pair resemblance for warmth provided was entirely genetic with a moderate heritability (38%). These results reflect genetic effects on the *provision of parenting* whereby parental behavior is directly influenced by genetically mediated characteristics of the parent.[2]

Interpretation of Parenting Studies

The most plausible interpretation of these results is that genetic factors have significant impact on both the provision of parental warmth and its elicitation. It seems likely that these genetic influences act through temperament and personality. In other words, some parents are, by their natures, more loving and caring than others, and some children are, by their natures, easier to love and care for.

Our results are similar to those obtained by other twin studies of parenting received. Of particular interest are the results from two studies of separated identical twins (Hur & Bouchard, 1995; Plomin, McClearn, Pedersen, Nesselroade, & Bergeman, 1988). Although the twins within a pair were reared by different sets of parents, the twin–cotwin ratings of parental warmth received correlated from 0.30 to 0.37. These results provide compelling evidence for a role of genetic factors in the *elicitation* of parental warmth. Our findings are also consistent with most prior studies in suggesting that genetic factors play a larger role in maternal than in paternal warmth. If true, this finding would suggest that parenting provided by mothers, perhaps due to more intense contact with children in their early years, is more sensitive to the genetically influenced temperament of their children than is the parenting provided by fathers.

Evidence from an observational study of young twins confirms the existence of genetic influences on elicited parenting. In responding to twin behavior, parents treated MZ pairs more similarly than DZ pairs. However, for the subset of "parent-initiated actions" (parenting behavior that was not a response to twin behavior), there was no difference between the similarity of treatment received by MZ and DZ pairs (Lytton, 1977). That is, the greater similarity of parental treatment of MZ twins resulted entirely from actions that the parents made *in response to behavior of the twins*. These results provide further support for the idea that parental behavior is influenced by the genetic predispositions of children.

We are aware of one other study that has examined parenting provided by twins. More than 1,000 elderly twins provided ratings on a short form of the PBI. The heritability of a construct similar to parental warmth was estimated to be between 23 and 39%. As with our study, no evidence was found for shared environmental effects (Perusse, Neale, Heath, & Eaves, 1994).

A major methodological issue in the interpretation of the findings from our studies of parenting is the validity of retrospective self-report measures. Perhaps our results reflect only the *perception* of twins as parents or as children and tell us little about what really happens between parents and offspring. However, other evidence suggests that these results cannot be entirely due to perceptions. Significant heritability has been found for measures of parental warmth obtained from external sources, including ratings by cotwins in our study, and from trained raters in a study of videotaped parent–adolescent interactions (O'Connor, Hetherington, Reiss, & Plomin, 1995).

Interestingly, our results for two other dimensions of parenting, protectiveness and authoritarianism, suggest that shared environmental influences are more important than genetic factors in influencing how parents treat their children (see Kendler, 1996b). This finding suggests that, unlike warmth, parental discipline style and willingness to allow children to be independent appear to originate in the beliefs of parents about how children should be raised and are not as sensitive to the behavior of the children themselves.

SUMMARY

In this chapter, we have taken three key "environmental" risk factors frequently used in studies of psychiatric disorders (SLEs, low levels of social support, and poor parenting) and studied them through the eyes of geneticists. We have found strong evidence, bolstered by similar findings from other research groups, that genetic factors significantly influence the probability that an individual will be exposed to these experiences. There are, in other words, *genetic influences on exposure to the environment* (Kendler & Eaves, 1986). In the traditional view of gene action, depicted in Figure 13.6, genetic expression that affects disease susceptibility takes place in a physiological internal milieu—that is, inside the skin. For example, it has long been postu-

Organism

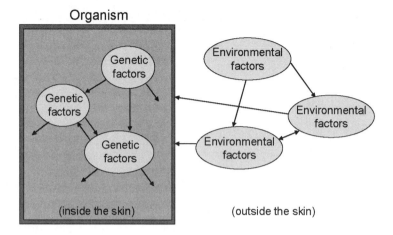

FIGURE 13.6. Traditional model of gene and environmental action.

lated that the risk for psychiatric disorders may be influenced by genetic variation coding for the synthesis, metabolism, and receptor sites for key brain neurotransmitter systems. This is a classic example of an "inside the skin" genetic pathway. Two other features of this traditional model are that the environment (which is conceived of as outside the skin) also influences disease susceptibility and that the causal relationship flows entirely in one direction: from the environment to the person.

Our findings suggest that this model is overly simplistic. For an animal as quintessentially social as Homo sapiens, our genes often reach "beyond the skin" to influence the interpersonal environment. Many examples in the animal and plant kingdom illustrate such an outside-the-skin pathway for genetic effects. For example, human cold viruses have probably evolved to tickle the human nose so that a sneeze can pass the virus to its next host. Certain butterflies, which taste good to birds, have evolved wing patterns that mimic the appearance of butterflies that birds do not like, providing protection from their avian predators. The target of this aspect of butterfly evolution is outside the butterfly—on the visual systems of their predators.

Let us illustrate the concepts of *genetic control of exposure to the environment* and *outside the skin* pathways with an example from general medicine. Assume that a cancer geneticist has collected a sample of 400 patients with lung cancer and 400 control participants. She scans a chromosome looking for gene variants that differentiate the two groups and finds a gene that is much more common among the lung cancer patients. With great excitement, she writes up her results and submits them to a major scientific journal, claiming to have found a new oncogene (i.e., a gene that can cause cancer). However, unbeknownst to her, the gene has no effect on the risk for cancer at a physiological level. Instead, it exerts an indirect effect, through behavior, on the risk for chronic cigarette smoking. For example, genetically controlled variation in nicotine receptors, which stimulate the pleasure centers in the brain, might affect the chances that individuals will seek repeated exposure to carcinogenic compounds.

Has this researcher really found a new oncogene? Yes and no. Traditional oncogenes act via inside-the-skin pathways (e.g., by influencing cell division), whereas this oncogene acts via an outside-the-skin pathway. This oncogene will have a few unusual properties not possessed by traditional oncogenes. In a culture in which tobacco is not smoked, it will have no effect on cancer risk. Any social process that reduces the frequency of heavy tobacco smoking (such as reduced social acceptability or increased taxation) will reduce the impact of the oncogene on risk for lung cancer.

When considering something as flexible as human behavior, a revised view of gene action is indicated. A schematic of an interactionist model is depicted in Figure 13.7. By influencing behavior, genetic factors affect the external social milieu via a pathway outside the skin. Here, environmental influences also reach back across the skin. One example is that taking psycho-active substances can alter the activity of genes that code for neurotransmitters. The results of our studies suggest the need to conceptualize gene action more broadly than the inside-the-skin pathway depicted in Figure 13.6. Genes may act on the brain to alter risk directly via neurobiological mechanisms and/or indirectly by acting on the brain to produce behavior that alters the environment. These environmental changes in turn alter environmental stress or affect social environments in ways that increase (or decrease) disease susceptibility. When we consider genetic effects on risk for psychiatric disorders, we should keep in mind that such outside-the-skin pathways supplement the traditional inside-the-skin pathways.[3]

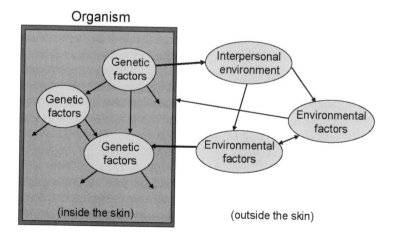

FIGURE 13.7. Interactionist model of gene and environmental action.

NOTES

1. The number of pairs is lower in this study, as it included only pairs whose children were at least 4 years old. We added this requirement because parental relations with infants and toddlers might be somewhat different from those established with older children.

2. The astute reader might have detected what is a slight confound to our analyses of the "genetic" effect of providing parenting. Because the offspring of MZ twins are more closely related genetically than the offspring of DZ pairs, some of the detected genetic effect on provision could be due to a genetic effect on elicitation. However, the effect from elicitation (due to correlations—for a perfectly heritable trait—of 0.125 and 0.0625 in offspring of MZ and DZ pairs, respectively) would explain only a small part of what we observed.

3. The model depicted in Figure 13.7 is consistent with a long body of research in the social and psychological sciences that supports an interactionist model of human behavior in which there is a bidirectional causal relationship between persons and their social and physical environments (Endler, 1983; Magnusson, 1988).

CHAPTER FOURTEEN

Mechanisms for Genetic Control of Exposure to the Environment

In Chapter 13 we showed that genetic factors can influence the risk for experiencing environmental adversity. In this chapter, we explore two sets of questions raised by these findings. First, through what mechanisms might genes influence the probability of exposure to environmental stress? What psychological processes might mediate the effect of genes on the environment? Second, what is the relationship between the genetic risk factors that predispose to environmental adversity and those that predispose to psychopathology? In particular, could they in part be the same genes?

MECHANISMS THROUGH WHICH GENETIC FACTORS INFLUENCE EXPOSURE TO ENVIRONMENTAL STRESS

How could genetic risk factors affect the probability of our exposure to environmental adversities such as SLEs or conflictual interpersonal relationships? Clearly, genes do not "directly" code for the probability of our experiencing such adversities. Instead, genes probably influence a wide range of traits that in turn contribute, via a complex set of pathways, to the risk for environmental adversities.

Despite this complexity, we wanted to gain some insight into the processes by which genes influence exposure to environmental adversities. We chose to focus on personality as a possible mediator and, in particular, the personality trait of neuroticism (see Sidebar 11.3). We selected neuroticism for three reasons. First, it is moderately heritable, with most estimates of heritability ranging from 30 to 45% (Loehlin, 1992; Lake, Eaves, Maes, Heath, & Martin, 2000). Second, in adults, measures of neuroticism are quite stable over time (McCrae & Costa, 1990). Third, we thought it was psychologically plausible that individuals who are low on neuroticism and are characterized by emotional stability and an "easy" temperament would be less prone to "getting into trouble" in life than those who have high levels of neuroticism and tend to manifest emotional instability, dysphoria, and irritability.

We conducted analyses to examine the causal relationship between neuroticism and future SLEs and social support. As we discussed in Chapter 8, causal inferences are subject to a number of biases, especially when all the measures are collected at the same time from the same person. Our approach was to use time, multiple informants, and family factors to help clarify the causal relationships. We describe in detail the strategy we applied for SLEs, then discuss the results for predicting SLEs and social support.

Stressful Life Events

The strategy we used is illustrated in Figure 14.1. The outcome being predicted is the number of SLEs experienced during the past year, as reported by twins during the FF3 interview.[1] We predicted SLEs from three measures of neuroticism. The first of these was based on the twins' self-reports obtained at the beginning of the FF study, on average about 6 years prior to the FF3 interview. Such a large time interval between the predictor and the outcome removes the possibility that recent SLEs caused an increase in neuroticism (rather than our hypothesis that higher neuroticism increases risk for SLEs).

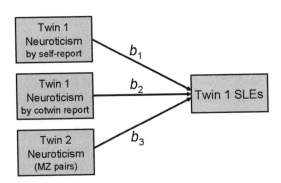

FIGURE 14.1. Twin model for studying genetic control of exposure to stressful life events (SLEs). We predict SLEs reported by twin 1 from three different reports of neuroticism: twin 1's neuroticism reported by twin 1 (path b_1), twin 1's neuroticism reported by twin 2 (path b_2), and twin 2's neuroticism reported by twin 2 in MZ pairs only.

The second variable used to predict SLEs was neuroticism as reported by the respondents' cotwin. We used this *cross-twin prediction* to help us evaluate the plausible hypothesis that the association between neuroticism and adversities is artifactual, resulting from reporting bias. How might such a bias arise? Imagine that people are divisible into those with a "plaintive set" and those with "rose-colored glasses." The former view everything in a negative light, exaggerating their own level of personality dysfunction, overreporting the number and severity of their SLEs (e.g., reporting as a major relationship difficulty what was in reality a minor disagreement), and judging all their relationships as being worse then they really are. Those with rose-colored glasses do the reverse, seeing their own personalities and the world around them more favorably than is actually the case. If lots of people have these sorts of biases, we would find a strong correlation between neuroticism and measures of adversity even if there were no true causal link between the two.

However, this type of reporting bias occurs only when the *same person* reports on her own personality and adversities. If *different individuals* report on these two variables, the hypothesis predicts that any artificial association should disappear. We asked each twin to rate her own personality and the personality of her cotwin. If the association between SLEs and neuroticism as reported by the cotwin (path b_2 in Figure 14.1) is less than that for SLEs and self-reported neuroticism (path b_1), this is evidence for reporting bias.

The third variable used to predict SLEs is the MZ cotwin's report of her own neuroticism (path b_3).[2] This variable was included to determine the role of *familial* factors in the association between neuroticism and SLEs. Because neuroticism and SLEs are influenced modestly by genetic factors, it is possible that there are familial factors that influence both of these traits. Because MZ twins share both their genotypes and their rearing environment, the contribution of familial factors to the association between neuroticism and adversities can be approximated by comparing the magnitude of path b_3 with those of paths b_1 and b_2. For example, if familial factors were entirely responsible for the relationship between neuroticism and adversities, then the adversities experienced by twin 1 in an MZ pair could be equally predicted from twin 1's neuroticism (as indicated by path b_1 or b_2) or from twin 2's neuroticism (path b_3).

We first predicted total SLEs from self-reported neuroticism and got an estimate of $0.09 \pm .02$. This analysis used a technique called Poisson regression, so these estimates do not have a simple meaning. Suffice it to say that the relationship is modest but highly statistically significant ($p < 0.0001$). Then we looked at neuroticism reported by the cotwin and, to our surprise, got a number that was slightly higher ($0.11 \pm .02$; $p < 0.0001$). The finding that the path for neuroticism as reported by the cotwin (path b_2) was not lower than that obtained for neuroticism by self-report (path b_1) suggests that the association we observed was not due to reporting bias. Finally, we looked at the neuroticism score of one MZ twin as a predictor of the SLEs reported 4 years later by her cotwin and obtained a very similar estimate ($0.08 \pm .02$; $p < 0.01$). This result indicates that most of the association is due to familial factors that contribute to both neuroticism and SLEs.

Social Support

We then predicted our aggregate measure of social support (see Sidebar 8.5) from the three different measures of neuroticism. High levels of self-reported neuroticism rather strongly predicted lower levels of social support 6 years later (-0.20 ± 0.03, $p < 0.0001$). (Here we used standard regression, so the estimate has a simple meaning: the proportion of a standard deviation change in the aggregate social support measure that we observe for every standard deviation change in neuroticism). Neuroticism as reported by the cotwin also predicted social support (-0.15 ± 0.03, $p < 0.0001$), but not as strongly as did self-report, suggesting the existence of some reporting bias. Finally, neuroticism scores of one MZ twin predicted her cotwin's future social support at a level that was significant but not as strong as those based on twin 1's neuroticism (-0.11 ± 0.03, $p < 0.01$), indicating that some, but not all, of this association was due to familial factors.

Implications

Three points are worth emphasizing about these results. First, we showed rather conclusively that neuroticism has at least a modest relationship with two important classes of "environmental" risk factors: SLEs and social support. These results are impressive because such a long interval separated our measures of neuroticism and the reports of environmental adversity. People with highly emotional personalities report more frequent stressful events and more difficult, conflictual relationships than do individuals with more stable and less reactive temperaments. Second, we have good evidence that this association is not due to reporting bias to any substantial degree (although a modest bias may operate in the relationship between neuroticism and measures of social support). Third, familial factors strongly contribute to the association between neuroticism and these environmental adversities. These results are consistent with our original hypothesis that personality in general and neuroticism more specifically may partly mediate the effects of genetic risk factors on exposure to environmental adversities.

Several other studies have found that dimensions of personality—particularly neuroticism—correlate substantially with the tendency to experience social adversities (Headey & Wearing, 1989; Magnus, Diener, Fujita, & Pavot, 1993; Monroe & Steiner, 1986; Windle, 1992). One study of elderly twins from Sweden is especially relevant to our own. Saudino and colleagues examined SLEs and the three major personality traits of neuroticism, extroversion, and openness to experience (Saudino, Pedersen, Lichtenstein, McClearn, & Plomin, 1997). They found that all of the genetic influences on what we would call dependent SLEs (see Sidebar 8.3) were mediated through these personality dimensions. Although this result must be replicated in other samples before we can accept it with confidence, it appears likely that personality plays a substantial role in the complex pathway from genes to the liability to encounter high-risk psychosocial environments.

ARE THE GENETIC RISK FACTORS
FOR ENVIRONMENTAL ADVERSITIES RELATED
TO THOSE FOR PSYCHIATRIC DISORDERS?

We have demonstrated that genetic factors influence the risk for many psychiatric disorders. We have also shown that genetic factors influence the probability of exposure to several environmental factors that increase risk for these disorders. A logical next question is: What is the relationship between these two sets of genetic risk factors—those that predispose to psychiatric illness and those that predispose to environmental adversities?[3]

To attempt to answer this question for SLEs and the liability to MD and alcoholism, we again turned to our FF sample. These analyses were based on the first two waves of interviews with the FF sample and used the same categories of SLEs—those experienced over the preceding year—that we have examined previously (see Chapter 8). As with the analyses earlier in this chapter, we used regression with cross-twin prediction. The form of regression was the same event-history analysis using a discrete time approach (Allison, 1982; Kalbfleisch & Prentice, 1980; Laird & Olivier, 1981) that we described in Chapter 8. We wanted to know whether a lifetime history of MD in one twin predicted the occurrence of SLEs in her cotwin. We reasoned that if a history of MD in one twin significantly predicted the occurrence of a particular type of SLE in her cotwin, and if this relationship was stronger among MZ than DZ pairs, then we would have presumptive evidence that the genetic factors that influence risk for MD also influence risk for that class of SLEs.

The results for MD are depicted in Figure 14.2. The first bar in each pair shows the OR for MZ pairs between lifetime MD in one twin and the risk for a category of SLEs in her cotwin. For example, having an MZ cotwin with versus without a lifetime history of MD significantly increases a woman's risk for having a serious marital problem during the 2 years covered by these two interviews (OR = 1.50). Among DZ pairs, the results are also significant, but the OR is lower (OR = 1.38). For 7 of the 12 SLE classes (network conflict, job loss, marital problems, divorce or other breakup, assault, major financial problems, and illness/injury), we obtained evidence for overlapping genetic influence on MD and SLEs. That is, a history of MD in one twin significantly predicted the occurrence of an SLE class in her MZ cotwin, and this relationship was stronger among MZ than DZ pairs. It is noteworthy that most of these categories reflect interpersonal problems.[4]

To explore the specificity between the risk for SLEs and the liability to psychiatric illness, we also examined the relationship between risk for SLEs and cotwin history of alcoholism. The results are depicted in Figure 14.3.[5] Our genetic model indicated a significant relationship between genetic risk factors for alcoholism and four SLEs: network conflict, serious marital problems, serious legal problems, and being robbed. Of these four event categories, two are also significantly increased by risk for MD (marital problems and network conflict). The two that are unique to alcoholism (being robbed and serious legal problems) reflect more externalizing-like problems. These results

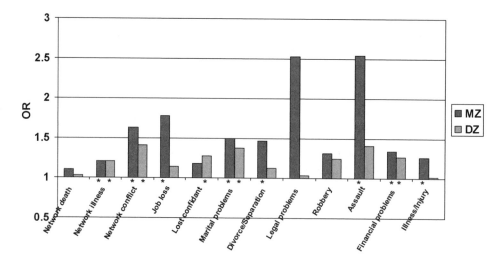

FIGURE 14.2. Odds ratios (OR) for the association between major depression in one twin and the 2-year occurrence of stressful life events in the other twin; MZ = monozygotic; DZ = dizygotic; *significantly different from 1.0 ($p < 0.05$). Data from Kendler and Karkowski-Shuman (1997, Table 2).

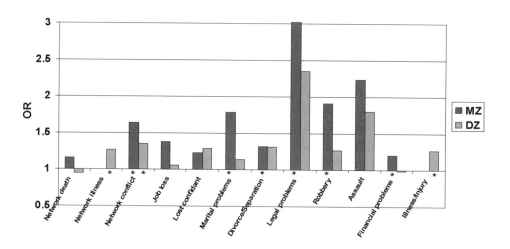

FIGURE 14.3. Odds ratios (OR) for the association between alcoholism in one twin and the 2-year occurrence of stressful life events in the other twin; *significantly different from 1.0 ($p < 0.05$). Data from Kendler and Karkowski-Shuman (1997, Table 2).

suggest that there is some specificity in the relationship between genetic risk for particular psychiatric and substance use disorders on the one hand and SLE categories on the other.

In summary, these analyses support the existence of an "outside the skin" genetic pathway, as discussed in Chapter 13 (see Figure 13.7). We suspect that similar associations exist for other disorders and risk factors.

SUMMARY

This chapter has presented a series of responses to the results of Chapter 13, which showed that several key "environmental" risk factors for psychiatric illness are in part "genetic." First, we explored the mechanisms whereby genes could influence exposure to environmental adversities. We showed that the personality trait of neuroticism is a good candidate for a mediating variable—one that lies between genes and risk of environmental exposure. Second, we demonstrated that the genetic risk factors for some psychiatric disorders are correlated with the genetic factors that influence SLEs—a key "environmental" risk factor.

The picture that is emerging from this work is a complex one. The clear dividing line between genetic and environmental risk factors for psychiatric disorders has become a lot blurrier. What we once saw as the neat and static categories of genetic and environmental risk factors are in reality dynamic, shifting, and interacting.

In the next chapter, we return to the question of the causal relationship between environmental adversities and risk for psychiatric and substance use disorders. We viewed this question in some detail with our "epidemiologist's hat" in Chapters 7 and 8. Now we need to examine it with our "geneticist's hat" to address the questions posed in this chapter. If genetic factors predispose to environmental exposure, and if some of these factors also influence risk of illness, then can we be sure that environmental exposure really causes illness? Or is it just a byproduct of having a high genetic risk? As it turns out, the most powerful way to address this key question about environmental risk factors is to use our genetic design.

NOTES

1. The original analysis reported results for different types of life events (see Kendler, Gardner, & Prescott, 2003b). For simplicity we combined across event types for the results reported here.

2. This part of the analysis was conducted only among MZ twin pairs.

3. The astute reader will note that two sets of results presented earlier in this book suggest that we ought to find a significant correlation between these two sets of genetic risk factors. We showed in Chapter 11 that genetic risk factors for MD and the personality trait of neuroticism are highly correlated; in this chapter we saw that

neuroticism predicts the occurrence of both SLEs and low levels of social support and that this association is largely mediated through familial factors. Nonetheless, we felt it important to try to demonstrate directly the relationship between genetic risk factors for psychiatric illness and those for environmental adversity.

4. The study was originally published in Kendler and Karkowski-Shuman (1997). We conducted several follow-up analyses to confirm and extend these findings. Briefly, (1) the genetic influences were confirmed using a different method; (2) the relationship between genetic risk for MD and exposure to SLEs was not due to individuals being depressed at the time of the SLE; and (3) standard bivariate twin analyses conducted for MD and the more common personal SLEs estimated the genetic correlation (with quite large standard errors!) between the liabilities to MD and these SLEs as: divorce/breakup, 1.00; serious illness, 0.53; and major financial problems, 0.41.

5. In these analyses, alcoholism was defined broadly to include alcohol dependence by DSM-III-R criteria or problem drinking. Data were not available on episodes of alcohol dependence in the preceding year, so it was not possible to control for the effect of "active" alcoholism in mediating the relationship between genetic risk for alcoholism and SLEs.

CHAPTER FIFTEEN

Is the Relation between Environmental Risk Factors and Psychiatric Disorders Causal?

In this book we have demonstrated that many of the putative environmental risk factors long studied by mental health researchers are influenced by genetic factors. Furthermore, there is some overlap between the genes that influence exposure to these risk factors and those that predispose to psychiatric illness. At this point, one might wonder whether there is any *causal* relationship between these environmental factors and risk for psychiatric illness. As illustrated in Figure 15.1, perhaps all that is happening is that the same set of genes influences both risk for psychiatric disorders (e.g., adult MD) and risk for environmental adversities (e.g., poor parenting). If this is true, we would expect environmental adversities and psychiatric illness to be highly correlated in the population, but these adversities would not necessarily have any causal impact on risk for psychiatric illness.

In Chapters 7 and 8, we presented a series of analyses, using standard epidemiological methods, to evaluate whether the correlations between environmental adversities and psychiatric illness were causal. In every instance, our results suggested some degree of causality: Environmental risk factors were, at least in part, truly increasing the risk for psychiatric illness. We now return to this critical issue using a complementary approach that takes advantage of our

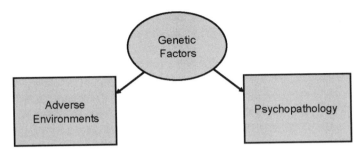

FIGURE 15.1. Genetic factors as the basis for the association between parenting received in childhood and adult depression.

genetic design. As we hope to convince the reader, this is a particularly powerful method for addressing this central conundrum in psychiatric research. Furthermore, its success demonstrates a central theme of this book: the interweaving of genetic and environmental risks for psychiatric illness. To show convincingly what the environment does, we have to be able to control for genetic effects.

In this chapter we use genetic strategies to evaluate the potential causal effects of five environmental risk factors: early alcohol use, SLEs, smoking, CSA, and childhood parental loss.

COTWIN-CONTROL DESIGN

At this point we introduce the *cotwin-control design*, which provides a powerful way to test for causality. Many studies in epidemiology begin with an *index* group of participants who have been exposed to a particular risk factor and a matched *control* group who have not been so exposed. The rates of a particular illness in the exposed and unexposed groups are compared to determine whether the risk factor is associated with increased risk for illness. A cotwin-control study is designed to achieve this same aim by selecting twin pairs in which one twin has been exposed to a risk factor and the other has not. Not only are such twins well matched for any background variables such as social class or environmental exposures in childhood but also, unlike with other designs, they are also matched for their genetic background. Therefore, an increased risk for disease in the exposed versus the unexposed twin can be taken as strong evidence that the risk factor is causally related to disease risk.

It is worth spending some time exploring why the cotwin-control method is so potentially powerful. After all, in Chapters 7 and 8 we presented a number of analyses that showed that environmental factors predicted risk of illness, even after controlling for possible confounding variables. Given these results, why should we apply other techniques? This question has a simple answer. The method we used previously works only for those confounding variables that we know about and are able to measure. Because in human genetics we do only observational science—we never conduct controlled experiments—we must also be concerned about the confounds that we do not know about. By studying pairs of twins who share their genetic and family backgrounds, we control for a whole host of such possible confounding variables—those we know about and, most important, those we do not.

A full cotwin-control design involves the comparison of the association between a risk factor and an outcome in three samples: (1) in the entire sample, (2) within DZ twin pairs discordant for exposure to the risk factor, and (3) within MZ pairs discordant for exposure to the risk factor. Three different patterns of results are illustrated in Figure 15.2. The results on the left side of the figure show the pattern obtained if the risk factor–outcome association is entirely causal. Controlling for family background or genetic factors makes no difference to the size of the association, and the three estimates are the same (within the limits of statistical fluctuation).

The middle set of results in Figure 15.2 shows an example in which part of the risk factor–outcome association is due to genetic factors that influence both the risk factor and the outcome (e.g., SLEs and MD). Here the association is strongest in the entire sample (in which genetic and causal effects are entirely confounded, as we control for neither genetic nor shared environmental factors), intermediate among discordant DZ twins (with whom we control for shared environmental factors and partly for genetic background), and lowest among discordant MZ pairs (with whom we control entirely for both shared environmental and genetic background). The degree to which the association declines from the entire sample to discordant MZ pairs is a rough measure of the proportion of the association that is genetic.

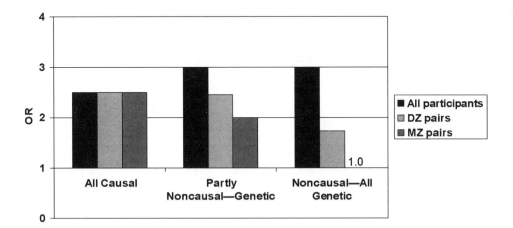

FIGURE 15.2. Interpretation of results obtained from studies using a cotwin-control design. OR = odds ratio for increased risk for a disorder given exposure to a risk factor; DZ = dizygotic; MZ = monozygotic.

The results on the right side of Figure 15.2 show the extreme case, in which *all* of the risk factor–outcome association is due to shared genetic effects and the risk factor has no real environmental effect on the outcome. Thus within discordant MZ pairs there will be no association between the risk factor and the outcome (i.e., an OR of 1.0), and the association within discordant DZ pairs is midway between 1 and the value for the entire sample.

Does Early Drinking Increase Risk for Alcoholism?

In general population samples, an early age at first drink has been consistently associated with an increased risk for developing alcoholism (Grant & Dawson, 1997). The prevalence of alcoholism among individuals who first try alcohol before age 15 is as high as 50% in some studies. Several studies that found this effect interpreted it to be a causal one—that early drinking *directly* produces an increased risk for later alcohol problems. On the basis of this interpretation, calls have been made to delay the age at first drink among early adolescents as a means of decreasing risk for adult alcohol problems (Pedersen & Skrondal, 1998).

However, as we have said before, correlation need not equal causation. There is another interpretation of these results (e.g., Jessor & Jessor, 1977). Early drinking could be just one manifestation of a broad liability to deviance that might be evident in a host of problem behaviors, such as use of illicit substances, antisocial behavior, lower educational achievement, and adult alcoholism. If this were the case, delaying the first exposure to alcohol use would not alter the underlying liability to adolescent problem behavior or to adult alcoholism.

We decided to use data from the VATSPSUD to test this important question: Does early drinking lead directly to alcoholism?[1] We found a strong association between lifetime prevalence of alcoholism and reported age at first drink among both males and females (Prescott & Kendler, 1999). As shown in Figure 15.3, males who began drinking before age 15 were twice as likely (OR = 2.0) to develop DSM-IV alcohol dependence (AD) as those who did not drink early. The value for females was even more dramatic: Early drinkers were more than four times as likely to develop AD as other women.

The information for testing causality comes from the twin pairs who were discordant for early drinking. Under the causal hypothesis, we would expect that the twins with earlier drinking onset would have higher risk for alcoholism than their later drinking cotwins and that the same pattern would hold for MZ and DZ pairs. But if early age at drinking is just an index of general deviance that influences (among other things) risk of developing alcoholism, we would expect that the prevalence would be similar for members of MZ discordant-onset pairs. The "unexposed" twins (those with a later onset of drinking) would be expected to share their cotwins' risk for behavioral deviance and thus have a higher risk for alcoholism than that seen in pairs in which neither twin drank early. The pattern observed in MZ versus DZ

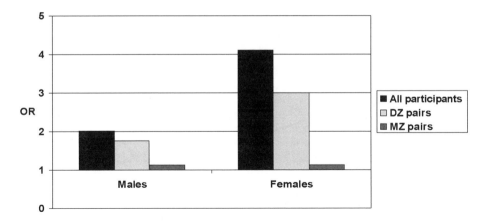

FIGURE 15.3. Odds ratios (OR) from cotwin-control analyses of the association between drinking before age 15 and later alcohol dependence.

discordant-onset pairs tells us to what degree familial resemblance for behavioral deviance is due to shared environmental versus genetic factors. If it is due to shared environmental factors, the risk for alcoholism among the unexposed twins from DZ discordant-onset pairs would be expected to be the same as that in the MZ pairs. However, if familial resemblance for deviance is due to genetic factors, the risk for alcoholism to an unexposed individual would be lower among DZ than MZ pairs.

As shown in Figure 15.3, the twin-pair resemblance was inconsistent with the causal hypothesis. Instead, the results suggested that early drinking and later alcoholism are both the result of a shared genetic liability. For example, among the 213 male and 69 female MZ pairs who were discordant for early drinking, there was only a slight difference in the prevalence of AD between the twins who drank early and the cotwins who did not. The ORs were 1.1 for both sexes, not statistically different from the 1.0 value predicted by the noncausal model for MZ pairs. The ORs for the DZ pairs were midway between those of the MZ pairs and the general sample, indicating that the source of the familial liability is genetic rather than environmental.

We then used our standard bivariate twin-pair model (e.g., Figure 11.1) to estimate the genetic and environmental overlap between drinking onset and risk for AD. We conducted this analysis so that we could treat drinking onset age as a continuous variable rather than relying on the (somewhat arbitrary) cutoff age of 15 (as we needed to do in order to calculate ORs). The results are depicted in Figure 15.4. Among males, 18% of the variation in liability to AD overlapped with age at first drink, and virtually all of this was due to shared genetic factors. The results were even stronger for females. About 29% of the liability in AD overlapped with drinking onset and, again, virtually all was due to overlapping genetic factors. As suggested by the patterns portrayed

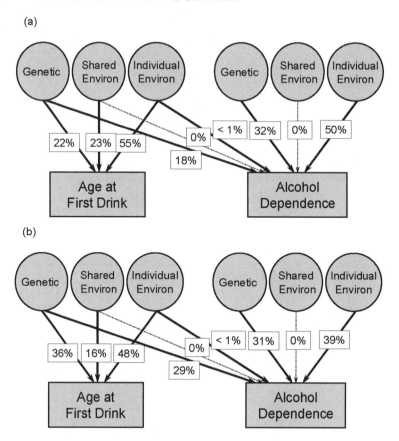

FIGURE 15.4. Results from twin analyses of the association between age at first drink and later alcohol dependence. (a) Males; (b) females. Data from Prescott and Kendler (1999, Table 3).

in Figure 15.3, the results were consistent with the behavioral deviance (correlated liability) hypothesis and completely inconsistent with the causal hypothesis.

This story of the association between age at first drink and alcoholism is one of the most striking examples we have come across of the problem with the following line of logic:

1. Investigators find a putative risk factor correlated with a given disorder.
2. They assume that the risk factor causes the disorder.
3. On the basis of this assumption, others attempt to reduce exposure to the risk factor, thereby expecting to reduce the rates of the disorder. However, if the assumption in step 2 is incorrect, step 3 is unlikely to be effective.

Lest we be misunderstood, we want to emphasize that we are not suggesting that drinking in early adolescence is benign or that efforts to reduce adolescent drinking are not worthwhile. Teenage drinking is associated with (and likely to be causal for) negative outcomes such as car accidents and other injuries. What our results do suggest is that prevention efforts aimed at delaying drinking may not be effective for reducing problem alcohol use in adulthood. Other behaviors, such as regular drinking or drinking to intoxication, may be better targets for intervention efforts.

Are Stressful Life Events Causal for Depression?

We used the cotwin-control method to examine the nature of the causal relationship between SLEs and the onset of major depression (Kendler, Karkowski, & Prescott, 1999b). As described in Chapter 8, we studied this question using our ratings of event dependence (the degree to which the SLE could have been influenced by the participant's own behavior). We found, after controlling for event severity, that independent SLEs were strongly associated with onset of MD. However, the magnitude of the association was weaker than that seen for dependent events. This is consistent with the hypothesis that at least some proportion of the SLE–MD association may be noncausal.

Among the nearly 1,900 women participating in the FF3 interview, the OR for a depressive onset in the month of the occurrence of a personal SLE was 5.64. Within pairs of DZ twins, a personal SLE was associated with an increased risk for an onset of MD, with an OR of 4.52, compared with the risk for the cotwin over the same interval. Within MZ twin pairs, the OR for this association was 3.58.[2]

These results tell us two important things about the association between SLEs and the onset of MD. First, within MZ twin pairs, who are matched for genotype and family environment, SLEs were strongly and significantly associated with subsequent episodes of MD. This finding provides strong evidence that the association observed between SLEs and MD is, at least in part, causal. Second, however, the strength of the association between SLEs and MD was lower in matched twin pairs than in the entire sample and lower in MZ than in DZ pairs. This is the middle pattern of results depicted in Figure 15.2, the one expected if only part of the observed association between SLEs and depressive onsets is mediated by shared genetic risk factors. In aggregate, these findings argue strongly that the association between SLEs and MD is also partly noncausal.

We can quantify these estimates in a commonsense way (although these estimates will not be as accurate—or elegant—as those obtained from structural equation modeling). The OR between SLEs and onsets of MD in the general sample includes all the sources of variation (a^2, c^2, and e^2), both causal (individual-specific) and noncausal (common genetic sources and family background). In contrast, the association for MZ pairs includes only the individual-specific portion (e^2). If the OR in MZ twin pairs accurately reflects the causal component of the association between onset of MD and SLEs, then the total proportion of the SLE–MD association that is causal can be estimated as the ratio of the OR in MZ pairs to the OR in the entire sample, 3.58/5.64, or 63%.[3]

Does Smoking Predispose to Depression?

We also used the cotwin-control method to look at another possible risk factor for MD: smoking. Smoking and depression are strongly associated (Anda et al., 1990). One plausible explanation is that smoking directly predisposes to depressive illness. Nicotine use and/or withdrawal could directly cause MD (Flanagan & Maany, 1982; Glassman et al., 1988) because nicotine affects several neurochemical systems in the brain that may be involved in the etiology of depression (Pomerleau & Pomerleau, 1984).

We studied the association between lifetime history of ever having smoked (as assessed in the FTQ; Fagerstrom & Schneider, 1989; see Sidebar 5.4) and lifetime history of MD (as measured at FF1) in female twin pairs (Kendler et al., 1993h). The results of the cotwin-control analysis are shown in Figure 15.5. In the entire sample, the OR for MD given a history of ever having smoked was 1.60, a value significantly greater than unity. Among the

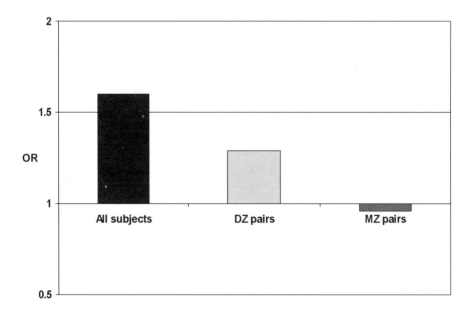

FIGURE 15.5. Odds ratios (OR) from a cotwin-control study of major depression and smoking history in women. Adapted from Kendler et al. (1993h, Figure 1). Copyright 1993 by the American Medical Association. Adapted by permission.

96 DZ twin pairs in which one had smoked and the other had not, the OR was 1.29, and among the 74 MZ twin pairs discordant for lifetime smoking, the OR was 0.96, neither of which differed significantly from unity. Most remarkably, among MZ twin pairs discordant for lifetime smoking, the rates of MD were virtually identical for the smoking twins (35.1%) and for the nonsmoking twins (36.5%). This result is completely inconsistent with smoking being a direct cause of MD.

Comparing these results with those depicted in Figure 15.2, it is clear that the pattern is exactly that predicted by the "noncausal all genetic" model. As we confirmed by several additional analyses, our results suggest that the association observed in our FF sample between lifetime smoking and lifetime MD was not causal but was instead due entirely to a shared set of genetic factors that predisposed to both conditions.

Is Childhood Sexual Abuse Causal for Psychiatric Disorders?

As we noted in Chapter 7, legitimate questions can be asked about the causal relationship between CSA and risk for psychiatric disorders. CSA does not occur at random within families, and it is often accompanied by other risk factors, including parental conflict, disrupted home environments, poor parenting, and parental psychopathology. We found that, after statistically adjusting for possible confounding effects, CSA was still strongly and significantly related to risk for nearly all of the disorders that we examined. Now we return to this question, using the more powerful cotwin-control method.

Because CSA was much less common than SLEs, we used a limited version of the cotwin-control design, focusing on 53 female twin pairs who were *broadly* discordant for severe CSA (Kendler et al., 2000c). These were pairs in which one twin reported severe CSA (attempted or completed intercourse, which was shown in Chapter 7 to be strongly associated with adult psychiatric illness) and the cotwin reported no CSA or a less severe form of CSA.[4]

Among these 53 pairs of twins, 24 pairs were discordant for having experienced lifetime MD. In 17 of those 24 pairs, the twin who had severe CSA was the one who had experienced MD, compared with 7 pairs in whom the unexposed twin was the one who developed MD. This ratio of 2.43:1 is statistically significant and similar to the results based on the entire sample of female twins. In that analysis, which treated the twins as individuals, the OR between CSA and MD was 2.79 (see Figure 7.8b). As shown in Figure 15.6, the ratios based on the case-control analyses were broadly similar to (and in some cases higher than) those based on standard regression analyses in the entire twin sample. Particularly noteworthy was the ratio found for AD: Among 11 of the 12 pairs discordant for both severe CSA and AD, the twin with alcoholism was the one who had experienced severe CSA. A strong association was also found for comorbidity—reporting at least two major lifetime psychiatric disorders. Among 19 of 22 doubly discordant pairs, the twin who

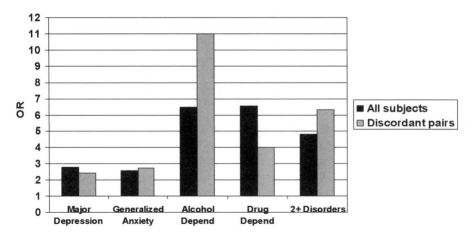

FIGURE 15.6. Odds ratios (OR) from standard regression and cotwin-control analyses of childhood sexual abuse and risk for psychiatric and substance use disorders in female twin pairs. Data from Kendler et al. (2000, Tables 5 and 6).

had experienced severe CSA was the one with two or more disorders. Even with the small sample size, we can conclude that these results are unlikely to have occurred by chance.

These results support a causal interpretation of the association between CSA and psychiatric and substance use disorders. Despite both twins' having been raised in the same family environment, having similar genetic backgrounds, and sharing exposure to other possible risk factors, the twin who experienced CSA had a consistently elevated risk for psychopathology compared with her unexposed cotwin.[5]

Two reports from the large Australian volunteer twin registry (Dinwiddie et al., 2000; Nelson et al., 2002) also used a cotwin-control approach to examine the association between CSA and adult psychiatric illness. As in our study, twins who experienced CSA had substantially higher rates for a range of disorders than their cotwins without CSA. The similarity of findings from two independent twin samples provides strong support for the hypothesis that part of the CSA–psychopathology association is causal.

Childhood Parental Loss and Risk for Alcoholism

In Chapter 7, we noted that the association between loss of a parent in childhood and adult psychopathology was not necessarily causal but could arise indirectly through noncausal means. We now take a closer look at this issue for the case of childhood parental loss and risk for alcoholism.

As we and others have demonstrated (see Chapter 5), the liability to AD is strongly influenced by genetic factors. This means that, on average, the parents of daughters who develop alcoholism will themselves have a higher than average risk for alcoholism. We also know that individuals with alcohol problems are at increased risk for premature death, marital separation, and divorce (Helzer, Burnam, & McEvoy, 1991; Vaillant, 1983). These observations lead to three plausible hypotheses about the nature of the association between parental loss and alcoholism. The first, or *causal*, hypothesis suggests that premature loss of a parent (or the family disruption that precedes or follows such loss) directly *causes* an increased liability to alcoholism among the girls who experience such a loss. This hypothesis is illustrated in Figure 15.7a. The second, or *noncausal*, hypothesis is that the parental loss–alcoholism association is not causal but arises because premature death or marital separation is an index of the liability to alcoholism in the parents, which, in turn, is genetically transmitted to their offspring (Figure 15.7b). A third hypothesis is that the association of parental loss with risk for alcoholism may result from a *combination* of both causal and noncausal mechanisms (Figure 15.7c).

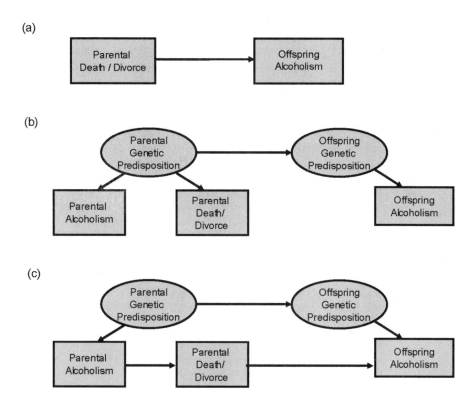

FIGURE 15.7. Alternative explanations for an association between parental loss and offspring alcoholism. (a) Causal association; (b) noncausal association; (c) combination.

To test which of these hypotheses was best supported by our data, we applied an extension of the parent–offspring model that we used to study the cross-generational transmission of liability to alcoholism (see Chapter 12). As shown in Figure 15.8, the major difference in the model is the addition of the measured parental-loss variable. The model posits that paternal and maternal alcoholism contribute directly to parental loss (through the j paths). Because early loss of a parent will always affect both twins, the loss directly contributes to the shared environment that may influence the liability to alcoholism (by path l). In addition, as in our standard twin–family model (see Figure 12.3), there are paths that reflect direct cultural transmission (parent to child environmental transmission [by path w]), which would occur if children acquired alcoholic behavior by observing their parents or from the environments created by their parents.

In this model, the causal hypothesis for the association between parental loss and risk for alcoholism in offspring is represented by the environmental path from childhood parental loss to the twins' shared environment to the twins' liability to alcoholism. This is illustrated by the bold arrows along

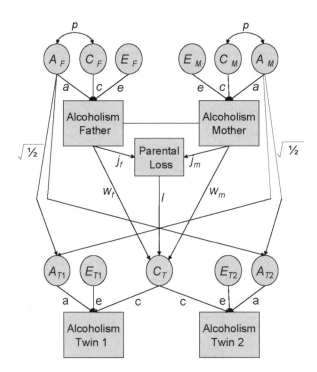

FIGURE 15.8. Parent–offspring model to test the sources of the association between childhood parental loss and alcoholism in offspring. Data from Kendler et al. (1996a, Figure 1).

paths l and c in Figure 15.9a. By contrast, the noncausal hypothesis is depicted as an indirect association between parental loss and risk for alcoholism in off-spring. This path is depicted by the bold arrows in Figure 15.9b (in this exam-ple, for paternal alcoholism). This association occurs through the connections from childhood parental loss to parental alcoholism to parental genetic risk factors for alcoholism to twin genetic risk factors for alcoholism to twin liabil-ity to alcoholism.[6]

Before we discuss the results of the analyses based on this model, let's examine the evidence supporting the noncausal hypothesis. The noncausal path has three parts: the connection from genetic liability to alcoholism (rep-resented by the a paths in Figure 15.9b), the genetic transmission between par-ents and offspring (represented by the path fixed to equal the square root of 0.5), and the path from parental alcoholism to parental loss (path j_f in Figure 15.9b). We already know from the results described in Chapter 5 that the a paths from the genetic factors to alcoholism will be significant. But what about the j paths from parental alcoholism to risk for childhood parental loss? Among the FF pairs whose parents were interviewed, paternal history of alco-hol dependence approximately doubled the chances that the twins had experi-enced childhood loss of father due to death (OR = 2.29) or to divorce (OR = 1.92). Maternal alcohol dependence, on the other hand, had no appreciable effect on risk for parental loss due to death (OR = 1.07) but strongly influ-enced parental loss due to divorce (OR = 2.66). These results suggest that it is possible that some of the association between loss and offspring alcoholism may be noncausal. To obtain a more precise picture, we turn to the results from our model fitting.

We fit a series of models based on that shown in Figure 15.8 to data from 1,030 FF twin pairs and, where available, their interviewed parents (853 mothers and 615 fathers).[7] We then compared how well each model ac-counted for the data (see Kendler et al., 1996a, for details).

The best-fitting model estimated the correlation between childhood parental loss and liability to AD to be rather substantial: 0.37. In this model, 84.7% of this total correlation was due to the causal pathway, and only 15.3% was due to the noncausal pathway. We tried several other analyses, but the proportion of the loss–alcoholism correlation accounted for by the noncausal path never exceeded 30%.[8] These results suggest that to a great degree the association between parental loss in childhood and the subsequent risk for AD in the twins was indeed causal. This result surprised some of our research team, but it demonstrates as clearly as could be expected how genetic designs can clarify the actions of environmental risk factors.

One word of caution is indicated. These analyses do not provide insight into what aspect of parental loss increases risk for alcoholism. The fact that the risk is quite a bit higher from parental divorce than from parental death (see Chapter 7) suggests that it may not be due to the loss itself but rather to the parental conflict and family dysfunction that often accompany divorce.

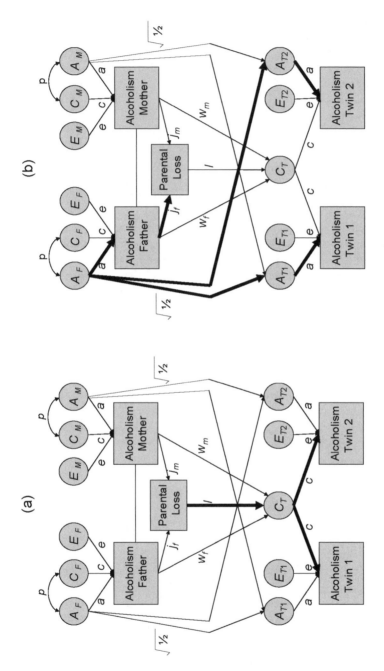

FIGURE 15.9. Explanations for the association between childhood parental loss and alcoholism. (a) Causal model, data from Kendler et al. (1996a, Figure 2); (b) noncausal model, data from Kendler et al. (1996a, Figure 3).

SUMMARY

This chapter has addressed the causal nature of the association between various environmental risk factors and psychiatric illness. In the five examples we explored (early drinking, SLEs, smoking, CSA, and parental loss), genetic designs helped clarify that three of them (SLEs, CSA, and parental loss) directly increase risk for illness. But these analyses also showed that for four of the five (all but CSA), some proportion of the correlation between the risk factors and psychiatric illness is noncausal—a result of genetic influences on exposure to environmental risk factors.

The results for CSA show strong evidence of causality, but the results presented in Chapter 7 suggest that there may also be some noncausal basis for the association between CSA and risk for internalizing disorders (e.g., compare the results of Figures 7.8a and 7.8b). In contrast to the other examples, noncausal effects explained all of the correlation between smoking and MD and between early onset of drinking and later risk for alcoholism.

The patterns of findings emerging from our work are complicated. The distinction between genetic and environmental risk factors for psychiatric disorders is not always straightforward. However, we are not yet done. The picture is about to get even more complex in Chapter 16, as we examine gene × environment interaction, or, as we prefer to call it, genetic control of sensitivity to the environment.

NOTES

1. The analyses use data from the fourth wave of interviews on female twin pairs and the first wave with male and male–female pairs. The results were similar when using alcohol dependence and alcohol abuse/dependence as outcomes. The analyses excluded twins who had never used alcohol.

2. This analysis was based on 1,898 twins with 24,648 individual person-months of exposure and 316 onsets of MD. These associations were quite substantial: For the entire sample, $\chi^2 = 171.2$; within DZ pairs, $\chi^2 = 44.9$; and within MZ twin pairs, $\chi^2 = 39.1$. (All tests had $df = 1$, $p < 0.0001$.)

3. We can also solve for the noncausal portions. The DZ:MZ ratio represents half the genetic variance, so the genetic proportion is $(4.52/3.58)^2$, or an OR of 1.58. This combines with the individual-specific estimate to give the total ($1.58*3.58 = 5.65$), indicating that the OR for shared environmental factors is about 1.0 and suggesting no additional risk.

4. We also examined narrow discordance, in which the cotwin had no CSA, and found broadly similar results.

5. A weakness of our analyses was our inability to separate our sample into MZ and DZ pairs due to the relatively small number of discordant pairs. Among discordant DZ pairs, part of the difference in rates of disorders may be due to genetic differences between the twins and not solely to differences in exposure to CSA.

6. For direct (causal) associations, the hypothesized path must run in the same direction as the arrows in the diagram. However, for indirect (correlational) associations, the path can run backward along the arrows.

7. These analyses included four family types: twins only (n = 129), twins and their fathers (n = 48), twins and their mothers (n = 286), and twins and both parents (n = 567). We used the DSM-III diagnosis of alcohol dependence derived at personal interview for both the twins and their parents.

8. The alternative analyses used several definitions of alcoholism and increased the number of parents by using information about alcoholism history provided by the twins whose parents were deceased or who did not consent to be interviewed.

CHAPTER SIXTEEN

Genetic Control of Sensitivity to the Environment

The commonsense model of how genes and environment combine to contribute to disease risk is that they add together. That is, the total risk for a given illness, such as heart disease, is the sum of the risk provided by genes and the risk created by various life experiences. For example, a man whose father had his first heart attack at age 42 might conclude: "I have a high genetic risk for heart disease. I need to reduce my risk by changing my environmental risk factors. I should stop smoking, follow a low-cholesterol diet, and exercise regularly."

This "additive model" is portrayed in Figure 16.1. The figure depicts the liability to develop a given illness for three hypothetical individuals with low, intermediate, and high genetic liability when exposed to varying levels of environmental risk. The key feature of this model is that the slopes of the lines of total liability are the same for each individual. That is, as individuals move from a low-risk ("protective") to a high-risk ("predisposing") environment, their liabilities increase the same amount, regardless of their level of genetic risk.

We want to contrast this additive model with the one depicted in Figure 16.2. Here, as in the additive model, the liability to illness increases for individuals with lower to higher genetic risk and with increasing levels of environmental risk. However, the slopes of the lines are no longer equal across individuals with different levels of genetic risk. Individuals with high genetic risk have the steepest slope, and those with low genetic risk the flattest slope. In

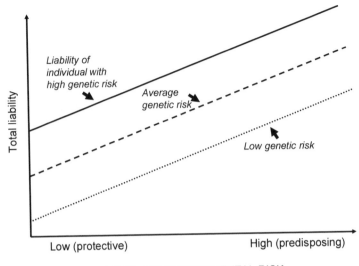

FIGURE 16.1. Schematic of additive model for the combination of genetic and environmental risk.

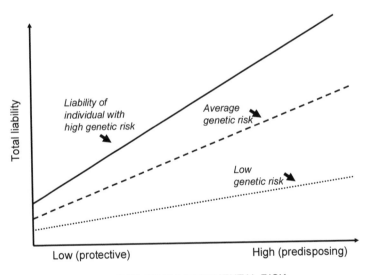

FIGURE 16.2. Schematic of genetic control of sensitivity to the environment (gene–environment interaction).

other words, the increase in liability that occurs in moving from a protective to a predisposing environment is itself related to genetic risk.

This is worth restating because of its central importance. In the model depicted in Figure 16.2, genetic risk contributes to disease liability in two fundamentally different ways: (1) it influences overall liability to illness, *and* () it alters the individual's sensitivity to the pathogenic effects of the environment. The pattern shown in Figure 16.2 is an example of what has been called *gene–environment interaction*. We find it more useful to call this *genetic control of sensitivity to the environment*.[1]

EXAMPLES OF GENETIC CONTROL OF SENSITIVITY TO THE ENVIRONMENT

General medicine provides many examples of genetic control of sensitivity to the environment. We briefly describe two. First, a variant of an important lipid transport protein called apolipoprotein E (apoE) increases sensitivity to environmental trauma. The ε-4 copy (technically termed an "allele") of this gene predisposes to the accumulation of a "garbage protein" (called amyloid) in the brain after head injury (Nicoll, Roberts, & Graham, 1995).[2] A study of the effects of head trauma among boxers (indexed by the number of times they had been knocked out!) found that those with low exposure had mild symptoms of organic brain damage, whereas individuals with greater trauma had more brain damage (Jordan et al., 1997). However, the level of brain damage was also related to their apoE genotype. Boxers with both the ε-4 allele and a high level of exposure to brain trauma had significantly more damage than those without the ε-4 allele but equally high exposure. So individuals with the ε-4 allele were more sensitive to the pathogenic effects of head trauma.

A second example is the relation between cancer and genetic variation in key liver metabolic/detoxification enzymes. Under most circumstances, genetic variation in these enzymes is unrelated to risk for cancer. However, in the presence of chemicals called polycyclic aromatic hydrocarbons (used in various industrial processes), some variants of these genes increase risk for lung, bladder, and breast cancer. This occurs because, depending on which variants a person has, the enzymes will either metabolize these industrial toxins into benign compounds that are easily excreted from the body or convert them into potent cancer-causing chemicals (Perera, 1997). Here again, we find genetic control of the sensitivity to environmental risk factors.

In both of these examples, the impact of a potential environmental risk factor (head injury or industrial toxin exposure) on the key outcome (organic brain damage or cancer risk) depends on genetic factors. In both instances, the sensitivity of the organism to the environmental exposure is modified by genes, which render the individual relatively vulnerable or relatively invulnerable to its effect.

Because of the importance of this topic, we illustrate it in yet another way, by clinical vignettes. Imagine two individuals, Charlie and Robert:

> Charlie has always been self-assured and quietly self-confident. He works as an emergency room physician in a large city hospital. He considers it to be a good night when he is kept very busy, moving quickly to treat individuals with heart attacks, motor vehicle accidents, stabbings, gunshot wounds, delirium tremens, and acute psychosis. In his free time, he likes to mountain climb and sky dive.

> Robert has been shy and withdrawn since adolescence. Despite years of therapy, he lacks self-confidence and feels awkward in social situations. He cannot avoid getting upset over the smallest perceived rejection, such as when a coworker makes a slightly critical comment or his therapist is a few minutes late for an appointment.

Charlie is like the low-risk individual in Figure 16.2. Stress rolls off him like water off a duck's back. Robert, on the other hand, is like the high-risk individual. He is very stress-sensitive.

The observation that individuals have important differences in their levels of stress responsivity is beautifully summarized by Burton in his classic text *The Anatomy of Melancholy*:

> . . . according as the humour itself is intended or remitted in men [and] their . . . rational soul is better able to make resistance; so are they more or less affected [by adversity]. For that which is but a flea-biting to one, causeth insufferable torment to another; and which one by his singular moderation and well-imposed carriage can happily overcome, a second is no whit able to sustain, but upon every small occasion of misconceived abuse, injury, grief, disgrace [and] loss . . . yields so far to passion, that . . . his digestion hindered, his sleep gone, his spirits obscured, and his heart heavy . . . he himself [is] overcome with melancholy. (Burton, 1621/ 1932)

EVIDENCE FOR GENETIC CONTROL OF SENSITIVITY TO THE ENVIRONMENT IN THE VATSPSUD

In this chapter, we present a range of examples from our research that tested for genetic control of sensitivity to the environment. These examples include several types of environmental risks, including SLEs, CSA, parental disciplinary practices, and family dysfunction, and several outcome variables, including MD, alcoholism, neuroticism, and smoking. In each case we asked how genetic and environmental risks combine to affect liability to the disorder or trait. We found some examples that were consistent with the additive model (as in Figure 16.1) and others in which genetic factors appear to alter sensitivity to the environment (Figure 16.2).[3]

Genes, Stressful Live Events, and Major Depression

We have seen, in the VATSPSUD and in many other studies, strong evidence that liability to MD is increased both by genetic risk factors (Chapter 4) and by SLEs (see Chapter 8). What has not been studied as extensively is how the two sets of risk factors combine. Do they add together, or do genetic factors modulate sensitivity to the depressogenic effects of SLEs?

During the course of our project we have addressed this question in several ways. Here we present the results from four series of analyses using different measures of life stress (recent SLE occurrence, SLE severity, and CSA) and different ways to index genetic risk (cotwin history of MD, neuroticism score, and measured genotype). The statistical methods ranged from simple to quite complex, but the results show a consistent pattern: Sensitivity to the environment is strongly influenced by genetic factors.

Interaction of Genetic Risk and Major Stressful Life Events in Major Depression

Our first approach to this problem was to study whether genetic risk interacts with the occurrence of SLEs to alter total liability to MD. To index genetic risk we used information about the MD history of both twins in a pair. As we described previously (Chapter 4), in our study resemblance between twins for MD is due almost entirely to genetic factors. Consequently, all twins can be conveniently assigned to one of four categories of increasing "genetic risk" for MD based on the history of MD in their cotwins: (1) MZ cotwin unaffected, (2) DZ cotwin unaffected, (3) DZ cotwin affected, and (4) MZ cotwin affected. For the present analysis, we assumed that the genetic effects in these four groups are proportional to −1.0, −0.5, +0.5, and +1.0, respectively.[4]

As described previously (see Figure 8.2), many types of SLEs were associated with increased risk for the onset of an episode of MD in the same month as the occurrence of an SLE. Here we focus on four event types that were particularly strongly associated with risk for depression. We created a new category, *major SLEs*, which included four events: death of a close relative, assault, serious marital problems, and divorce or romantic breakup. One or more of these events was reported to have occurred in 1,228 of the 51,268 person-months (2.4%) included in waves 1 and 2 of our FF study. Onsets of MD during the same period were relatively rare (476 onsets, or 0.9%), but they increased 12.2-fold in months containing one of these major events.

We then conducted an analysis to predict MD onset from our "genetic risk" index and our measure of major SLEs. The results are depicted in Figure 16.3.[5] Individuals with higher genetic risk were more likely to have had an episode of MD, regardless of whether a major SLE had occurred. Similarly,

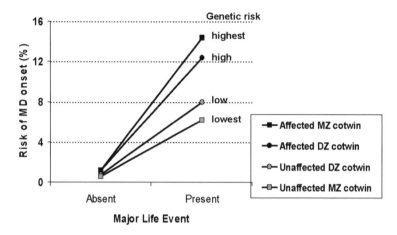

FIGURE 16.3. Risk of onset of major depression (MD) in a month as a function of inferred genetic risk and presence or absence of a major stressful life event (SLE) during that month. MZ = monozygotic; DZ = dizygotic. Adapted from Kendler et al. (1995a, Figure 1). Copyright 1995 by the American Psychiatric Association. Adapted by permission.

rates of MD increased for all groups when moving from a low- to a high-stress environment. These observations are consistent with the additive model. However, the results differ from the prediction of the additive model in that the *increase* in risk associated with moving from lower to higher stress was substantially greater among individuals at highest genetic risk and least in those at lowest genetic risk. Genetic factors appear to affect liability to MD in two different ways: (1) they influence overall liability (regardless of environmental risk) and (2) they alter the sensitivity of individuals to the depressogenic effects of high-stress environments.[6] This pattern of results fits the interactive model (Figure 16.2).

This study provided a reasonably clear answer to the question of how genetic risk and major SLEs interrelate in the etiology of MD. However, it had several limitations. First, the analyses included only women. Would we observe the same result for men? Other limitations were related to the statistical approach. We believed we could improve the analyses with the additional knowledge and better software that became available later in the project. Finally, the early work had been limited by the fact that our four-category measure of genetic risk was indirect and approximate. There were also important questions about the effects of stress: Do genetic factors influence the depressogenic effects of minor stressful events? Are the effects of recent stress altered by early exposure to traumatic events? The remaining three examples of the association between SLEs and MD illustrate the ways in which we addressed these issues.

Stressful Life Event Severity and Major Depression

Our initial analyses used only a "yes/no" measure (of whether a major life event had occurred) rather than a range of levels of stress. This made it impossible to examine how genetic or temperamental factors influence the "dose–response" relationship between stress and MD. Recalling the stories of Charlie and Robert, we might ask, is there a level of stress at which the Roberts of this world would have an increased chance of developing MD but the Charlies would remain largely immune? To answer this question, we used the finer grained measure of long-term contextual threat (LTCT) obtained for SLEs measured in the later waves of our study (see Sidebar 8.3).

Another refinement was to use a continuous index of each individual's genetic risk rather than the cotwin history of MD. We selected the personality trait of neuroticism (N). This was based on our results showing that neuroticism is a good indicator of genetic risk for MD (see Chapter 11).[7]

We examined the chance of developing an MD episode in a particular month associated with the level of stress experienced (LTCT ratings for events that occurred in that month or the few preceding months) and genetic risk (N level). These analyses were based on information from 7,517 individuals interviewed in FF wave 3 or 4 and MF wave 2. Figure 16.4 summarizes the results separately by sex.[8] The figure depicts the predicted chance of developing MD for 5 levels of LTCT (*no event* through *severe*) and 5 levels of N: very low (2 *SD* below the mean), low (1 *SD* below the mean), average (mean N), high (1 *SD* above the mean), and very high (2 *SD* above the mean). The values are hazard ratios representing the chance of developing MD associated with LTCT and N level relative to a reference group (which is assigned a value of 1.0). The reference group were males with an average level of N and an adversity level of zero (i.e., who had not experienced an SLE that month).

What are the take-home messages from these results? As we observed in the analyses described in Chapters 8 and 11, there were large "main effects" of both LTCT and neuroticism. The chance of developing an MD episode increased dramatically with higher levels of LTCT regardless of the level of neuroticism and was much greater among individuals with higher levels of neuroticism regardless of the LTCT level of the event they had experienced.

The most important result was to confirm, using superior methods, the results of the first example in this chapter. The effects of stress severity and neuroticism do not just add together. Instead, they interact. This can be seen most clearly in the way that the curves for the various levels of N "splay out" with increasing levels of adversity (as predicted by Figure 16.2). Higher levels of neuroticism magnify the impact of LTCT. Compared with individuals with low and very low neuroticism, those with very high neuroticism have a liability to MD that is shifted both *upward* and *to the left*. In other words, the higher the level of neuroticism, the more sensitive individuals are to the depressogenic effects of high levels of adversity. Among individuals with

(a)

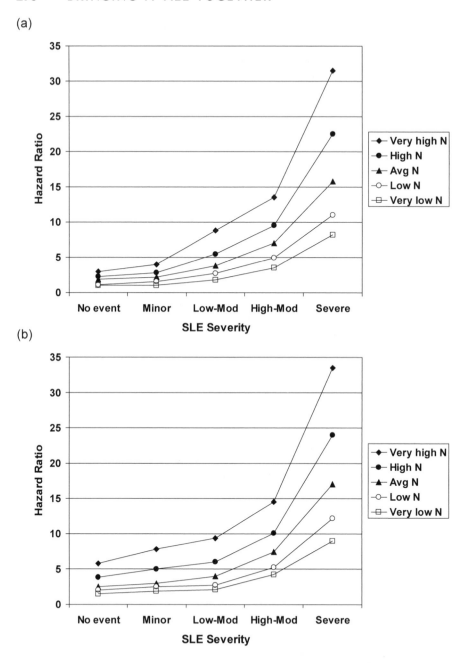

(b)

FIGURE 16.4. Risk of onset of major depression (MD) from neuroticism (N) level and stressful life event (SLE) severity. (a) Males; (b) females. Adapted from Kendler, Kuhn, and Prescott (2004b, Figure 1). Copyright 2004 by the American Psychiatric Association. Adapted by permission.

very low N, MD liability does not increase much with minor and low-moderate LTCT events; it takes greater stress to trigger depression in these individuals. However, among those with high and very high levels of neuroticism, the chance of developing MD starts to increase even at the lower levels of LTCT. Thus, as we predicted, there do seem to be levels of adversity at which some individuals (the Charlies of the world) are nearly immune, whereas others (the Roberts) are not.

A final conclusion, and one we did not anticipate, is that the pattern of results differed for men and women. As is typical, women were about twice as likely as men to develop a depressive episode.[9] However, there was a strong interaction between sex and levels of LTCT: Women had increased rates of MD relative to men for months when there was no event; for events with a minor LTCT, the rates of MD were about twice as high in women as in men; but at higher levels of adversity, the rates were similar across the sexes.

These results are consistent with those from several other studies. Five prior studies of the relationship of neuroticism and "life stress" to self-report symptoms of depression, anxiety, or distress all found that participants with high neuroticism had greater sensitivity to stress than did participants with low neuroticism (Avison & Turner, 1988; Bolger & Schilling, 1991; Ormel & Wohlfarth, 1991; Rijsdijk et al., 2001; Van Os & Jones, 1999). One study found that SLEs predisposed to MD only among individuals who had high levels of neuroticism or a prior long-term difficulty (Ormel, Oldehinkel, & Brilman, 2001). However, none of these studies reported sex differences such as we found, so this provocative finding awaits confirmation.

Is the Impact of Genetic Risk and Recent Stress on Depression Altered by Early Exposure to Trauma?

The previous two examples show that genetic or temperamental risk factors can influence, in a relatively enduring way, the sensitivity of individuals to the depressogenic effects of stress. As we pondered these findings, an obvious question emerged: Would a similar effect be seen for a history of childhood trauma? This question was stimulated by the results of an intriguing study of the effects of childhood abuse on stress reactivity in adulthood (Heim et al., 2000). Women with and without a history of childhood physical or sexual abuse were exposed to standard laboratory stressors (public speaking and solving arithmetic problems before a critical audience). Women with prior abuse displayed larger physiological and hormonal responses to this stress than did women from a control group. In the more naturalistic setting of our twin study, in which the stressors are life events rather than controlled laboratory experiences, would we also see increased stress responsivity in women with a history of abuse?

To answer this question, we used data on past history of CSA, levels of N, SLE severity (based on LTCT rating), and onsets of MD episodes from 1,404 women who had participated in waves 3 and 4 of the FF study. As described in Chapter 7 (see Sidebar 7.3), women who had experienced CSA were grouped into three categories reflecting increasing severity: (1) *nongenital* CSA (7.8%), (2) *genital* CSA (genital contact but no intercourse; 14.1%), and (3) *attempted or completed intercourse* (8.4%). The analyses were identical to those in the prior example except that the hazards for developing MD were estimated within each CSA group.

The results of the best-fitting model are summarized in Figure 16.5. The figure depicts the relationship between history of CSA, exposure to LTCT, and probability of a depressive onset in women with low levels of N (1 *SD*

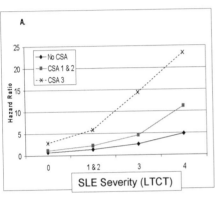

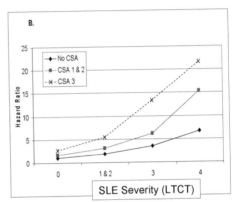

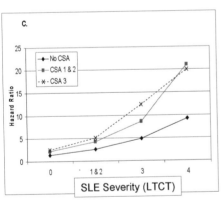

FIGURE 16.5. The effect of a history of childhood sexual abuse (CSA) and neuroticism (N) score on the association between severity of stressful life events (SLEs) and risk for major depression (MD) in women. Relative risk for developing MD among women with (A) neuroticism scores −1 *SD* below the sample mean; (B) neuroticism scores at the sample mean; (C) neuroticism scores +1 *SD* above the sample mean. Reference group is women with average N (panel B) with no CSA and long-term contextual threat (LTCT) = 0. CSA 1 and 2 = women who report nongenital or genital CSA; CSA 3 = women who report attempted or completed intercourse. Adapted from Kendler, Kuhn, and Prescott (2004c, Figure 1). Copyright 2004 by Cambridge University Press. Adapted by permission.

below the mean; Figure 16.5a), average levels of N (Figure 16.5b), and high levels of N (1 *SD* above the mean; Figure 16.5c). Each line represents a group defined by CSA history. The slopes of these lines index *stress sensitivity*, the change in the chances of developing MD associated with increasing levels of LTCT. The *steeper* this curve is, the greater is the sensitivity to the depressogenic effects of SLEs. The reference group (assigned a hazard of 1.0) is formed of women with an average level of neuroticism, no history of CSA, and no SLE exposure (i.e., an LTCT of zero). The hazards for the other groups are scaled relative to this one. (Our analyses found no significant differences for minor versus low-moderate LTCT or for nongenital versus genital CSA, so these categories were combined in the figures).

The figure illustrates clearly the main effects of N, CSA, and LTCT in the prediction of depressive onsets. The chance of experiencing a depressive episode in the prior year was substantially increased by high N, by SLEs with high LTCT, and by a history of CSA. In addition to all these effects, we see unambiguous evidence that CSA influences sensitivity to the depressogenic effects of recent stress: The slopes of the lines are substantially greater among women with a history of CSA. The CSA "dose–response" relationship is particularly clear among women with average or low levels of N. The level of stress sensitivity is relatively modest for women with no history of CSA, intermediate for those whose CSA did not involve intercourse, and high for those with exposure to CSA that included attempted or completed intercourse.[10]

Our more naturalistic study replicated the results found in a controlled laboratory environment. Women with a history of CSA showed substantial increases in stress responsivity. These findings suggest that not only genetic factors but also early environmental traumas can produce long-term changes in sensitivity to stress.

These results are congruent with several other lines of research. First, women with a history of childhood sexual or physical abuse demonstrate structural brain changes, notably in the shrinkage of the hippocampus—a portion of the brain particularly involved in memory formation (Bremner et al., 1997; Stein, Koverola, Hanna, Torchia, & McClarty, 1997; Vythilingam et al., 2002). Second, a large body of work in both rodents and nonhuman primates shows that certain early environmental stressors augment later behavioral and hormonal sensitivity to stressors (Heim & Nemeroff, 2001). Third, some forms of early childhood stress, including parental loss, may also increase sensitivity to the depressogenic effects of SLEs (Bifulco, Brown, & Harris, 1987; Brown & Harris, 1978).

A Measured Gene Example of Gene–Environment Interaction

The results described so far suggest that aggregate genetic effects influence stress responsivity. However, these studies provide no insight into the nature or identity of the specific genes involved. In our next example, we describe a similar analysis using a measured gene rather than inferred genetic risk.

First, we provide some background to this study. In 2003, in the journal *Science*, Caspi and coworkers (2003) reported that a variant in the serotonin transporter gene moderated the influence of SLEs on MD in a large epidemiological sample from New Zealand. This gene was of interest because it codes for the protein that removes serotonin from the synapse, thereby terminating its activity. This protein is the site of action of the widely used class of antidepressant drugs termed serotonin-specific reuptake inhibitors (SSRIs), including the widely used drugs Prozac and Zoloft. Furthermore, this gene comes in two common variants that result in different amounts of functional protein being produced. These two variants are called, simply, short (S) and long (L), with the S version producing less functional protein. Everyone has two copies (or alleles) of these genes, one received from the mother and one from the father. Thus the possible combinations of these variants are SS, LL, and LS. Caspi et al. (2003) showed that individuals with one or two short alleles (i.e., SS or LS) were more stress sensitive than those with two copies of the long allele (LL).

This exciting report had two potentially important limitations. First, the SLE measure was simply the count of the number of SLEs experienced (out of 14 possible) in the prior 5 years. The analyses did not include any information about event type or severity. As we have seen, both of these dimensions are related to MD liability. Additionally, the impact of SLEs on MD episodes is typically of short duration, usually lasting 1 to 3 months and nearly always less than a year. However, Caspi and colleagues (2003) predicted the risk for MD in the last year from SLEs in the preceding 5 years. It is thus possible that the study results do not reflect the direct effects of SLEs on depressive episodes but are due to some other indirect association (e.g., higher neuroticism in individuals with the SS and LS genotypes influences risk for both SLEs and depressive episodes).

With the help of our molecular geneticist colleague, Brien Riley, we attempted to replicate the Caspi et al. (2003) findings using data from the VATSPSUD, including our ratings of SLEs and LTCT (Kendler, Kuhn, Vittum, Prescott, & Riley, 2005b). We obtained genotypes of the serotonin transporter variants for 572 randomly selected participants from our FF and MM/MF studies (284 males, 288 females) for whom DNA was available. (Genotyping the entire sample would have been very costly and was not necessary to address this question.) We then attempted to predict the onset of MD from the sex of the twin, the LTCT of the SLEs to which the twin had been exposed (with the effect at "full strength" in the month of the event and then decaying over the subsequent 2 months), the serotonin transporter variant, and the interaction between LTCT and the transporter variant. The results are illustrated in Figure 16.6a, which shows the overall results of the best-fit model, and Figure 16.6b, which shows a close-up of the critical part of the curve. In these analyses we assigned males with an SS genotype and no life-event exposure to be our reference group (i.e., hazard ratio [HR] = 1.0).[11]

Two of these results should be familiar. The HR for MD increases with higher levels of LTCT, with the effect being particularly marked when moving

(a)

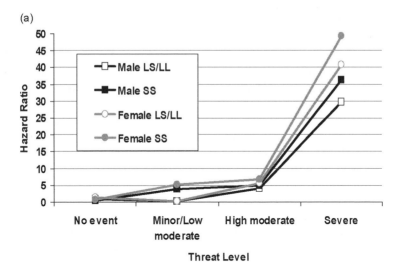

FIGURE 16.6a. Hazard ratio for major depression (MD) by serotonin transporter genotype, sex, and stressful life event (SLE) severity. SS = two short alleles; LL = two long alleles; LS = one long and one short allele. Adapted from Kendler, Kuhn, Vittum, Prescott, and Riley (2005b, Figure 2). Copyright 2005 by the American Medical Association. Adapted by permission.

(b)

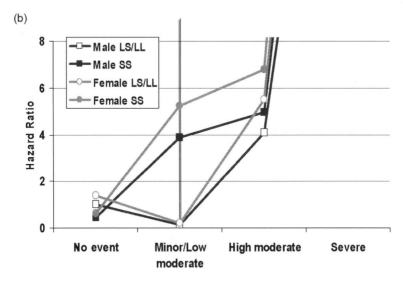

FIGURE 16.6b. Close-up of hazard ratio for MD by serotonin transporter genotype, sex, and SLE severity. Adapted from Kendler, Kuhn, Vittum, Prescott, and Riley (2005b, Figure 2). Copyright 2005 by the American Medical Association. Adapted by permission.

from high-moderate to severe levels of LTCT. Further, at every level of threat and genotype, the HR for MD is greater for females than for males. However, two results are new. At high-moderate and severe LTCT levels, the HR for MD is greater for males and females with the SS than with the LS or LL genotypes, but the difference is small. By contrast (as most clearly seen in Figure 16.6b), at minor and low-moderate levels of threat, the differences in risk between those with the SS versus the LS or LL genotypes is substantial. For individuals with an SS genotype, the risk for an episode of MD is more than eight times greater in the presence of a minor or low-moderate threat event compared with months with no reported SLE.

To summarize, we broadly replicated the key findings of Caspi et al. (2003) that the length polymorphism in the serotonin promoter modified the depressogenic effects of SLEs. By examining the occurrence of SLEs and onsets of MD to the nearest month, our analyses had greater temporal resolution than their original findings. But our findings revealed a subtle relationship between genotype and stress not predicted by the results of Caspi et al. That is, the genotype–environment interaction we observed was due to a "leftward" shift in the dose–response curve. For individuals with the protective LS or LL genotype (perhaps Charlie has this genotype), mild SLEs produced no appreciable change in MD. However, for those with the predisposing SS genotype (perhaps like Robert), even modest levels of adversity produced a substantial increase in rates of depression. Replication of these findings is certainly needed. If correct, they suggest that the unraveling of the pathways to psychiatric illness may require not only measures of specific genetic risk factors but also detailed and careful assessment of environmental risks.

Are the Effects of Parental Alcoholism Moderated by Parental Rearing Style?

As we described in Chapter 12, rates of AD were higher among women who had a parent with alcoholism. We also found that alcoholism was more common among women who had received cold and authoritarian parenting (Figure 7.2). We decided to put these pieces together to study how parenting practices and parental alcoholism combine to influence problem drinking in offspring.

These analyses were based on information collected from 1,887 women during our second wave of interviews with female twin pairs. We first looked at the association of twin problem drinking with three measures of parent–child relationship quality, three measures of parenting style, and three measures of disciplinary practices (see Sidebar 16.1). Figure 16.7 summarizes these results. Women who had a history of problem drinking were more likely to rate their relationships with their mothers and fathers as being distant, cold, and conflictual. They were also more likely to report that their parents used physical punishment, administered punishment based on their moods, and used withholding of privileges as punishment. However, problem drink-

SIDEBAR 16.1. Measures Used for Study of Parenting and Problem Drinking

We used self- and (when available) cotwin reports of parenting. We included three measures of relationship quality (distance, coldness, and conflict) and three measures of parenting style (discouraging independence, overprotectiveness, and inconsistency). Coldness, discouraging independence. and overprotectiveness were taken from the Parental Bonding Instrument (PBI; Parker et al., 1979; see Sidebar 7.1). The other measures came from the Home Environment Interview (Robins et al., 1985). We also obtained three measures of disciplinary practices: physical punishment, withholding privileges, and mood dependence. These were assessed by asking twins what their parents would do when, as a child, "you were misbehaving." Items that assessed physical punishment included those that asked about spanking, slapping, and hitting the twin with a brush, belt, or stick. Items that assessed withholding privileges included those that asked about taking away privileges, sending the twin to her room, or grounding her. We also asked how much the way twins were disciplined by their mothers and fathers depended on the parent's mood at the time. Twins rated each of the nine items on a 4-point scale from *often* to *never*.

Problem drinking in the twins was based on responses to the first FF interview (see Sidebar 5.3). Parental diagnosis of alcoholism was based on a combination of information from personal interviews (available for 76% of mothers and 55% of fathers) and reports by twins and interviewed spouses. Family members were asked to report whether their relatives had been treated for a drinking problem or had experienced problems arising from drinking in five areas: legal, health, marital or family, social, and work. According to their daughters, alcohol-related problems were more common among parents who were not interviewed than among those who were. Therefore, we decided it was important to include information about the alcoholism history of parents who had not been interviewed. We classified parents as having alcoholism if they were positive for AD based on personal interview, if any family member reported that they were treated for alcoholism, or if three of the five problem areas were reported by at least one family member. Twins were classified as family history positive if either parent met these criteria for alcoholism and as family history negative if neither parent met criteria.

ing was not significantly associated with parenting styles of discouraging independence, being overprotective, or being inconsistent.[12]

We then examined whether these factors interacted with presumed genetic liability for alcoholism based on having a parent with a history of alcohol-related problems. The results are summarized in Figure 16.8. We found significant interactions for two measures, whereby the ORs for women with a positive family history (FH+) were significantly *lower* than those for women with a negative family history (FH–). In both cases the interaction was in a protective direction: Among women with a family history of alcoholism, risk for developing problem drinking was *reduced* among those who had close relationships with their parents or whose parents punished them by withholding privileges (i.e., a less punitive punishment strategy).

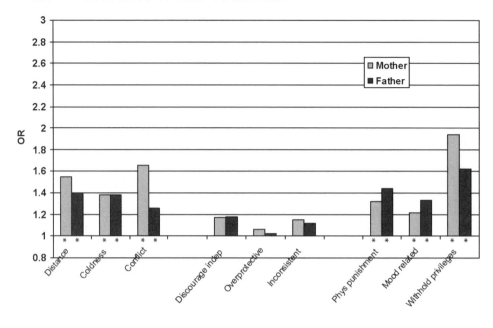

FIGURE 16.7. Odds ratios (OR) for the association between problem drinking in female twins and parenting received; *significantly greater than 1.0 (p < 0.05). Adapted with permission of the authors from Prescott et al. (1993).

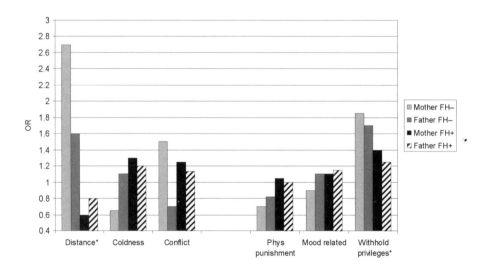

FIGURE 16.8. Odds ratios (OR) for the association between problem drinking in female twins and parenting received by parental alcoholism history; *OR of FH+ (positive family history) and FH– (negative family history) significantly different (p < 0.05) for *Distance* and *Withhold Privileges*. Adapted with permission of the authors from Prescott et al. (1993).

These results provide a slightly different example of how genetic and environmental factors can interact. Looking once again at the model shown in Figure 16.2, we can see that when individuals with high genetic risk are raised in protective environments, their genetic liability is less likely to be expressed.[13] Similar findings have been reported in longitudinal studies of children and adolescent offspring of alcoholics. Among these high-risk individuals, those who received supportive parenting were less likely to develop substance use disorders (King & Chassin, 2004; Werner & Johnson, 2004).

MODERATION OF GENETIC EFFECTS BY ENVIRONMENTAL RISK FACTORS

All of the analyses presented in this chapter so far have been based on the models depicted in Figures 16.1 and 16.2. We now introduce a complementary approach to thinking about how genes and environmental risk factors can interrelate. This model, illustrated in Figure 16.9 and implemented in the Mx program developed by our colleague, Mike Neale, allows us to ask whether genetic and background (i.e., unmeasured) environmental factors are *moderated* by the level of the specified environmental risk factor. The top part of the model should be familiar, as it is identical to models we have used pre-

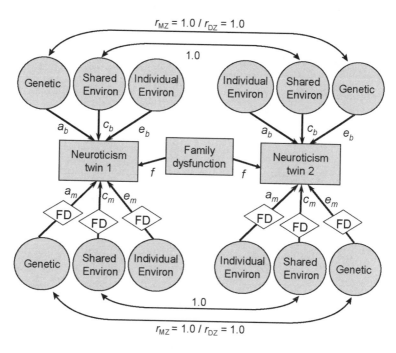

FIGURE 16.9. Twin model for estimating moderated effects. FD = family dysnfunction.

viously in this book. However, the bottom part of the model is new. What makes this model different from our previous approaches to analyzing twin-pair data is that it allows us to separate genetic and environmental risk factors into two sets, which we call *basal* and *moderated*. *Basal* factors (depicted by the subscript $_b$) represent the expected impact of genes and background environment on our trait of interest when the specified environmental risk factor is at a minimal level. *Moderated* genetic and background environmental factors are so named because they are moderated (or altered) by the level of the specified environmental risk factor. These moderated factors are indicated in the figure by the subscript $_m$ and also by the diamonds on these paths. It is critical to be clear about what we mean by the term "moderated." In this model, "moderated" means that the genetic and environmental effects on the trait of interest are directly influenced by the level of the specified environmental risk factor. (See Sidebar 16.2 for more details about the model.)

This approach provides a more detailed picture of how risk factors influence liability to a disorder or trait because we can examine the impact of the specified risk factor not only on genetic effects but also on shared background and individual-specific environment. We applied this model to examine how family dysfunction combines with genetic and environmental risk to affect two outcomes: neuroticism and smoking.

Family Dysfunction and the Heritability of Neuroticism

As we reviewed in Chapter 7, many studies have shown that different kinds of dysfunction in the home environment have a *direct* effect on risk for later psychopathology (Burbach & Borduin, 1986; Gerlsma, Emmelkamp, & Arrindell, 1990; Holmes & Robins, 1988; Moffitt et al., 2001; Parker, 1990; Perris et al., 1994). We now want to ask a more subtle question. Could the home environment influence later indices of mental health *by moderating the effects of genetic influences?*

Evidence for such a mechanism (which could be called a *genetic-by-shared-environment interaction*) has come from adoption studies of several forms of psychopathology, including CD (Cadoret, Yates, Troughton, Woodworth, & Stewart, 1995), ASP (Cadoret, Cain, & Crowe, 1983), schizophrenia (Tienari, 1991), and some subtypes of alcoholism (Cloninger et al., 1981; Sigvardsson, Bohman, & Cloninger, 1996). All of these studies suggest that genetic effects on the outcome are *increased* among individuals who were exposed to a pathogenic rearing environment. A family-environment-by-genetic interaction has also been found for the trait of disinhibition, with stronger genetic effects observed in families with a "laid-back" rather than a restrictive style of child rearing (Boomsma, deGeus, van Baal, & Koopmans, 1999).

Why might we think that families can modify the impact of genes on a personality trait such as neuroticism, which reflects emotionality or vulnerability to negative affect? One influential model of family development

SIDEBAR 16.2. Model for Moderated Genetic and Environmental Effects

The model shown in Figure 16.9 allows us to separate genetic and environmental risk factors into two sets, which we call *basal* (depicted by the subscript $_b$) and *moderated* (subscript $_m$). Mathematically, the values of A_m, C_m, and E_m are multiplied by the value of the measured risk factor (here, level of family dysfunction, FD). At the lowest level of the measured environmental risk (when FD = 0), the genes in the A_m factor are completely "silent," exerting no effect on the trait of interest (neuroticism). By contrast, as the values of the measured environmental risk factor increase, these genes will have more and more effect on the trait.

It might help to think of the diamonds as spigots on a water line. If the spigot is nearly closed (e.g., the level of the measured environmental risk is very low), only a small amount of the moderated effects gets through to influence the outcome. However, if the spigot is wide open (e.g., a high level of the measured environmental risk), then the moderated factors have a greater influence on the development of the trait.

This model has four noteworthy differences from the model depicted in Figures 16.1 and 16.2. First, it is designed to handle a continuous environmental risk factor rather than one that is either present or absent (such as parental alcoholism) or that can be graded into a small number of categories (such as LTCT). Second, this new model works best when the trait being studied is also continuous—such as a personality trait—rather than dichotomous—such as a diagnosis. Third, our previous analyses examined whether genetic risk factors *moderated* the impact of environmental risks. This model turns the problem around and explores whether exposure to an environmental risk factor *moderates* the impact of genes and unmeasured environmental factors. Fourth, our previous model was a form of regression analysis in which the goal was to predict liability to illness. The current approach instead involves structural equation modeling, in which we decompose risk into its genetic and environmental components. This approach provides a richer picture of what is going on. For example, we can examine the impact of the specified risk factor not only on genetic effects but also on the impact of background shared and individual-specific environment.

The model allows two kinds of relationships between the measured risk factor and the outcome:

1. A simple "main effect" (as in standard regression analysis) in which the risk factor affects the mean levels of the outcome (and the variance is constant). This is represented by path f in Figure 16.9.
2. A "moderated" effect, in which the risk factor moderates the impact of genetic and environmental risk factors and affects the variance of outcome.

(Bronfenbrenner & Ceci, 1994), which has been supported by several recent empirical studies (Rowe, Jacobson, & van den Oord, 1999; Turkheimer, Haley, Waldron, D'Onofrio, & Gottesman, 2003), suggests that rearing environments that allow full expression of a child's innate potential will increase the genetic variation of a trait. For example, parents who provide an intellectually stimulating environment (e.g., by encouraging their children to read or taking them to libraries or museums) might increase the chances that their children's genetically influenced abilities will be fully expressed. Would the same model work for neuroticism?

If a child with a genetic predisposition to high levels of neuroticism grows up in a family that expresses little conflict or infrequent negative emotion, it is possible that the child will not express this predisposition. Or, to consider the converse, a child growing up in a family with lots of fighting and conflict might have the opportunity to fully express (or "actualize") his or her "genes for neuroticism."

In most of our previous analyses, the degree of variability (or spread) of our data was not a subject of concern. However, in some cases, differences in variability among subgroups can be informative. In Chapter 10 we considered an example in which different age groups showed different variances in frequency and quantity of alcohol consumption (see Figure 10.7). Like that example, the moderator model makes predictions about variation. If moderation is occurring, the *variance* of neuroticism should be higher among groups with higher levels of family dysfunction. The reason is that new sources of individual differences (e.g., the A_m genetic factor) that are quiescent at low levels of family dysfunction are active at higher levels.

We tested three alternative models for the association between family dysfunction (FD) and neuroticism. Each of these is based on the path model shown in Figure 16.9, and each makes a different prediction about the values of genetic and environmental variation in neuroticism across different levels of family dysfunction. Figure 16.10 illustrates the patterns of data that would be predicted by each of the three models.

The simplest is the *standard* model (shown in the left portion of Figure 16.10), in which the moderated paths are all set to zero. This is equivalent to our usual twin model (e.g., Figure 3.3) and estimates a single set of values: the proportions of variance in neuroticism due to a^2, c^2, and e^2. Under this model, which is equivalent to the additive model in Figure 16.1, these variance proportions and the total variance of N (obtained by adding together the a^2, c^2, and e^2 components) are constant across different levels of FD.

The *proportional* model predicts that the variance of neuroticism changes as a function of family dysfunction but that the *proportion* of variance in family dysfunction that is due to a^2, c^2, and e^2 does not change. Because genetic variance changes proportionally with total variance in this model, heritability remains constant. This is shown in the middle portion of Figure 16.10: All three sources of variance increase proportionally with increasing levels of FD.

The third alternative is the *moderator* model. The variance that is due to a^2, c^2, and e^2 changes as a function of the level of family dysfunction, but the different sources do not have to be proportional to each other, and the total variance can change across levels of dysfunction. One possible pattern from a moderated model is illustrated in the right portion of Figure 16.10. Here, higher levels of FD "activate" a new set of genes that influence N, resulting in an increase in genetic variance with increasing levels of dysfunction.

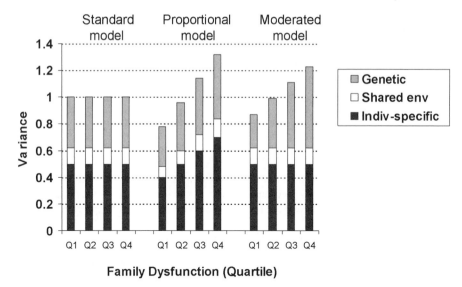

FIGURE 16.10. Expected results from standard, proportional, and moderated twin models of the relationship between sources of variance in neuroticism scores and level of family dysfunction. Env = environment.

In testing these models, we used information obtained from 957 female twin pairs from the FF sample, from whom we had collected parental as well as twin assessments of family dysfunction (see Sidebar 16.3). We divided the sample into quartiles based on level of FD and examined, for each quartile, the estimated genetic and environmental sources of variance (Figure 16.11). The total variance of neuroticism increased across the increasing levels of FD, as is predicted by the proportional and moderator models. However, the variance proportions were clearly inconsistent with those predicted from the moderator model because the total proportion of variance due to genetic effects did not change with increasing levels of family dysfunction.

As suggested by these results, when the data were formally tested using the moderator model, we found little evidence that level of family dysfunction moderated the impact of genetic or environmental risk factors on levels of neuroticism. Genetic risk factors and FD both influenced levels of N. However, the genetic effects were not moderated by pathogenic rearing environment. As shown in Figure 16.11, there was a tendency for the genetic and individual-specific environmental variance to increase slightly across levels of family dysfunction, so we cannot clearly reject the proportional model. However, the pattern of results was closest to an additive model of genetic and environmental action (Figure 16.1).

These results may seem a bit anticlimactic, but they provide at least two lessons. First, there may be many situations in which genetic and environmen-

SIDEBAR 16.3. Assessment of Family Dysfunction

Family dysfunction (FD) was measured using 14 items from the Family Environment Scale (Moos & Moos, 1986), which reflected the general emotional tone of the home. Two sample items are:

> Family members really helped and supported one another.
> Family members would get so angry sometimes that they would throw things or hit each other.

Twins and their parents (for the FF sample) were asked the frequency with which each of the preceding conditions existed during the period when the twins were growing up (defined as until age 16). There were four response choices for each item, ranging from *often* to *never*.

We formed a single score for each individual by taking the first principal component of these items. The number of reporters per family ranged from one to four. About 50% of the time, ratings were available from all four family members (two twins and their parents). Three ratings (most commonly, twin, cotwin, and mother) were available for 32%, two ratings (usually twin and cotwin) were obtained for 13%, and one rating (self) for 5%. We formed a composite score for each family by averaging the scores across all available informants. The correlations between raters for family dysfunction scores were moderate, ranging from 0.35 to 0.58.

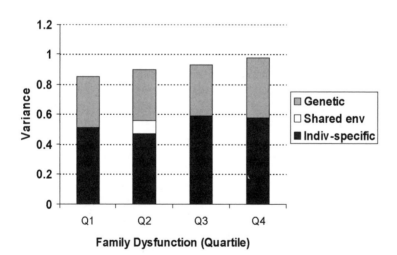

FIGURE 16.11. Relation of neuroticism score proportions of variance to level of family dysfunction. Env = environment. Data from Kendler, Aggen, Jacobson, and Neale (2003a).

tal factors really do add together. Searching for genotype–environment inter-actions has become trendy in psychiatric and behavioral genetics, but they may be the exception more often than the rule. It is instructive that with organisms such as plants and fruit flies, in which genetic and environmental effects can be studied using experimental controls, there are many situations in which genes and environments do no more than add together (Mather & Jinks, 1982).

A second lesson is that the ways in which genetic factors influence a per-sonality trait such as neuroticism may be different from the ways they affect liability to a psychiatric disorder such as major depression. As anyone who has been a parent can attest, personality traits feel "hardwired" and do not seem easily amenable to environmental interventions. Among adults, person-ality tends to be quite stable, even over long periods of time (McCrae & Costa, 1990). By contrast, depression is an episodic and often "reactive" con-dition that is frequently precipitated by environmental stressors. From this perspective, it is perhaps not surprising that the pathway from genes to per-sonality may be less "perturbable" by the environment than is the case for the pathways to major depression or other psychiatric disorders.

A final consideration is that, although our result represents a failure to reject the null hypothesis, this is not the same as proving the null hypothesis. We can conclude only that we could not detect any moderation effects with our sample size and our statistical methods. Detecting statistical interactions (the basis of the moderator model) requires larger sample sizes than does detecting main effects (Wahlsten, 1990).[14]

Family Dysfunction and the Heritability of Cigarette Smoking

In our final example, we apply the moderator model to examine the rela-tionships between family functioning and risk for smoking. We chose cigarette smoking because it is a common, highly heritable behavior (Li et al., 2003; Sullivan & Kendler, 1998) that can be accurately assessed by self-report (Luepker, Pallonen, Murray, & Pirie, 1989; Slattery, Hunt, French, Ford, & Williams, 1989). There is strong evidence that a disrupted home environment is associated with an increased risk for smoking (Tyas & Pederson, 1998). This is generally assumed to be an environmental effect. However, we hypoth-esized that the home environment might also influence smoking through a dif-ferent mechanism—by moderating the effects of genetic influences.

We hypothesized that the genetic influences on smoking would be higher among individuals who had experienced higher levels of dysfunction in their homes of origin. This was suggested by an adoption study of alcoholism in which genetic risk factors were more important among women who experi-enced greater family conflict in their adoptive homes (Cutrona et al., 1994). Although this is (to our knowledge) the only prior study of substance use showing this kind of gene-by-environment interaction, it is quite persuasive because of its use of the adoption design. Here, family conflict was clearly an environmental risk factor because it arose in an adoptive home among adoptive relatives genetically unrelated to the participant.

To test for moderation of the genetic influences on smoking of family dysfunction, we used information on smoking among 1,676 female twins who had participated in our second and third interview waves. We formed a six-category variable reflecting cigarette use at the time of heaviest smoking.[15] Our measure of family dysfunction was the same as that used in the analysis of neuroticism described earlier. The statistical methods we employed were also nearly identical.

When we fit the moderator model (similar to Figure 16.9) and a model without moderated effects, we found that the statistical differences between the models were not large but that, overall, the moderator model was the most parsimonious. The results are summarized in Figure 16.12. The values are scaled relative to the results for individuals in the lowest quartile of family dysfunction. The results show that (1) the magnitude of the genetic variance was constant across levels of family dysfunction, (2) the effect of shared family environment was estimated to be zero in all conditions,[16] and (3) the individual-specific environmental variance in liability to smoking was higher at higher levels of family dysfunction. Thus we found some evidence for moderation, but it was on the individual-specific environmental factor, not on the genetic factor as we had predicted.

These results can be reexpressed in terms of heritability (which again is the *ratio* of genetic to total variance in liability). Heritability of smoking was

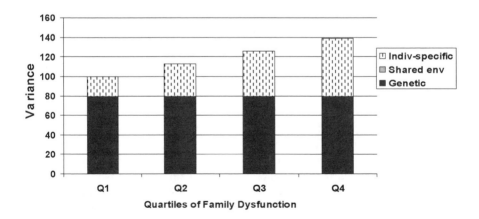

FIGURE 16.12. Effects of childhood family dysfunction on estimated genetic and environmental contributions to variation in smoking. Env = environment. Data from Kendler, Aggen, Prescott, Jacobson, and Neale (2004a).

higher when levels of family dysfunction were at a minimum ($a^2 = 0.79$) than when they were at a maximum ($a^2 = 0.57$). Individual-specific environment showed the reverse pattern—being relatively more important at maximum ($e^2 = 0.43$) than minimum ($e^2 = 0.21$) levels of family dysfunction. These results show, as we have stated elsewhere, that heritability is not a constant property of a trait or a population. Under different environmental conditions, heritability estimates can change.

We have pondered the interpretation of these results. Because so little is known about the role of gene–environment interactions in drug use, the literature is not of much help. At the simplest level, these findings suggest caution in the articulation of broad pronouncements about the nature of these interactions. We might be tempted to declare for all phenotypes that exposure to a broader range of environments will permit expression of a broader range of genetic variation, but the reality is likely to be much more complex.

Although these results can be expressed as a declining heritability of smoking with increasing family dysfunction, it is important to emphasize that the level of genetic variance is not changing. Instead, as shown in Figure 16.12, these findings reflect a systematic increase in individual-specific environmental effects on smoking as the level of family dysfunction increases.[17] What might be happening? Imagine a set of extrafamilial environmental factors that in adolescence increase the risk for heavy smoking. An example of such a "prosmoking" influence would be hanging around with the "bad kids" after school. High-functioning families are relatively effective at protecting their children from these kinds of influences, whereas in dysfunctional families parental monitoring of children's activities may be lower. In these families it might be more likely that one of the twins would encounter situations in which she would be exposed to these prosmoking influences and, by chance, the cotwin would not be similarly exposed. This situation—greater "random" exposure to smoking-related social influences for twins growing up in poorly functioning families—would explain the results we have observed. Although speculative and in need of further empirical testing, this explanation of the findings is at least a plausible one.

SUMMARY

A major goal of this book is to try to understand how genetic and environmental risk factors interrelate in the etiological pathways to psychiatric and substance use disorders. Although the work presented in this chapter is preliminary, it represents an important step toward addressing this fundamental question. Essentially, we have tried to address whether we can assume that genetic and environmental factors add together to influence these outcomes or whether they may combine in more complex ways.

To address this fundamental question, we used two different conceptual and statistical approaches, illustrated by Figures 16.1, 16.2, and 16.9, respectively. These models addressed different permutations of the same question. Our first model asked whether genes moderate the sensitivity of individuals to the pathogenic effects of the environment, such as SLEs. The second model examined whether specified environments, such as family dysfunction, can moderate the effects of genes.

The results of our examples are summarized in Table 16.1. These findings show convincingly that, in at least some circumstances, we cannot assume that genetic and environmental risk simply add together. Using three varying approaches, we found evidence that genetic factors (expressed as a function of cotwin history of MD, level of neuroticism, or variants of the serotonin transporter) influenced the sensitivity of individuals to the depressogenic effects of life events. We also saw that positive rearing styles protected against genetic risk for drinking problems. More tentatively, we found that family dysfunction altered the environmental variance (and thus the heritability) of smoking. However, we also found that sometimes the additive model is probably the correct one. In particular, genetic effects on the key personality trait of neuroticism were not altered or moderated by the effects of family dysfunction.

We have tested models for gene–environment interaction in only a small handful of the disorders and environmental risk factors included in the VATSPSUD. Much more work needs to be done. But our results so far allow us to conclude that for at least some risk factors and disorders we cannot assume that an individual's total liability to illness is just the sum of his or her genetic risk plus adverse environmental experiences. The etiology is more complex than that. Our risk emerges over time through the interweaving of genes and environment.

NOTES

1. The terms *gene–environment interaction* and *genetic control of sensitivity to the environment* are broadly synonymous, and we use both in this book. However, the second term focuses on the key issue we wish to illustrate: how genetic factors alter the response of the organism to environmental stressors. It would be equally valid to describe "gene–environment interaction" as "environmental control of gene expression." Another consideration is that the use of the term *interaction* in its statistical sense (as here) is often confusing, because it has a broader meaning in everyday usage.

2. This is the same allele that has been implicated in increased risk for Alzheimer's disease (Lendon, Ashall, & Goate, 1997). One theory for the mechanism is that having the ε-4 allele increases the buildup of amyloid plaques as a response to even mild head trauma.

3. As discussed in Chapters 13 and 14, these events and experiences are probably influenced to some degree by genetic factors, so they are not strictly "environmental" risk factors.

4. This index of genetic risk was strongly associated with risk for an episode of MD, confirming its usefulness. Compared with the lowest risk group (MZ twin with cotwin unaffected), the proportional increase in risk for MD in any given month

TABLE 16.1. Results from Studies of Genetic Influences on Environmental Sensitivity

Environmental risk						
Factor	Type	Outcome	Index of genetic risk	Main effects	Gene–environment interaction?	Conclusion
Major SLE	Proximal	MD	Cotwin history of MD	G, E	Yes	Sensitivity to environment varies with genetic risk.
Severity of SLE	Proximal	MD	Neuroticism score	G, E	Yes	Sensitivity to environment varies with genetic risk.
CSA Severity of SLE	Distal Proximal	MD	Neuroticism score	G, E	Genetic × distal × proximal interaction	Sensitivity to recent stress varies with genetic risk and early trauma.
Severity of SLE	Proximal	MD	Serotonin transporter genotype	G, E	Yes	Sensitivity to minor and low-moderate stress varies by genotype.
Parenting received	Distal	Problem drinking	Parental history of alcoholism	G, E	Yes	Genetic risk is moderated by favorable parenting.
Family dysfunction	Distal	Neuroticism	Twin-pair resemblance	G, E	No	Genetic and environmental influences on neuroticism are not moderated by family dysfunction.
Family dysfunction	Distal	Smoking amount	Twin-pair resemblance	G, E	No, but E × E	Environmental influences on smoking are moderated by family dysfunction.

was 27% for a woman with an unaffected DZ cotwin, 103% for a woman with an affected DZ cotwin, and 158% for a woman with an affected MZ cotwin. These results were originally published in Kendler et al. (1995a).

5. The interaction suggested by Figure 16.3 was confirmed statistically using a standard linear regression model.

6. Although the group differences were small when a major event was absent, they were statistically significant in our large sample. For example, MD onset in the absence of a major SLE occurred 0.5% of the time in the lowest genetic risk group (women whose MZ cotwins were unaffected) versus 1.1% in the highest risk group (women whose MZ cotwins had a history of MD).

7. To reduce the possibility of state effects of MD on neuroticism scores, the measures of neuroticism used in these analyses were obtained prior to the period for which SLEs and depressive onsets were assessed. In using neuroticism instead of an index of genetic risk, these analyses technically reflect "temperamental control of sensitivity to the environment" rather than "genetic control of sensitivity to the environment."

8. These analyses were based on person-month data and conducted with a Cox proportional hazards model using the SAS procedure PHREG (Allison, 1995; Cox, 1972). Three predictor variables were used: N, sex, and LTCT. The dependent variable was the onset of a depressive episode. These individuals reported a total of 1,194 onsets of MD. The final model was developed based on nine strata. Each stratum consisted of data for participants from the FF3, FF4, or MF2 interviews with zero, one, or two prior onsets in the previous 13 months. N was standardized to have a mean of 0 and standard deviation of 1, allowing easy interpretation and a meaningful quadratic term. LTCT was coded so that 0 meant no SLE occurrence in the month and 1 through 4 meant the occurrence of a SLE with minor, low-moderate, high-moderate, and severe LTCT. As in the previous analyses presented in this chapter, there is the problem of the scale of interaction, especially when the dependent variable—a depressive episode—is dichotomous. We confirmed, using additive models, that the result presented in Figure 16.4 is indeed a statistical interaction. Details can be found in the original publication by Kendler, Kuhn, and Prescott (2004b).

9. The main effect of sex is not easily apparent from the figures because they do not reflect sex differences in the frequency of the LTCT categories (women have more minor and low-moderate LTCT events) or in neuroticism (on average, women have higher N scores).

10. The astute observer will note that the curves differ somewhat across levels of neuroticism. Our final model contained one interaction: between neuroticism and CSA with intercourse. This interaction meant that liability for MD among individuals with high N and CSA with intercourse was less than predicted by the main effects of these two factors. This study was originally published in Kendler, Kuhn, and Prescott (2004b).

11. In our best-fitting model, the main effects of serotonin genotype ($\chi_1^2 = 2.04$, NS) and LTCT ≥ 1 ($\chi_1^2 = 3.31$, NS) were nonsignificant. By contrast, the main effects of both levels of stress remained significant: LTCT ≥ 3 ($\chi_1^2 = 9.89$, $p = 0.002$) and LTCT = 4 ($\chi_1^2 = 18.66$, $p < 0.0001$). Most important, we observed a significant *positive* interaction between genotype and LTCT ≥ 1 ($\chi_1^2 = 10.74$, $p = 0.001$) such that individuals with the SS genotype had greater sensitivity to the depressogenic effects of SLEs with mild or greater LTCT levels than did individuals with the SL or LL genotypes. Furthermore, we also saw a significant *negative* and nearly balancing interaction

between genotype and LTCT ≥ 3 (χ_1^2 = 6.47, p = 0.001). That is, at high levels of stress, individuals with LL and LS genotypes were at about the same risk for MD as those with SS genotype.

12. It is possible that women who develop problem drinking have biased perceptions of their early family life. We addressed this possibility by repeating the analyses using cotwin reports of parenting received. The effects were somewhat weaker, but the pattern was consistent with that observed based on self-reports. These results were originally presented at the 1993 meeting of the World Congress on Psychiatric Genetics (Prescott et al., 1993).

13. As we saw in Chapter 13, parenting given is not a completely "environmental" variable. It is possible that the results we observed occurred because alcoholic parents who are able to provide good parenting may themselves have lower genetic liability and are thus providing "better" genes along with better environments. This would represent gene–environment correlation rather than gene–environment interaction. We are not able to distinguish the two, as we do not have much information on the severity of parental alcoholism.

14. An inspection of our raw data in a number of different ways detected no hints of moderation effects. Thus, we were not in a situation, as sometimes occurs, of seeing a strong trend that falls short of statistical significance. We really saw no trend toward moderation in our data at all. The study was originally published in Kendler, Aggen, Jacobson, & Neale, 2003a.

15. The categories of weekly smoking were (1) zero cigarettes per week (34.5% of the sample), (2) 1–2 (16.2%), (3) 3–20 (15.7%), (4) 21–120 (11.1%), (5) 121–200 (14.7%), and (6) > 200 (7.8%). Because this variable was not normally distributed, we analyzed it as an ordered polychotomous variable assuming a multiple-threshold liability model. Twin-pair resemblance was based on a polychoric correlation. Additional information about our assessment of smoking history can be found in Sidebar 5.4. The study was originally published in Kendler, Aggen, Prescott, Jacobson, and Neale (2004a).

16. In fact, the true "best-fit" model was a reduced moderator model with all the shared environmental pathways set to zero.

17. The psychometrically astute reader might now be asking, "Could all these results just be due to increased error in the assessment of smoking at higher levels of smoking?" This is a viable explanation, because mean smoking levels increase with increasing family dysfunction. However, the short-term test–retest reliability of our smoking measure was very high (weighted κ = 0.87; 95% CI = 0.83, 0.90) with no evidence that degree of agreement was related to the level of reported smoking. We also tested whether the level of family dysfunction affected the stability of our cross-time maximal smoking measures. It did not (χ_1^2 = 0.19, p = 0.66). These results suggest that higher error variance for our smoking measure among twins with higher family dysfunction is an unlikely explanation for the observed results.

CHAPTER SEVENTEEN

Integrative Models

$\mathbf{A}$s we are nearing the end of this book, the goal of this chapter is a daunting one: to pull together the various themes taken up in earlier sections of the book by developing a truly integrated etiological model for a disorder—MD. We will fail at this task, because there are complexities in the etiological pathways to psychiatric and substance use disorders that are beyond our data and beyond our current ability to conceptualize and model.[1] Readers will therefore need to see this effort as a "rough draft" toward a final model that will take years—if not decades—to achieve. Nonetheless, it is worth trying. For too long, review papers in psychiatry and abnormal psychology have proposed such "integrative models" for particular disorders based solely on literature reviews and/or the authors' own speculations. However, such models were never tested against real data, both because there are substantial methodological issues about how to incorporate the required complexity and because few data sets contain good measures on a wide variety of risk factors. At some point, it is critical for one group of investigators with one data set to try to set out a preliminary integrative model. We began with MD in females.

INTEGRATIVE MODEL FOR MAJOR DEPRESSION IN WOMEN

The goal of our analyses was to understand how genetic background, early risk factors, and proximal stressors combine to influence risk for MD in females. Our model predicts the occurrence of an episode of MD in the 1-year period prior to the fourth wave of interviews with our female–female twin sample. Of the 1,940 female twins who participated in FF4, 176 (9.1%) reported symptoms of a past-year depressive episode that met DSM-III-R criteria. We set out to understand what was different about the background and experiences of these women that may have led to their depressive episodes.

This large analytic task required us to make several critical decisions about our approach. First, we decided to use a structural equation modeling approach to understanding the connections among the variables. Because this was an exploratory analysis, we decided to keep the model as simple as possible and include only *additive* relationships between variables.

Second, we took a developmental approach to our analysis, organizing our model along temporal lines, moving from risk factors expressed early in life to those that occurred in the "outcome" year. We selected five developmental "tiers" for our risk factors: childhood, early adolescence, late adolescence, adulthood, and the past year.

Third, after many preliminary analyses, some reflected in an earlier published attempt at an integrative model (Kendler, Kessler, Neale, Heath, & Eaves, 1993a), we selected a set of 18 predictor variables organized into the five developmental tiers as follows:

1. *Childhood*: genetic risk factors, disturbed family environment, CSA, and childhood parental loss.
2. *Early adolescence*: neuroticism, low self-esteem, early-onset anxiety, and conduct disorder.
3. *Late adolescence*: low educational attainment, lifetime traumas, low social support, and substance misuse.
4. *Adulthood*: divorce and history of MD.
5. *Past year*: past-year marital problems, total difficulties, and two types of SLEs: dependent and independent.

Fourth, not all twins completed all interviews and questionnaires. Because we could not assume that people drop out of the study at random, we did not want to base the analyses only on women for whom complete information was available. We therefore employed methods of data imputation so we could include as much information from as many respondents as possible.

Fifth, we wanted to obtain the best measures of our constructs. For six out of the 18 variables, we were able to construct latent variables that either were based on several measures of the construct or on the same scale administered at more than one interview. This should have the net effect of improving both the reliability and the validity of our predictor variables (see Sidebar 17.1).

Once we had selected our variables and their initial order within the model, we began the process of model simplification. As in all such model fitting, our goal was to achieve a balance of explanatory power and parsimony. After much work (done with great care by our colleague Charles Gardner), we arrived at a final model that accounted for 52.1% of the variance in liability

SIDEBAR 17.1. Predictor Variables

Complete details of the measures are available in the original publication (Kendler et al., 2002a). Briefly:

Genetic Risk was assessed by a composite measure of the lifetime history of MD in cotwin and the mother and father.

A *Disturbed Family Environment* factor was indicated by two manifest continuous variables: parental warmth, measured using a modified version of the Parental Bonding Instrument (Parker et al., 1979; see Sidebar 7.1) and family environment scores, measured by 14 items chosen from the Family Environment Scale (Moos & Moos, 1986; see Sidebar 16.3). For each scale, an aggregate measure was formed by combining the reports from both twins and any interviewed parents.

Childhood Sexual Abuse was a binary variable that was coded 1 if the twin reported experiencing prior to age 17: (1) unwelcome genital contact or (2) attempted or completed intercourse (see Chapter 7).

Parental Loss was a binary measure that was scored 1 if the twin reported that, prior to the twin reaching age 17, one or more parents left the nuclear home due to death, divorce, or parental separation.

The *Neuroticism* factor was indicated by the 12-item version from the EPQ-R (Eysenck et al., 1985, see Sidebar 11.2) assessed at up to three separate waves.

The *Self-Esteem* factor was based on Rosenberg's scale (Rosenberg, 1969) obtained at the wave 1 and wave 3 interviews.

Early-Onset Anxiety Disorder was a binary variable that was scored 1 for subjects with an onset of panic disorder, GAD (with 1 month minimal duration), or phobia prior to age 18.

Conduct Disorder was treated as an ordinal variable that reflected the number of DSM-IV CD criteria met prior to age 18 that were endorsed at FF4.

Years of Education was treated as a continuous variable.

Lifetime Traumas was the number of lifetime traumatic events (out of 10, including physical assault, unexpected death of a loved one, and abortion) reported at the initial questionnaire.

The *Social Support* factor was based on a combined score from the first- and third-wave interviews. We summed those dimensions of social support that related most strongly to risk for depression: problems with relatives and church/club attendance (Kendler et al., 2002a).

Substance Misuse was a factor of three binary manifest variables: (1) a lifetime diagnosis of DSM-III-R alcohol abuse or dependence; (2) a lifetime diagnosis of DSM-IV drug abuse or dependence; and (3) lifetime nicotine dependence as assessed by a score of ≥ 7 on the Fagerstrom Tolerance Questionnaire (Fagerstrom & Schneider, 1989; see Sidebar 5.4).

Ever Divorced was a binary measure that scored 1 for women who reported ever being divorced at any of our interviews.

History of MD was a binary measure reflecting the presence or absence of one or more episodes of DSM-III-R MD occurring at least 1 year prior to the first wave interview.

(continued)

SIDEBAR 17.1. *(continued)*

Past-Year Marital Problems was constructed as a three-level ordinal variable based on seven items assessing the level of marital satisfaction in the year prior to FF4 obtained from the Social Interaction Scale (Schuster, Kessler, & Aseltine, 1990). A piecewise regression indicated that an elevated risk for onset of MD was associated with levels of satisfaction in the lower 20%. The variable was constructed as: 0 = upper 80% of marital satisfaction, 1 = unmarried, and 2 = lower 20%.

Dependent and Independent Stressful Life Events (SLEs) were dichotomized into those clearly or probably independent versus clearly or probably dependent (see Chapter 8). For individuals experiencing a new onset of MD in the year preceding their FF4 interview, we counted the number of dependent and independent life events occurring in that month and the 2 preceding months. For individuals reporting no depressive onset, a random 3-month window was used to assess the occurrence of SLEs.

Past-Year Difficulties reflected the sum of all SLEs reported at other times during the year prior to the FF4 interview.

to develop an episode of MD. As reflected by standard statistical indices, the model fit quite well.[2]

This final model is depicted in Figure 17.1. This is a complex figure, but we think it is worth the effort to understand. The path coefficients depicted in the figure reflect the *unique relationship between variables, adjusting for all the other possible connections through other variables in the model.* That is, a pair of variables will be connected both by a direct path and, typically, by several indirect paths that pass through other variables. One-headed arrows are used to indicate causal paths. Two-headed arrows represent correlations—in which the variables are associated but we cannot assume that one causes the other. (See Chapter 3 for details of path diagrams.) It is also important to keep in mind that the path coefficients represent the "average" relationships among variables *in the whole sample.* They do not tell us about the individual pathways that particular people may take on their journey to developing depression.

In considering our final model, we first describe the variables and paths one by one. Then we step back and comment on the big picture.

Childhood Risk Factors

We begin with the four childhood risk factors, shown in the top tier of Figure 17.1. All four variables are moderately and positively correlated. The level of a woman's genetic risk for MD was positively correlated with her exposure to childhood environmental risk factors. Furthermore, having been exposed to one of these risk factors was associated with increased chances of exposure to the others. These results illustrate the difficulty of studying typical nuclear families: genetic risk and environmental risk tend to occur together (or, more technically, are statistically *confounded*).

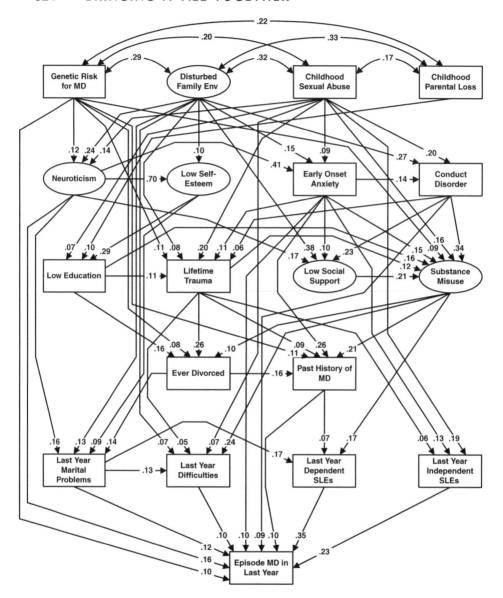

FIGURE 17.1. Results from integrative model for MD in women. Adapted from Kendler, Gardner, and Prescott (2002a, Figure 1). Copyright 2002 by the American Psychiatric Association. Adapted by permission.

Now let's turn to the childhood risk factors one at a time. As shown in Figure 17.2, high *genetic risk* for MD was directly predictive of elevated levels of neuroticism (a key temperamental risk factor for later depression), substance misuse, traumatic experiences, and divorce. The level of genetic risk for MD also directly predicted both MD prior to the past year and the probability of a depressive episode in the past year.

We illustrate direct and indirect paths by examining the relationship between genetic risk and episodes of MD in the past year. As noted, genetic risk directly predicted risk for a depressive episode. However, high genetic risk also directly predicted high levels of neuroticism and a history of depression, which in turn directly predicted risk for MD in the past year. Furthermore, a number of more complex, indirect pathways from genetic risk to past year MD can be seen in the figure. Two of them are: (1) genetic risk ⇒ neuroticism ⇒ early-onset anxiety ⇒ past-year MD and (2) genetic risk ⇒ substance misuse ⇒ history of MD ⇒ past-year MD. Thus, for any two variables in the model, it makes sense to think about direct paths, indirect paths, and (if you have the patience to trace them all out and add them up) the total association, which is the sum of all the direct and indirect connections.

Returning to Figure 17.1, a *disturbed family environment* uniquely predicted all four early adolescent risk factors, with the strongest effect on CD, followed by neuroticism. A disturbed family background also strongly predicted low levels of social support, as well as an increased risk for lifetime traumas, past-year marital problems, and past-year difficulties.

Childhood sexual abuse (CSA) uniquely predicted three of the four early-adolescent and three of the four late-adolescent risk factors, with its strongest effects on CD and lifetime trauma. In addition, CSA also predicted both difficulties and independent SLEs in the past year.

Childhood parental loss uniquely predicted only low educational attainment.

Of the three childhood "environmental" risk factors, a disturbed family environment had the most extensive effect on downstream variables, whereas childhood parental loss had by far the least. Consistent with the results of our previous analyses of CSA (see Chapter 7), it is clear that the experience of sexual abuse has a potent impact on future risk factors, even after adjusting for the impact of family dysfunction and genetic risk.

Risk Factors of Early Adolescence

We turn now to the four early-adolescent risk factors, shown in the second tier of Figure 17.1. *Neuroticism* had a particularly strong effect on low self-esteem and early-onset anxiety disorders. High levels of neuroticism also predicted low levels of social support and past-year marital problems.

Low self-esteem had a substantial influence on low educational attainment and also predicted past-year marital problems.

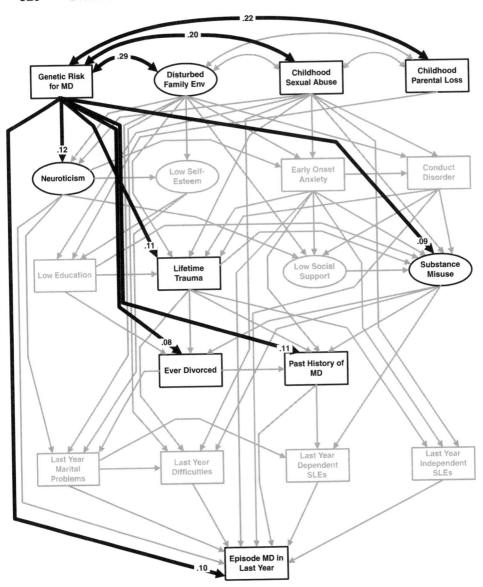

FIGURE 17.2. Risk factors significantly associated with genetic risk for depression in women. Adapted from Kendler, Gardner, and Prescott (2002a, Figure 2). Copyright 2002 by the American Psychiatric Association. Adapted by permission.

Early-onset anxiety disorder increased the risk for CD, low social support, substance misuse, and past history of MD, as well as exposure to lifetime trauma and preceding-year independent SLEs.

CD symptoms increased the risk for lifetime traumas, low social support, and, especially strongly, substance misuse.

Of note, three of these four early-adolescent risk factors—neuroticism, early-onset anxiety and CD—had a direct and independent impact on risk for the onset of MD in the past year.

Risk Factors of Late Adolescence

Looking now at the third tier of Figure 17.1, *low educational attainment* uniquely predicted only lifetime traumas and the risk for divorce. *Lifetime trauma* also predicted divorce, as well as history of MD, past year difficulties, and independent SLEs. *Low social support* was a unique predictor only of substance misuse.

Substance misuse was the most "connected" variable in the model. It was the second strongest predictor of a history of MD and it also predicted exposure to three later environmental risk factors: divorce, past-year difficulties, and dependent SLEs.

Adult Risk Factors

Moving down another tier, both *ever divorced* and *past history of MD* were predicted by an array of upstream variables. Having ever been divorced uniquely predicted only past history of MD and past-year marital problems, whereas past MD predicted past-year dependent SLEs and risk for an episode of MD in the past year.

Past-Year Risk Factors

Finally, our model included four measures of environmental adversity occurring in the past year. Two of these, *past-year marital problems* and *past-year difficulties*, were not timed relative to episode onset, whereas *dependent* and *independent SLEs* had to have occurred in temporal proximity to the onset of MD. All four of these risk factors were uniquely related to risk for MD, with SLEs having a stronger impact than difficulties.

Episode of Major Depression in the Past Year

As depicted in Figure 17.3, the unique influences on risk for MD in the past year are diverse and include genetic risk, three risk factors from early adolescence, history of MD, and all four past-year risk factors. Quantitatively, the three strongest risk factors were past-year dependent SLEs, independent SLEs, and neuroticism.

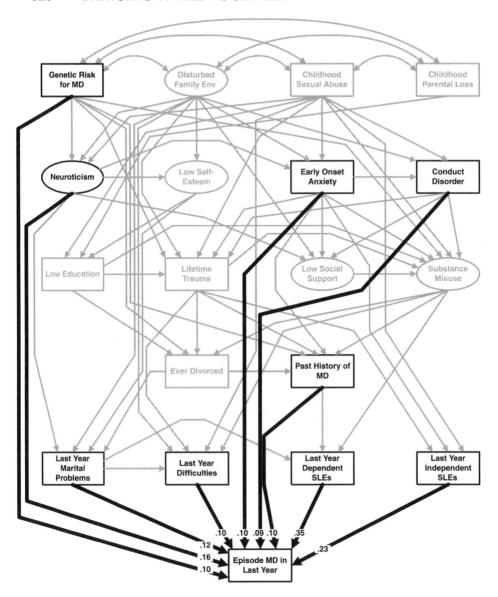

FIGURE 17.3. Risk factors associated with past-year MD in women. Adapted from Kendler, Gardner, and Prescott (2002a, Figure 3). Copyright 2002 by the American Psychiatric Association. Adapted by permission.

Interpretation of Results

Looking beyond the mass of individual path coefficients, what are the broader implications of these results? Certainly they demonstrate what it means to say that MD is a complex, multifactorial disorder! They also show the potential power of using a developmental perspective to understand the emergence of vulnerability to psychopathology.

The results suggest that there are three sets of paths connecting early risk factors to the development of an MD episode and that these paths are identifiable based on both their theoretical associations and the strength of their statistical connections. We term these paths *internalizing, externalizing,* and *adversity.* The set of internalizing paths, depicted in Figure 17.4, is anchored by two variables: neuroticism and early-onset anxiety disorders. The externalizing portion of the model (Figure 17.5) is also anchored by two variables: CD and substance misuse. By contrast, the adversity paths (Figure 17.6) are more extensive, beginning with the three childhood risk factors of disturbed family environment, CSA , and parental loss; flowing through low education, lifetime trauma, and low social support to being divorced; and then influencing all four of the past-year environmental risk factors. This last set of paths might be more accurately termed *adversity/interpersonal difficulties,* because many of the depressogenic consequences of the earlier adversities appear to occur through troubled interpersonal relationships.

It would be incorrect to give the impression that these pieces of the model represent three distinct pathways to illness. Rather, they are interlinked in a number of ways. Genetic risk factors for MD contribute to all three, having a unique predictive relation to neuroticism (internalizing), substance misuse (externalizing), and lifetime traumas and divorce (adversity). Childhood adversities are strong risk factors for externalizing disorders, which in turn predict later adversity. Finally, to a lesser extent, internalizing variables also predispose to future adversity.

Two further points about these analyses are noteworthy. First, the results illustrate the intricacy of the "gene-to-phenotype" pathway for complex psychiatric disorders such as MD. Two paths involve what we have termed *genetic control of exposure to the environment* (see Chapter 13), by which individuals at high genetic risk for MD choose situations associated with events (such as traumas and divorce) that increase risk for depressive episodes. Consistent with our earlier work (Kendler et al., 1993b; see Chapter 11), one path suggests that genetic risk factors for MD act in part by influencing personality. Substance misuse is also an important intervening variable between genetic factors and MD. Finally, in addition to all these indirect pathways, genetic risk factors directly increase the probability for both prior and past year episodes of MD. Genetic factors were the *only childhood risk factor* to directly influence past year episodes; all the others acted through indirect paths.

A second point worth noting is that the present results suggest that a disturbed family environment may play an important role in the developmental

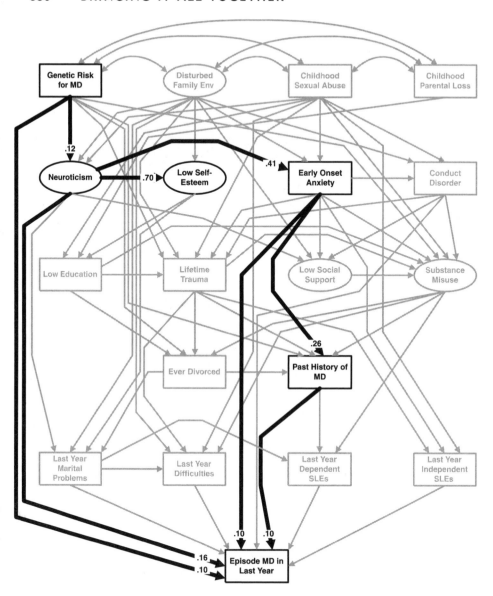

FIGURE 17.4. *Internalizing* risk factors associated with past-year MD in women. Adapted from Kendler, Gardner, and Prescott (2002a, Figure 4). Copyright 2002 by the American Psychiatric Association. Adapted by permission.

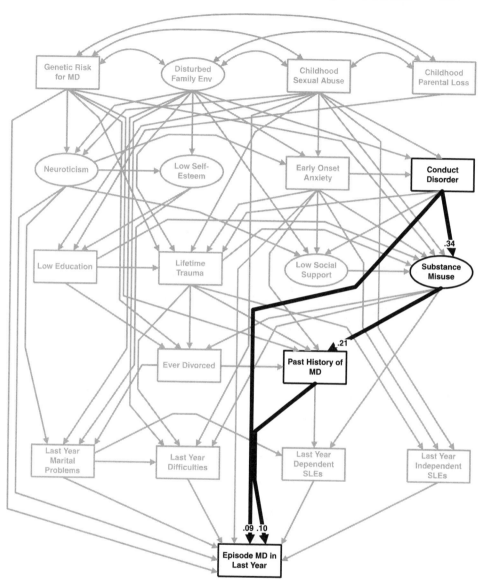

FIGURE 17.5. *Externalizing* risk factors associated with past-year MD in women. Adapted from Kendler, Gardner, and Prescott (2002a, Figure 5). Copyright 2002 by the American Psychiatric Association. Adapted by permission.

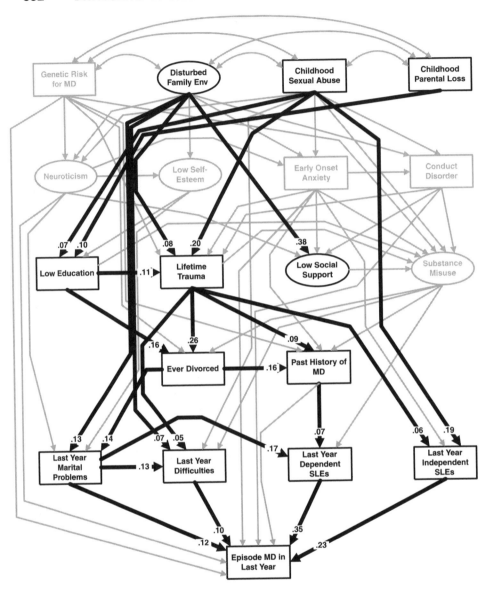

FIGURE 17.6. *Adversity* factors associated with past-year MD in women. Adapted from Kendler, Gardner, and Prescott (2002a, Figure 6). Copyright 2002 by the American Psychiatric Association. Adapted by permission.

cascade leading to depression. This finding is in opposition to the results from our twin analyses, which showed no evidence for a familial-environmental contribution to the etiology of MD (see Chapter 4), There are several possible explanations for this apparent contradiction. First, disturbed family environment could be a manifestation of familial genetic risk for MD. For example, a father's genetic liability to MD could cause him to exhibit lack of warmth. Second, these could be true environmental effects that we had limited power to detect in our twin modeling. Third, as we noted earlier (Chapter 3) the shared environment factor estimated in standard twin models includes only environmental factors that make members of a twin pair more similar. Many aspects of the family are likely to have a different impact on siblings within a family, either because one child is singled out or because children of differing temperaments or maturity react differently to the same stressor. Thus the effects of a disturbed family environment could appear in twin models as part of the individual-specific environmental factor. A final consideration is that detecting small shared environmental effects in the presence of genetic effects requires much larger samples than ours (see Sidebar 3.2).

INTEGRATIVE MODEL FOR MAJOR DEPRESSION IN MEN

Nearly 2 years after completing our integrative model for MD in women, we set about trying to replicate, as closely as possible, the same analyses in men. Numerous studies have examined sex differences in the prevalence and risk factors for MD (Bebbington, 1998; Nolen-Hoeksema, 1990). Although higher rates of MD in women have been consistently reported, finding robust and replicable differences between the two sexes in risk factors for MD has been more difficult. Most studies have compared only a small number of risk factors. To our knowledge, no prior attempts have been made to compare comprehensive etiological models for MD in the two sexes.

For the analyses of males, we used data from 2,935 members of male–male pairs who had completed both the MF1 and MF2 interviews, making this sample over 50% larger than that used in our model for women. Of these individuals, 2,394 came from 1,197 complete pairs and 541 were single twins whose cotwins did not complete both interview waves. A depressive episode meeting DSM-III-R criteria in the year prior to the MF2 interview was reported by 179 (7.5%) of these men.

The variables that we included in the model with men were, insofar as possible, identical to those used with women. Some differences were unavoidable, as we interviewed the men only twice (compared to four times for the women) and did not interview their parents.[3] The model-fitting procedures used with the male data were also nearly identical to those used with the women and produced similar results, indicating a very good balance of explanatory power and parsimony.[4]

Our best-fit model, which predicted 48.7% of the variance in liability to past year MD, is shown in Figure 17.7. We will not go through a variable-by-variable description of these results. Instead, we discuss six broad conclusions that emerge from a comparison of this model with that obtained in women.

First, and most important, the overall similarities in the two models far outweigh the differences. The general pattern of risk factors and their relationships through developmental time were broadly congruent in the two sexes. We are impressed with the degree of replication of our previous findings in women that emerged from our entirely independent sample of men.

Second, the results suggested that in men, as in women, there were three broad pathways to MD characterized by internalizing symptoms (genetic risk factors, neuroticism, low self-esteem, early-onset anxiety, and history of MD), externalizing symptoms (genetic risk factors, CD, and substance misuse) and adversity/interpersonal difficulties (low parental warmth, CSA, parental loss, low education, lifetime trauma, low social support, history of divorce, history of MD, marital problems, and SLEs). As in women, a number of cross-influences were seen among the three pathways. Genetic risk factors for MD contributed to all three. Several other variables in the internalizing and externalizing pathways predicted increased interpersonal difficulties. Early adversity (i.e., childhood sexual abuse and parental loss) was strongly related to later externalizing symptoms and more weakly related to later internalizing symptoms.

Third, there were important similarities and differences across men and women in how genetic factors influenced risk for MD. In both sexes, the final model contained paths from genetic risk factors to neuroticism, substance misuse, lifetime traumas, history of MD, and past year MD. Across genders, genetic risk for depression is partly mediated by effects on personality, increased exposure to traumatic events, and substance misuse. Furthermore, in both men and women, after controlling for the impact of genetic factors on prior episodes, individuals at high genetic risk remain at increased risk for further episodes into middle-adult life. In men, but not in women, genetic risk factors for MD uniquely predicted risk for early-onset anxiety and CD. Whereas in women genetic risk factors for MD increased risk for divorce, in men they increased exposure to difficulties and SLEs in the preceding year. Perhaps due to greater statistical power in the larger male sample, we detected a broader array of genetic influences on MD in men than in women.

Fourth, childhood parental loss had more diverse and potent effects in men than in women. Whereas in women parental loss uniquely contributed solely to risk for substance misuse, in men such loss predicted all four early-adolescent risk factors, as well as low educational achievement, social support, and dependent SLEs.

Fifth, low self-esteem appears to be a more potent variable in men than in women. In women, low self-esteem predicted only low educational attainment; in men, it increased risk for five downstream variables, including lifetime and past-year MD.

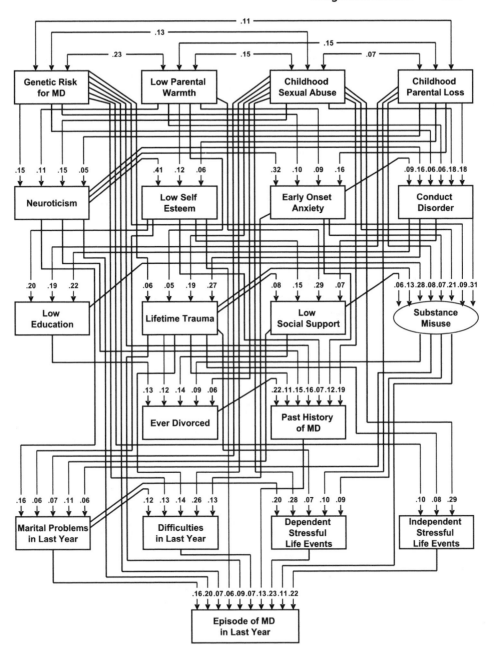

FIGURE 17.7. Results from integrative model for MD in men. Adapted from Kendler, Gardner, and Prescott (2006, Figure 1). Copyright 2006 by the American Psychiatric Association. Adapted by permission.

Sixth, two plausible hypotheses with which we began this study were not supported. We expected CSA to have more potent effects in women than in men. This was not seen. We also predicted that the pathway to MD running through conduct disorder and substance misuse would be more prominent in men than in women, but this was not strongly supported. In men, the best-fit model contained a direct path from substance misuse to past year MD that was not present in women. However, in women, the model contained a direct path from CD to past year MD and a direct path from substance misuse to history of MD, both of which were lacking in the males.

In summary, MD in men is a complex, multifactorial disorder, the liability to which is influenced by a broad array of risk factors that act at different stages of development. Variables that influence risk for MD in men include genetic and temperamental factors, psychosocial adversity both early in life and in adulthood, childhood anxiety and CD, and substance misuse. These results suggest that, from an etiological perspective, MD is largely the same disorder in men and women. As in women, the results in men further illustrate the complexity of the "gene-to-phenotype" pathway. Individuals at elevated genetic risk for MD are likely to be exposed to increased rates of childhood adversity, to have higher levels of neuroticism, to be at greater risk for early-onset anxiety disorder and substance misuse, and to choose or create environments that lead to more difficulties and SLEs in adulthood—all of which increase risk for a depressive episode.

METHODOLOGICAL LIMITATIONS

A few caveats are in order lest we overinterpret the results of these analyses. First, our interpretation of the results implies a causal relationship between upstream and downstream variables. The validity of this assumption varies across different parts of the model. For example, the path from genetic risk to neuroticism could only plausibly go in one direction. By contrast, the relationship between low self-esteem and low educational attainment or between divorce and history of MD is likely to be bidirectional. After the completion of our model, we experimented with shifting the order of variables. The overall fit of the model consistently declined, and little change was seen in path estimates. It is unlikely, therefore, that our parameter estimates are far off due to our assumptions about direction of causality. It is probable, however, that in some parts of our model the relationships between variables that we assume take the form of A → B may be truly either A ← B or, more likely, A ⇄ B.

Second, the models we employed assume that multiple independent variables act additively and linearly in their impact on risk for MD. We know for some variables that this assumption is not true. For example, neuroticism and SLEs interact nonadditively in the prediction of risk for MD (see Chapter 16). We could have included interactions in our model, but the large number of possible interactions was more than our data set could support.[5]

Third, our analyses predicted onset of a recent episode of MD. Most individuals who reported recent episodes had a prior history of MD. Therefore, the findings in this model relative to past year difficulties might be viewed as indicating the proximal triggers for new episodes among individuals who were vulnerable.

Fourth, our model underestimates the impact of genetic factors on the etiology of MD in two ways:

1. Our measure of genetic risk for MD was indirect and did not incorporate the most powerful aspect of the twin model—the direct comparison of correlations between monozygotic and dizygotic twins.
2. Our model did not reflect the known genetic influences on neuroticism, anxiety disorders, CD, or substance use. Part of the risk contributed by these variables to risk for MD is likely to be attributable to genetic factors.

Fifth, in the evaluation of direct paths to past year depression, a model of this complexity has a built-in bias. Upstream variables (such as childhood risk factors) have many more possible indirect pathways to risk for MD than do downstream variables. Thus, all other factors being equal, direct paths will tend to be weaker for upstream variables and become progressively stronger for downstream variables closer in the model to the depressive onsets.

Finally, a number of variables in our model were assessed by long-term retrospective recall. Such data are subject to recall bias, which is more likely to overestimate than underestimate causal relationships (Bradburn, Rips, & Shevell, 1987; Henry, Moffitt, Caspi, Langley, & Silva, 1994; Maughan & Rutter, 1997). Ideally, this study would be done prospectively with a twin cohort followed from birth, but no such studies exist (for obvious financial and logistical reasons). Within the limits of a longitudinal design beginning with a cohort in early to mid-adulthood, we have done several things to reduce retrospective bias and other measurement error, including: combining reports of multiple raters, assessing variables in a prospective fashion (using measures from interviews *prior to* the one at which past year MD was assessed), and combining data from assessments at multiple waves. We look forward to the collection of adult outcomes by our colleagues conducting longitudinal studies of adolescent twins to see whether their results will replicate our findings.

NOTES

1. For example, we lack any information about risk factors that are reflected in brain structure or function or in hormonal or autonomic regulation.
2. We began with a fully saturated model and used a combination of three approaches to produce a model with the optimal balance of explanatory power and parsimony. First, observing the significance levels of individual paths, we fixed sets of

paths to zero when the associated z value was < 1.96. Second, because our sample size was so large, some paths remained significant that in our judgment were too small to be meaningful. Therefore, we set all paths to zero with a regression weight of < 0.05, regardless of z value. In our third step, we further trimmed our model by setting individual paths to zero to test whether removing them increased model χ^2 more than 3.84 (i.e., significant at $p < 0.05$). If it did not, they were removed. As a last check, taking final results from an earlier iteration of the model, we added and subtracted a number of paths that were marginal by significance and/or magnitude to see if we could arrive at a better overall fit; this indeed produced a modest improvement in fit and explanatory power. We utilized three indices of model fit. All three indices had values that are generally considered good fit: CFI = 0.951 (Bentler & Bonett, 1980), TLI = 0.950 (Bentler, 1990), and RMSEA = 0.033 (Steiger, 1990). For the original study see Kendler, Gardner, and Prescott (2002a).

3. Only one variable was substantially different in the two samples. What we termed *disturbed family environment* in the female sample had to be renamed *low parental warmth* in our male sample because we lacked family environment scores and reports from parents. Several other variables were measured differently: CSA was evaluated with a single item, and we used only a single measurement of neuroticism, self-esteem, and social support (instead of the two occasions used in our female sample).

4. The values of the three fit indices for the male analyses were: CFI = 0.948, TLI = 0.951, and RMSEA = 0.019. For the original study see Kendler, Gardner, and Prescott (2006).

5. A sample size of nearly 2,000 would be adequate to test more complex relations among variables if the variables were all continuous. However, many of our variables were binary and of low frequency, features that reduce power to detect such relations among variables.

CHAPTER EIGHTEEN

Conclusions

We have now come a long way. It is time to step back from the welter of detail and draw some broad conclusions. What have we learned? We have organized our response in terms of the answers to the questions we posed in the Introduction. First we address the *four central themes* of this book.

1. The first question we asked in the Introduction was:

What can we learn about the role of genetic factors in the etiology of psychiatric and substance use disorders? To this, our answer is: *Genetic risk factors are important in determining susceptibility to psychiatric and substance use disorders.*

Our results and those from other studies provide strong and consistent evidence that genetic risk factors play a significant role in the etiology of the common disorders studied in the VATSPSUD. Working from the principle of "inference to the best explanation," it is difficult for us to conceive of a viable alternative explanation for this pattern of findings. We do not claim that our results are without error or bias, as they almost certainly have some of both. Nonexperimental studies in humans always will. But we believe it is very unlikely that our conclusions are horribly wrong. Given our attention to possible biases (e.g., in subject ascertainment, diagnostic reliability, and violations of the equal environment assumption) and the similarity of our findings to those from comparable studies, we are relatively confident that, at a broad level, we got things about right.

It is critical to emphasize that, although the magnitude of genetic effects for common psychiatric and substance use disorders is not overwhelming, neither is it trivial. It is too large to be ignored by anyone who wants to truly understand the etiology of these disorders. To restate this important point: We cannot come to a deep, integrative understanding of the causal pathways to psychiatric and substance abuse disorders in humans without taking genetic factors into account. This is a brute fact of our world. It will not be changed by whether it does or does not fit our ideological, philosophical, or religious views about the nature of personhood.

However, it is also worth stating that the implications of genetic influences can be exaggerated. The disorders we have studied are *not* classical genetic disorders such as cystic fibrosis or Huntington's disease, in which individuals who have the disease gene (or genes) inevitably develop the illness. Genetic risk factors for psychiatric and substance use disorders act probabilistically and not deterministically. What is inherited is a vulnerability or liability. Even when correcting for errors of measurement, we found that heritability estimates were typically less than 50% and always less than 65%.

There have now been enough genetically informative studies of common psychiatric and substance use disorders to enable us to reach the conclusion that our findings are not limited to residents of the Commonwealth of Virginia. It is probably justified to extrapolate these results to other white populations in Europe, North America, and Australia. We know much less about the role of genetic factors in psychiatric illness in other ethnic groups, making this an important area of future research.

2. Our second question was:

Can we clarify the nature of the associations between key environmental factors and the risk for psychopathology? To this, we respond: *Environmental risk factors are of critical etiological importance for the common psychiatric and substance use disorders.*

By studying MZ and DZ twin pairs, we can estimate the aggregate effect of all genes on twin resemblance. It is not quite so easy with the environment. In particular, there are no two individuals who have shared all of their environments in the way that MZ twins share all of their genes. Also, the environment does not distribute itself in populations according to the nice, clean algebraic laws of Mendel (e.g., there is a 50% chance that the maternal or paternal copy of each gene will be transmitted to the offspring). Genes come in relatively discrete "packets." You get one of a small number of distinct versions. The environment is just messier. Take, for example, two male adolescent twins. They "share" their family environment, which encourages participation in community activities. One of them spends years in the Boy Scouts, whereas the other is active in after-school sports. They have both engaged in structured activities outside the home, but have they had the "same" environment? Well, yes and no. Imagine that in early adulthood, they have both experienced romantic rejection that would be rated as a moderately severe SLE. From a research perspective, you might judge that they have experienced the "same" event. But is this degree of similarity like having the "same" genes? Probably not, as there will always be unique features of these life experiences that defy our ability to classify them.

Studying the role of the environment in psychiatric disorders is harder than studying the role of genes for another reason. Being psychiatrically ill does not influence one's genes. All the causal effect goes in one direction. But this is not the case with the environment; being psychiatrically ill can plausibly affect many aspects of one's environment. So the key problem of causal inference in relating environmental factors to risk of psychiatric and substance use disorders does not arise for the study of genetic factors.

In the VATSPSUD, we have studied the role of environmental risk factors in two quite different ways. First, using latent variable modeling, we have examined the aggregate effects of two broad classes of unobserved environment—that which is shared by members of a twin pair and that which is unique to each member of a pair. Results of our twin analyses, especially those models in which we eliminated the effect of errors of measurement, provide strong evidence for the importance of nongenetic factors in the etiology of these disorders. In no case did genetic factors come close to explaining all the variability in risk.

Second, we examined in the VATSPSUD a range of specific environmental risk factors. We do not claim to have examined all of the environmental experiences of etiological importance for psychiatric and substance use disorders. That is probably impossible. But we did study in at least moderate detail key risk factors, particularly parenting, parent–child separation, CSA, social support, and SLEs. Repeatedly, we found significant associations between these environmental factors and risk for psychiatric and substance use disorders. Sometimes the associations were modest, as for parenting, and sometimes they were quite strong, as for certain classes of SLEs.

These results led us to face the critical problem of causal inference. It is not sufficient to demonstrate that a given risk factor is associated with a psychiatric outcome. We must try to determine whether the association is a causal one. Using a combination of methods, including multiple informants, longitudinal sampling, and the cotwin control design, we have produced compelling results that environmental factors are causally related to risk for disorders. We have found evidence for the causal effects of distal risk factors, particularly CSA, and of proximal risk factors, particularly SLEs.

So our two methods of studying the environment, latent variables in twin models and measured specific risk factors, lead us to the same conclusion: Environmental experiences make important differences in the risk of developing the common psychiatric and substance use disorders we studied in the VATSPSUD.

3. The third question that we posed in the Introduction was:

Can we begin to understand how genetic and environmental factors together contribute to risk for psychiatric and substance use disorders? Our reply to this rather complex question begins as follows: *To come to a deeper understanding of the etiological pathways to psychiatric and substance use disorders, it is insufficient to think of genetic and environmental risk factors as simply "adding together."*

Instead, these two broad classes of factors are "woven" together into a complex fabric to determine an individual's overall level of risk. We do not pretend to understand the process completely, but we have good evidence that at least two major mechanisms are at play.

The first of these we have termed *genetic control of sensitivity to the environment*. So far we have demonstrated this mechanism in a limited number of cases. However, we suspect that it is more widespread in its effects. Genetic risk factors for psychiatric and substance use disorders do not just influence the overall level of liability. Rather, an important part of their mode of action is to render individuals more or less vulnerable to the pathogenic effects of environmental risk factors.

The second of these mechanisms is *genetic control of exposure to the environment*. Within the population, environmental and genetic risk factors are not randomly distributed with respect to one another. Instead, there is some correlation. Genetic factors affect the probability of entering or creating stressful environments, be they life events or low social support.

A boating metaphor may help to illustrate these points:

We all know individuals who go through life like a canoe through still water. Their passage is quiet, leaving only a few ripples in their wake. These individuals typically are lovable, have easy temperaments, and rarely get into conflict. They usually have long and successful marriages and are satisfied with their work.

We also know individuals who pass through life like a noisy paddleboat, kicking up lots of waves, leaving a wide and tumultuous wake. Such people are typically "difficult" and have unstable or conflict-ridden relationships and work histories.

Obviously, the paddleboats are more likely to be seen in mental health settings than are the canoes. Our results suggest that in part the vulnerability to being a paddleboat—of encountering stressful social environments—is due to genetic factors. Thus, when we think about gene action for psychiatric disorders, we have to consider two types of pathways. The obvious type is physiological, via "inside the skin" pathways, the nature of which is being uncovered through advances in cognitive and affective neuroscience. But there are also important "outside the skin" pathways, which, partly as a result of genes, can lead individuals to experience adversity.

The idea that individuals play a critical role in shaping their own environments—in part as a result of their own genetic heritage—is not new to evolutionary biology. A substantial literature explores "niche construction," in which animals influence their own physical environment through the building of nests, burrows, dams, or webs (Day, Laland, & Odling-Smee, 2003). We humans do this more than any other creature; we have now reshaped much of the world's landscape to our own ends. In fact, each of us not only affects the physical environment but also determines the structure of our social environment. Because many of the risk factors for psychiatric and substance use disorders emerge from this social environment, it is clear that this "outside the skin" pathway is an important mechanism whereby genes influence risk of illness.

4. The final question that we asked in the Introduction was:

How do genes and environments combine over development to influence risk for psychiatric and substance use disorders? We do not yet have a simple, clear answer to this critical but very difficult question.

As became clear to us when working on our integrative model for MD (Chapter 17), it is vital to understand the "dance through time" of genetic and environmental risk factors. Time is the key element missing from many formulations of the etiology of psychiatric and substance use disorders. Development is the fabric through which these risk factors play out—the process by which the cloth of our lives is woven.

The VATSPSUD was not ideally designed to study developmental processes, as the youngest participants were already in late adolescence or young adulthood when we first studied them. We used careful retrospective measures to ask about events earlier in life. However, this is not as powerful a method as a true prospective study, which tracks individuals through the key years of late childhood and adolescence. Other research groups are now engaging in such studies, and we await with great interest their fine-grained analyses of how genetic and environmental risk factors interact through developmental time.

Several important developmental lessons did emerge from analyses that we were able to conduct. As described in Chapter 10, we showed that in adulthood, genetic risk factors for MD were stable at least over periods of a few years. By contrast, environmental risk factors had time-limited effects. This is particularly interesting because it suggests that the "time profile" of these two major classes of risk factors may differ substantially. Although we are sure this is an oversimplification, it does seem that much of what causes the temporally stable liability to depression comes from our genes, whereas environmental factors create the large but relatively brief spikes in risk that induce episodes in vulnerable individuals.

Also in Chapter 10, we showed how genes and environment affect antisocial behavior over developmental time. Again, the story was an interesting one. Family environment plays a critical role early in development but then fades in importance as adolescents leave home. At the same time, genetic factors grow in importance.

These are only small insights into the broad developmental landscape. But we can see enough to conclude that the interrelationships of genetic and environmental risk factors are complex, dynamic, and critical to an understanding of how these disorders emerge.

Now, at the end of this book, we also want to summarize what we have learned about the *minor themes* that we listed in the Introduction. We again provide our responses to the questions initially asked there.

1. *To what degree are the genetic and environmental risk factors for psychiatric and substance use disorders specific or nonspecific to disorders in their effect?* We have learned a fair amount about levels of specificity, the degree to which genetic and environmental risk factors affect one and only one diagnostic category. Nonspecificity was more common than was specificity. It was rare to find a set of genetic risk factors or a particular environmental risk factor that affected only one disorder. However, there were notable exceptions. Parental death increased the risk only for MD. We found evidence of genetic risk factors that were specific to each phobia subtype. In our multivariate model of seven disorders, drug abuse/dependence and AD were influenced by sets of genes specific to these disorders. Other risk factors, including CSA and poor parenting, were largely nonspecific in their effects, increasing the risk for virtually all disorders that we examined. Overall, with respect to specificity, our genetic findings were nuanced. Our results do not indicate that "DSM got it right" in suggesting that there are specific sets of genetic factors for each disorder. However, we also did not find complete diagnostic nonspecificity. The results from our most complete multivariate model (Chapter 11) suggest that a substantial proportion of the genetic risk factors for common psychiatric and substance use disorders belong to two broad sets of factors that predispose to internalizing and externalizing disorders. Certainly this is not the complete story, but it is a start.

2. *How important are shared or family environmental factors—those environments that affect the members of a twin pair in the same way?* Contrary to what we expected when we began this study, we uncovered little evidence that environmental factors shared by members of a twin pair have substantial impact on risk for psychiatric disorders. In interpreting these results, it is important to recall our discussion from Chapter 3 about the difference between *effective* and *objective* impact. That is, in twin studies we detect the effects of family environment only if they effectively influence both twins to a similar degree. If parents are abusive to one twin in a way that has a strong impact on later risk for psychopathology but are not abusive to the other twin, it might seem logical that this effect—which certainly occurs within the

family—would be identified in a twin analysis as part of the "family environment." But it will not be. Instead, it will appear as an individual-specific effect because it affects only one member of the twin pair. Alternatively, the twins might be exposed to the same adversity but, because of prior differences in experience (or, among DZ twins, of genetic differences), one twin may be much more vulnerable to its pathogenic effects than the other. Again, in a twin design, this will appear as an individual-specific, not a shared environmental, effect. Thus obtaining low estimates of shared environment in a twin study does not mean that families and peers do not substantially affect risk. It does mean that if these factors are important, they are not affecting the two members of a twin pair in the same way.

In the first years of the VATSPSUD, when we focused largely on depression and anxiety disorders, our results caused us some concern. For most of the disorders we examined, we found little evidence of shared environmental effects. Two sets of findings that came later in our study were reassuring. First, using our standard models, we detected substantial shared environmental effects for conduct disorder and illicit drug use. The results from our study were reassuringly consistent with other findings in the genetic and sociological literature indicating that environmental effects shared by siblings influence risk for CD and use of illicit substances. The twin method proved capable of detecting shared environmental effects.

Second, as described in Chapter 7, our analyses of parenting behavior were very illuminating. At first glance, our evidence that parenting behavior affects risk for anxiety and depressive disorders seemed at odds with our inability to detect shared environmental effects for these disorders in our twin analyses. However, further examination of this question resolved the apparent paradox. The magnitude of resemblance expected in siblings for risk for key psychiatric disorders due to their experiences of shared parenting was modest and too small to be detected by standard twin modeling.

We offer the following conclusions about shared environmental effects as measured in twin studies as a latent variable. For most of the disorders that we studied, such effects probably exist but are of minor impact, accounting for 10% or less of total variance in liability. This is too small an effect to be reliably detected using standard twin analysis, even with samples larger than ours. Detecting the effects of many aspects of the family environment probably requires that they be included explicitly in twin models. For a small set of traits, especially CD and illicit substance use, the effects of shared environment are quite a bit larger and can be detected with our standard modeling.

3. How does unreliability of measurement alter the interpretation of our results? With our new "technology" of structured psychiatric interviews, mental health researchers are prone, through what we consider a touch of hubris, to think that we have solved our problems of measurement. However, as analyses from the VATSPSUD and other studies show, when assessing lifetime prevalence of psychiatric and substance use disorders in community samples, this is not so. Unreliability of measurement remains a real problem. A substantial proportion of individuals give inconsistent answers when asked, by well-trained professional interviewers, the same set of questions on two different occasions about their lifetime history of psychiatric or substance use disorders.

One approach to this problem is to accept the problem as intractable and give up trying to assess lifetime history of psychiatric disorders. Several distinguished psychiatric epidemiologists have taken just this line and assess illness only over briefer periods of time, such as the last year. But for those studying psychiatric genetics, in which an entire lifetime is really the period of interest, this is not a good solution. Another approach is to assume that there is error and to understand that the risk factor–outcome associations will appear less strong than they really are. But the magnitude of the error is not small, and it can hurt our power to detect critical effects. With foresight in data collection and the use of proper analytic tools, it is possible to do better than this. Measuring people twice or getting reports from participants and informants who know them well are two methods that can go a long way toward offsetting the effects of the unreliability of our assessments.

4. *Do men and women have the same or different genetic and environmental risk factors for psychiatric and substance use disorders?* Sex probably has a large impact on risk for psychopathology, but there is still a great deal we do not understand about its effects. In the design of our second major study in the VATSPSUD, we included opposite-sex twin pairs. We did so because we wanted to understand more about how sex affects the pathways to risk for psychiatric and substance use disorders. Although we are only part of the way toward completing this line of research, several results are already worthy of emphasis. First, the genes that predispose to depression, several forms of phobia, and alcohol dependence are at least partly different in males and females. We consider these results to be quite significant, as they mean that the biological or cultural milieus are sufficiently different for men and women that they modify the pathway from genes to phenotype. Second, the depressogenic effects of low social support are much stronger in women than in men.

5. *How can we progress from initial findings that a risk factor and a disorder are **correlated** with each other to the much more difficult and important problem of clarifying whether the relationship between them is a **causal** one?* We have illustrated the potential dangers in moving quickly from the observation of correlation to the inference of causality. This is not merely an academic question, because broad policy questions might be decided on such a basis. We have described in this book a cautionary tale involving substance use. Our research in the VATSPSUD is in keeping with that of other researchers in showing that early onset of drinking is strongly related to subsequent drinking problems. However, further analyses suggested that the bulk of the associa-

tion is not a causal one. Early onset of drinking does not cause subsequent alcohol problems. Rather, both traits appear to reflect an underlying genetically influenced liability. Although we do not claim that such results are definitive, they do suggest an important point. It is naive to assume that in something as complex as human behavior you can easily move from correlation to causation. Furthermore, it is inefficient and expensive to base intervention attempts on such conclusions. If our inferences are correct, a great deal could be invested in trying to prevent high school students from gaining access to alcohol, with little payoff in reduction in rates of alcohol problems later in life.

These results can be usefully contrasted with our findings for CSA and SLEs, in which the cotwin-control method provided strong support for the hypothesis that these environmental experiences truly increased the risk for disorder. We do not claim that our methods to demonstrate causality are foolproof. They are not. But they do provide important insight into the critical question of the discrimination between correlation and causation.

6. *Can we develop indices of genetic risk and/or identify the "intervening" or "mediating" variables that sit in the pathway from genes (or environmental risk factors) to the outcome of illness?* It hardly needs repeating that genes do not directly code for depression, anxiety, or substance misuse. Viewed either from the perspective of biology (expressed in brain) or psychology (expressed in mind), we are woefully ignorant about the steps in the pathway connecting genes to psychiatric and substance use disorders. The VATSPSUD has made a few contributions to this issue. Our results suggest that the personality trait of neuroticism is an important intermediate phenotype for MD and that drinking motivations may be a useful intermediate phenotype for alcoholism. Future genetically informed studies that incorporate measures missing from VATSPSUD, such as those from neuropsychology, affective neuroscience, and imaging, will likely make important advances in this area.

7. *Some disorders are best understood as a series of stages. For example, it is not possible to abuse a substance until you have used it. Do genetic and environmental risk factors differ across these stages?* Typical models of gene action for psychiatric and substance use disorders assume a "one-stage" process. Although this might be an appropriate model for certain disorders, it is clearly not for others. Using data from the VATSPSUD and applying new models that we developed (with the invaluable help of our colleague Michael Neale), we were able to show how additional important knowledge could come from the application of multiple-stage models to the problems of substance use. The crucial insight came in our analyses of substance abuse/ dependence, when we realized that we were classifying as unaffected two quite different sorts of individuals—those who had tried illicit drugs but never developed problems and those who had never tried them. Although individu-

als from both groups are technically "unaffected," they are really quite different from one another. Critically, the latter group (those who had never tried these drugs) have an unknown level of liability to abuse/dependence. In a series of analyses, we were able to show that indeed the genetic and environmental factors that influence risk for initiation of substance use are not entirely the same as those that influence the risk for progression from use to abuse or dependence. Our multistage model could be applied to other "conditional" processes in psychopathology. One example includes studying the factors that underlie the emergence of an irrational fear versus those factors that lead someone with such a fear to develop impairment and thus meet criteria for a phobia. In another example, our colleague Debra Foley applied this model to study whether the factors that lead to depression differ from those that determine the degree of impairment among people who are depressed (Foley, Neale, Gardner, Pickles, & Kendler, 2003).

8. *Do parents convey risk to their children only through the genes they pass on to them or also through the environments they provide for them?* One real limitation of the twin method is that members of a twin pair are, by necessity, of the same generation and therefore studying twins alone provides only limited insight into the mechanisms whereby risk of illness is transmitted from parents to children. In the VATSPSUD, we studied the parents of the FF twin pairs. In this book, we have examined only one disorder, alcohol dependence, using a twin-family design. The critical question that we sought to address was how the vulnerability to alcoholism was passed across generations from parents to their children. Could alcoholism be taught as you might teach children a language or a set of social attitudes? Our results argue strongly against this hypothesis. However, our studies also suggest that other aspects of parental beahvior (such as the relationship quality of parents and children) can affect risk for psychiatric and substance use disorders.

THE VATSPSUD AND THE NEW MOLECULAR GENETICS

When this study began, the central paradigms in psychiatric genetics were the old "workhorses" of family, twin, and adoption studies. The application of molecular genetics to psychiatric and substance use disorders was still largely a twinkle in the eyes of a small handful of researchers. But during the years in which we were conducting interviews for the VATSPSUD, the shape of psychiatric genetics began to change. Center stage has been taken by gene-finding studies using molecular methods. Some researchers have come to regard studies such as the VATSPSUD as old-fashioned and even antiquated.

It will not surprise the reader to learn that we do not share this view. Both of us are heavily involved in molecular genetic studies of psychiatric disorders, so we can comment on research from both sides of this fence.

Studies such as the VATSPSUD—an example of the hybrid field of genetic epidemiology—are quite different from gene-finding molecular genetic investigations in their design, focus, strengths, and limitations (see Kendler, 2005b, for a more complete discussion of these issues). Briefly, studies such as ours can be best understood as consisting of basic and advanced stages. The goal of the basic stage is to quantify the degree to which individual differences in risk for illness result from genetic and environmental factors. Given the demonstration of significant heritability, the goal of the advanced stage is to explore the nature and mode of action of these aggregate genetic risk factors.

The goal of gene-finding studies, by contrast, is to determine the location of the genes on the genome (or, more technically, *loci*), variation in which influences liability to psychiatric disorders. A further and more refined goal for such studies is to clarify the history of the pathogenic variant or variants in the susceptibility gene by determining the background pieces of DNA (termed *haplotypes*) on which these variants are found.

Although predicting the future of science is a risky business, it is our guess that the techniques of genetic epidemiology (as illustrated in our study) and those of molecular genetics will begin to merge as we move forward in psychiatric genetics. One illustration of this synthesis is our study of the interaction between variants in the serotonin transporter gene and SLEs in the etiology of major depression (described in Chapter 16). The results of this analysis illustrate that understanding the action of genes on risk for psychiatric disorders may require high-quality measures of environmental risk factors, as well as of specific genes. Just as we saw from the results of our more traditional twin analyses, if the goal is to understand etiological pathways to psychiatric illness, it will be hard to study genes and environments in isolation from one another. Because they often interrelate so closely in causing disorder, good measures of genetic risk will help to clarify the action of environmental risk factors and vice versa.

We are sure that in the years ahead molecular genetics will come to play an increasing role in psychiatric genetics. But we predict that the lessons we learned from the VATSPSUD will hold true. Genetic effects, at least for the common disorders we have studied here, will tend to be moderate for most disorders, and pathways to illness will be complex, involving, in important ways, pathogenic environments.

PHILOSOPHICAL IMPLICATIONS

The main purpose of this book was to present the results of the VATSPSUD without much attention to the conceptual and philosophical issues that swirl about the analysis of human behavior. However, a few such thoughts are in order as we conclude.

Our findings provide substantial support for the hypothesis that genetic factors—expressed of necessity through biological mechanisms—are an important risk factor for all major forms of adult psychopathology. These results lead directly to the conclusion that biological factors must play a central role in the causal pathways to psychiatric and substance use disorders. Despite this, our results do not support the "hard" reductionist position that psychiatric and substance use disorders can be entirely understood within a neurobiological and molecular framework. Our experiences as social beings existing in a complex world also contribute in important ways to our risk of illness. For example, we found that SLEs strongly predicted the onset of episodes of MD. When we attempted to characterize the important dimensions of these events, we found that those that involved both loss and humiliation were especially depressogenic. It is hard to conceive of a more classical mental construct, or one that would be harder to reduce to biological phenomena, than that of humiliation. These results strongly suggest that how we humans experience and interpret the psychological and social world around us alters our risk for illness.

Our results show that the pathway from genes to disorder is not always a purely biological one. The impact of genetic risk factors can depend on environmental exposure. The pathway from genes to illness can go outside the skin to affect aspects of the social environment such as social support and interpersonal SLEs. These then feed back to the organism to influence risk of illness.

Thus we end with a nuanced view of the human organism. Risk factors for illness come from both genetic/biological and social/psychological realms. Furthermore, these realms interact in complex ways within individuals, within social groups, and across time. This picture is neither simple nor elegant. But it is realistic. To ignore any of these perspectives will limit our ability to alleviate the suffering caused by mental disorders and, ultimately, to understand and appreciate the essential aspects of being human.

References

Agid, O., Shapira, B., Zislin, J., Ritsner, M., Hanin, B., Murad, H., Troudart, T., Bloch, M., Heresco-Levy, U., & Lerer, B. (1999). Environment and vulnerability to major psychiatric illness: A case control study of early parental loss in major depression, bipolar disorder and schizophrenia. *Molecular Psychiatry*, **4**: 163–172.

Agrawal, A., Jacobson, K. C., Prescott, C. A., & Kendler, K. S. (2004). A twin study of personality and illicit drug use and abuse/dependence. *Twin Research*, **7**: 72–81.

Agrawal, A., Neale, M. C., Jacobson, K. C., Prescott, C. A., & Kendler, K. S. (2005). Illicit drug use and abuse/dependence: Modeling of two-stage variables using the CCC approach. *Addictive Behaviors*, **30**: 1043–1048.

Akaike, H. (1987). Factor analysis and AIC. *Psychometrika*, **52**: 317–332.

Allison, P. D. (1982). Discrete-time methods for the analysis of event histories. In S. Leinhardt (Ed.), *Sociological methodology* (pp. 61–98). San Francisco: Josey-Bass.

Allison, P. D. (1995). *Survival analysis using the SAS system: A practical guide.* Cary, NC: SAS Institute.

American Psychiatric Association. (1980). *Diagnostic and statistical manual of mental disorders* (3rd ed.). Washington, DC: Author.

American Psychiatric Association. (1987). *Diagnostic and statistical manual of mental disorders* (3rd ed., rev.). Washington, DC: Author.

American Psychiatric Association. (1994). *Diagnostic and statistical manual of mental disorders* (4th ed.). Washington, DC: Author.

Anda, R. F., Williamson, D. F., Escobedo, L. G., Mast, E. E., Giovino, G. A., & Remington, P. L. (1990). Depression and the dynamics of smoking: A national perspective. *Journal of the American Medical Association*, **264**: 1541–1545.

Andrews, G. (1981). A prospective study of life events and psychological symptoms. *Psychological Medicine*, **11**: 795–801.

Aneshensel, C. S., Estrada, A. L., Hansell, M. J., & Clark, V. A. (1987). Social psychological aspects of reporting behavior: Lifetime depressive episode reports. *Journal of Health and Social Behavior*, 28: 232–246.

Anthony, J. C., Warner, L. A., & Kessler, R. C. (1994). Comparative epidemiology of dependence on tobacco, alcohol, controlled substances, and inhalants: Basic findings from the National Comorbidity Survey. *Experimental and Clinical Psychopharmacology*, 2: 244–268.

Antonucci, T. C. (1985). Personal characteristics, social support, and social behavior. In R. H. Binstock & E. Shanas (Eds.), *Handbook of aging and the social sciences* (pp. 94–128). New York: Van Nostrand Reinhold.

Antonucci, T. C., & Jackson, J. S. (1990). The role of reciprocity in social support. In B. R. Sarason, I. G. Sarason, & G. R. Pierce (Eds.), *Social support: An interactional view* (pp. 173–198). New York: Wiley.

Argyle, N., & Roth, M. (1989). The definition of panic attacks: Part I. *Psychiatric Developments*, 3: 175–186.

Avison, W. R., & Turner, R. J. (1988). Stressful life events and depressive symptoms: Disaggregating the effects of acute stressors and chronic strains. *Journal of Health and Social Behavior*, 29: 253–264.

Bandura, A. (1986). *Social foundations of thought and action: A social cognitive theory*. Englewood Cliffs, NJ: Prentice Hall.

Beardslee, W. R., Son, L., & Vaillant, G. E. (1986). Exposure to parental alcoholism during childhood and outcome in adulthood: A prospective longitudinal study. *British Journal of Psychiatry*, 149: 584–591.

Bebbington, P. (1996). The origins of sex differences in depressive disorder: Bridging the gap. *International Review of Psychiatry*, 8: 295–332.

Bebbington, P. E. (1998). Sex and depression [Editorial]. *Psychological Medicine*, 28: 1–8.

Becker, A. E., Burwell, R. A., Gilman, S. E., Herzog, D. B., & Hamburg, P. (2002). Eating behaviors and attitudes following prolonged exposure to television among ethnic Fijian adolescent girls. *British Journal of Psychiatry*, 180: 509–514.

Bell, R. Q. (1968). A reinterpretation of the direction of effects in studies of socialization. *Psychological Review*, 75: 81–95.

Bentler, P. M. (1990). Comparative fit indexes in structural models. *Psychological Bulletin*, 107: 238–246.

Bentler, P. M., & Bonett, D. G. (1980). Significance tests and goodness of fit in the analysis of covariance structures. *Psychological Bulletin*, 88: 588–606.

Bergeman, C. S., Neiderhiser, J. M., Pedersen, N. L., & Plomin, R. (2001). Genetic and environmental influences on social support in later life: A longitudinal analysis. *International Journal of Aging and Human Development*, 53: 107–135.

Bertelsen, A., Harvald, B., & Hauge, M. (1977). A Danish twin study of manic-depressive disorders. *British Journal of Psychiatry*, 130: 330–351.

Bierut, L. J., Dinwiddie, S. H., Begleiter, H., Crowe, R. R., Hesselbrock, V., Nurnberger, J. I., Porjesz, B., Schuckit, M., & Reich, T. (1998). Familial transmission of substance dependence: Alcohol, marijuana, cocaine, and habitual smoking. *Archives of General Psychiatry*, 55: 982–988.

Bierut, L. J., Heath, A. C., Phil, D., Bucholz, K. K., Dinwiddie, S. H., Madden, P. A. F., Statham, D. J., Dunne, M. P., & Martin, N. G. (1999). Major depressive disorder in a community-based twin sample. *Archives of General Psychiatry*, 56: 557–563.

Bifulco, A. T., Brown, G. W., & Harris, T. O. (1987). Childhood loss of parent, lack of adequate parental care and adult depression: A replication. *Journal of Affective Disorders*, **12**: 115–128.

Birtchnell, J. (1980). Women whose mothers died in childhood: An outcome study. *Psychological Medicine*, **10**: 699–713.

Bolger, N., & Schilling, E. A. (1991). Personality and the problems of everyday life: The role of neuroticism in exposure and reactivity to daily stressors. *Journal of Personality*, **59**: 355–386.

Boomsma, D. I., de Geus, E. J. C., van Baal, G. C. M., & Koopmans, J. R. (1999). A religious upbringing reduces the influence of genetic factors on disinhibition: Evidence for interaction between genotype and environment on personality. *Twin Research*, **2**: 115–125.

Bower, G. H. (1987). Commentary on mood and memory. *Behaviour Research and Therapy*, **25**: 443–455.

Bowlby, J. (1980). *Attachment and loss: Vol. 3. Loss: Sadness and depression.* New York: Basic Books.

Boyd, J. H., Burke, J. D., Gruenberg, E., Holzer, C. E., III, Rae, D. S., George, L. K., Karno, M., Stoltzman, R., McEvoy, L., & Nestadt, G. (1984). Exclusion criteria of DSM-III: A study of co-occurrence of hierarchy-free syndromes. *Archives of General Psychiatry*, **41**: 983–989.

Boyd, J. H., & Weissman, M. M. (1981). Epidemiology of affective disorders: A reexamination and future directions. *Archives of General Psychiatry*, **38**: 1039–1046.

Bradburn, N., Rips, L. J., & Shevell, S. K. (1987). Answering autobiographical questions: The impact of memory and inference on surveys. *Science*, **236**: 157–161.

Breier, A., Kelsoe, J. R., Jr., Kirwin, P. D., Beller, S. A., Wolkowitz, O. M., & Pickar, D. (1988). Early parental loss and development of adult psychopathology. *Archives of General Psychiatry*, **45**: 987–993.

Bremner, J. D., Randall, P., Vermetten, E., Staib, L., Bronen, R. A., Mazure, C., Capelli, S., McCarthy, G., Innis, R. B., & Charney, D. S. (1997). Magnetic resonance imaging-based measurement of hippocampal volume in posttraumatic stress disorder related to childhood physical and sexual abuse: A preliminary report. *Biological Psychiatry*, **41**: 23–32.

Brennan, P. A., Raine, A., Schulsinger, F., Kirkegaard-Sorensen, L., Knop, J., Hutchings, B., Rosenberg, R., & Mednick, S. A. (1997). Psychophysiological protective factors for male subjects at high risk for criminal behavior. *American Journal of Psychiatry*, **154**: 853–855.

Breslau, N., Davis, G. C., & Prabucki, K. (1987). Depressed mothers as informants in family history research: Are they accurate? *Psychiatric Research*, **24**: 345–359.

Breslau, N., Johnson, E. O., Hiripi, E., & Kessler, R. (2001). Nicotine dependence in the United States: Prevalence, trends, and smoking persistence. *Archives of General Psychiatry*, **58**: 810–816.

Brett, J. F., Brief, A. P., Burke, M. J., George, J. M., & Webster, J. (1990). Negative affectivity and the reporting of stressful life events. *Health Psychology*, **9**: 57–68.

Bromet, E. J., Dunn, L. O., Connell, M. M., Dew, M. A., & Schulberg, H. C. (1986). Long-term reliability of diagnosing lifetime major depression in a community sample. *Archives of General Psychiatry*, **43**: 435–440.

Bronfenbrenner, U., & Ceci, S. J. (1994). Nature–nurture reconceptualized in developmental perspective: A bioecological model. *Psychological Review*, **101**(4): 568–586.

Brown, G. W. (1989). Life events and measurement. In G. W. Brown & T. O. Harris (Eds.), *Life events and illness* (pp. 3–45). New York: Guilford Press.

Brown, G. W. (1996). *Guidelines, examples, and LEDS-2 notes on rating for a new classification scheme for humiliation, loss, and danger.* London: Department of Social Policy and Social Sciences, University of London.

Brown, G. W., & Harris, T. O. (1978). *Social origins of depression: A study of psychiatric disorder in women.* London: Tavistock.

Brown, G. W., & Harris, T. O. (Eds.). (1989). *Life events and illness.* New York: Guilford Press.

Brown, G. W., Harris, T. O., & Hepworth, C. (1995). Loss, humiliation and entrapment among women developing depression: A patient and non-patient comparison. *Psychological Medicine,* 25: 7–21.

Burbach, D. J., & Borduin, C. M. (1986). Parent-child relations and the etiology of depression: A review of methods and findings. *Clinical Psychology Review,* 6: 133–153.

Burke, C. B., Burke, J. D., Regier, D. A., & Rae, D. S. (1990). Age at onset of selected mental disorders in five community populations. *Archives of General Psychiatry,* 47: 511–518.

Burton, R. (1932). *The anatomy of melancholy* (Vol. 1). New York: Dutton. (Original work published 1621)

Cadoret, R. J., Cain, C. A., & Crowe, R. R. (1983). Evidence for gene–environment interaction in the development of adolescent antisocial behavior. *Behavior Genetics,* 13: 301–310.

Cadoret, R. J., Cain, C. A., & Grove, W. M. (1980). Development of alcoholism in adoptees raised apart from alcoholic biologic relatives. *Archives of General Psychiatry,* 37: 561–563.

Cadoret, R. J., O'Gorman, T. W., Troughton, E., & Heywood, E. (1985). Alcoholism and antisocial personality: Interrelationships, genetic and environmental factors. *Archives of General Psychiatry,* 42: 161–167.

Cadoret, R. J., Troughton, E., & O'Gorman, T. W. (1987). Genetic and environmental factors in alcohol abuse and antisocial personality. *Journal of Studies on Alcohol,* 48: 1–8.

Cadoret, R. J., Yates, W. R., Troughton, E., Woodworth, G., & Stewart, M. A. (1995). Gene–environment interaction in genesis of aggressivity and conduct disorders. *Archives of General Psychiatry,* 52: 916–924.

Carey, G., & Gottesman, I. I. (1981). Twin and family studies of anxiety, phobic and obsessive disorders. In D. F. Klein & J. G. Rabkin (Eds.), *Anxiety: New research and changing concepts* (pp. 117–136). New York: Raven Press.

Carlson, E. A. (1966). *The gene: A critical history.* Philadelphia: Saunders.

Carmelli, D., Swan, G. E., Robinette, D., & Fabsitz, R. R. (1990). Heritability of substance use in the NAS-NRC twin registry. *Acta Genetica Medica et Gemellologia,* 39: 91–98.

Caspi, A., Sugden, K., Moffitt, T. E., Taylor, A., Craig, I. W., Harrington, H., McClay, J., Mill, J., Martin, J., Braithwaite, A., & Poulton, R. (2003). Influence of life stress on depression: Moderation by a polymorphism in the 5-HTT gene. *Science,* 301: 386–389.

Chapman, T. F., Mannuzza, S., Klein, D. F., & Fyer, A. J. (1994). Effects of informant mental disorder on psychiatric family history data. *American Journal of Psychiatry,* 151: 574–579.

Chitkara, B., MacDonald, A., & Reveley, A. M. (1988). Twin birth and adult psychiatric disorder: An examination of the case records of the Maudsley hospital. *British Journal of Psychiatry*, 152: 391–398.

Christiansen, B. A., Smith, G. T., Roehling, P. V., & Goldman, M. S. (1989). Using alcohol expectancies to predict adolescent drinking behavior after one year. *Journal of Consulting and Clinical Psychology*, 51: 93–99.

Cleckley, H. (1982). *The mask of sanity* (rev. ed.). St. Louis, MO: Mosby.

Clifford, C. A., Hopper, J. L., Fulker, D., & Murray, R. M. (1984). A genetic and environmental analysis of a twin family study of alcohol use, anxiety, and depression. *Genetic Epidemiology*, 1: 63–79.

Cloninger, C. R. (1987b). Neurogenetic adaptive mechanisms in alcoholism. *Science*, 236: 410–416.

Cloninger, C. R., Bohman, M., & Sigvardsson, S. (1981). Inheritance of alcohol abuse: Cross-fostering analysis of adopted men. *Archives of General Psychiatry*, 38: 861–868.

Cloninger, C. R., & Gottesman, I. I. (1987). Genetic and environmental factors in antisocial behavior disorder. In S. A. Mednick, T. E. Moffitt, & S. A. Stack (Eds.), *The causes of crime: New biological approaches* (pp. 92–109). Cambridge, UK: Cambridge University Press.

Cloninger, C. R., Przybeck, T. R., Svrakic, D. M., & Wetzel, R. D. (1994). *The Temperament and Character Inventory (TCI): A guide to its development and use*. St. Louis, MO: Washington University, Center for Psychobiology of Personality.

Cohen, S., & Wills, T. A. (1985). Stress, social support, and the buffering hypothesis. *Psychological Bulletin*, 98: 310–357.

Collaer, M., & Hines, M. (1995). Human behavioral sex differences: A role for gonadal hormones during early development. *Psychological Bulletin*, 118: 55–107.

Coryell, W., Winokur, G., Keller, M., Scheftner, W., & Endicott, J. (1992). Alcoholism and primary major depression: A family study approach to co-existing disorders. *Journal of Affective Disorders*, 24: 93–99.

Cox, D. R. (1972). Regression models and life tables [with discussion]. *Journal of the Royal Statistical Society (Series B*, 34: 187–220.

Crook, T., & Eliot, J. (1980). Parental death during childhood and adult depression: A critical review of the literature. *Psychological Bulletin*, 87: 252–259.

Crowe, R. R. (1990). Panic disorder: Genetic considerations. *Journal of Psychiatric Research*, 24(Suppl. 2): 129–134.

Crowe, R. R., Noyes, R., Pauls, D., & Slymen, D. (1983). A family study of panic disorder. *Archives of General Psychiatry*, 40: 1065–1069.

Crowe, R. R., Noyes, R. Jr., Persico, T., Wilson, A. F., & Elston, R. C. (1988). Genetic studies of panic disorder and related conditions. In D. L. Dunner, E. S. Gershon, & J. E. Barrett (Eds.), *Relatives at risk for mental disorder* (pp. 73–85). New York: Raven Press.

Cunningham, F. G., MacDonald, P. C., & Gant, N. F. (1989). *Williams obstetrics* (18th ed.). Norwalk, CT: Appleton & Lange.

Cutrona, C. E., Cadoret, R. J., Suhr, J. A., Richards, C. C., Troughton, E., Schutte, K., & Woodworth, G. (1994). Interpersonal variables in the prediction of alcoholism among adoptees: Evidence for gene–environment interactions. *Comprehensive Psychiatry*, 35: 171–179.

Darwin, C. (1859). *The origin of species*. London: Murray.

Darwin, C. (1877). A biographical sketch of an infant. *Mind*, 2: 285–294.

Day, R. L., Laland, K. N., & Odling-Smee, F. J. (2003). Rethinking adaptation: The niche-construction perspective. *Perspective Biological Medicine*, 46: 80–95.

DiLalla, L. F., & Gottesman, I. I. (1989). Heterogeneity of causes for delinquency and criminality: Lifespan perspectives. *Development and Psychopathology*, 1: 339–349.

Dinwiddie, S., Heath, A. C., Dunne, M. P., Bucholz, K. K., Madden, P. A. F., Slutske, W. S., Bierut, L. J., Statham, D. B., & Martin, N. G. (2000). Early sexual abuse and lifetime psychopathology: A co-twin-control study. *Psychological Medicine*, 30: 41–52.

Dohrenwend, B. P. (1995). "The problem of validity in field studies of psychological disorders" revisited. In M. T. Tsuang, M. Tohen, & G. E. Zahner (Eds.), *Textbook in psychiatric epidemiology* (pp. 3–20). New York: Wiley.

Dohrenwend, B. S. (1978). Exemplification of a method for scaling life events: The Peri Life Events Scale. *Journal of Health and Social Behavior*, 19: 205–229.

Dohrenwend, B. S., & Dohrenwend, B. P. (Eds.). (1984). *Stressful life events and their context*. New Brunswick, NJ: Rutgers University Press.

Eaton, W. W., Dryman, A., & Weissman, M. M. (1991). Panic and phobia. In L. N. Robins & D. A. Regier (Eds.), *Psychiatric disorders in America: The epidemiologic catchment area study* (pp. 155–179). New York: Free Press.

Eaves, L. J., Eysenck, H. J., Martin, N. G., Jardine, R., Heath, A. C., Feingold, L., Young, P. A., & Kendler, K. S. (1989). *Genes, culture and personality: An empirical approach*. London: Academic Press.

Eaves, L. J., Long, J., & Heath, A. C. (1986). A theory of developmental change in quantitative phenotypes applied to cognitive development. *Behavior Genetics*, 16: 143–162.

Eissenberg, T., & Balster, R. L. (2000). Initial tobacco use episodes in children and adolescents: Current knowledge, future directions. *Drug and Alcohol Dependence*, 59(Suppl 1): S41–S60.

Endler, N. S. (1983). Interactionism: A personality model, but not yet a theory. In M. M. Page (Ed.), *Nebraska Symposium on Motivation* (pp. 155–200). Lincoln: University of Nebraska Press.

Eysenck, H. J. (1979). The conditioning model of neurosis. *Behavior and Brain Science*, 2: 155–166.

Eysenck, H. J., & Eysenck, S. B. G. (1964). *Manual of the Eysenck Personality Inventory*. London: London University Press.

Eysenck, H. J., & Eysenck, S. B. G. (1975). *Manual of the Eysenck Personality Questionnaire*. London: Hodder & Stoughton.

Eysenck, S. B. G., Eysenck, H. J., & Barrett, P. (1985). A revised version of the psychoticism scale. *Personality and Individual Differences*, 6: 21–29.

Fabsitz, R. R., Carmelli, D., & Hewitt, J. K. (1992). Evidence for independent genetic influences on obesity in middle age. *International Journal of Obesity-Related Metabolic Disorders*, 16: 657–666.

Fagerstrom, K. -O., & Schneider, N. G. (1989). Measuring nicotine dependence: A review of the Fagerstrom Tolerance Questionnaire. *Journal of Behavioral Medicine*, 12: 159–182.

Falconer, D. S. (1989). *Introduction to quantitative genetics*. New York: Wiley.

Fanous, A., Gardner, C. O., Prescott, C. A., Cancro, R., & Kendler, K. S. (2002). Neuroticism, major depression and gender: A population-based twin study. *Psychological Medicine*, **32**: 719–728.

Faraone, S. V., Lyons, M. J., & Tsuang, M. T. (1987). Sex differences in affective disorder: Genetic transmission. *Genetic Epidemiology*, **4**: 331–343.

Fendrich, M., Weissman, M. M., Warner, V., & Mufson, L. (1990). Two-year recall of lifetime diagnoses in offspring at high and low risk for major depression: The stability of offspring reports. *Archives of General Psychiatry*, **47**: 1121–1127.

Fergusson, D. M., & Horwood, L. J. (1984). Life events and depression in women: A structural equation model. *Psychological Medicine*, **14**: 881–889.

Fergusson, D. M., & Horwood, L. J. (2000). Cannabis use and dependence in a New Zealand birth cohort. *New Zealand Medical Journal*, **113**: 156–158.

Fergusson, D. M., & Horwood, L. J. (2002). Male and female offending trajectories. *Developmental Psychopathology*, **14**: 159–177.

Fergusson, D. M., Horwood, L. J., & Lynskey, M. T. (1993). Prevalence and comorbidity of DSM-III-R diagnoses in a birth cohort of 15-year-olds. *Journal of the American Academy of . Childhood and Adolescent Psychiatry*, **32**: 1127–1134.

Fergusson, D. M., Horwood, L. J., Lynskey, M. T., & Madden, P. A. (2003). Early reactions to cannabis predict later dependence. *Archives of General Psychiatry*, **60**: 1033–1039.

Fergusson, D. M., & Mullen, P. E. (1999). *Childhood sexual abuse: An evidence-based perspective*. Thousand Oaks, CA: Sage.

Finlay-Jones, R., & Brown, G. W. (1981). Types of stressful life events and the onset of anxiety and depressive disorders. *Psychological Medicine*, **11**: 803–815.

Fisher, R. A. (1918). On the correlation between relatives on the supposition of Mendelian inheritance. *Transactions of the Royal Society of Edinburgh*, **52**: 399–433.

Flanagan, J., & Maany, I. (1982). Smoking and depression. *American Journal of Psychiatry*, **139**: 541.

Foley, D. L., Neale, M. C., Gardner, C., Pickles, A., & Kendler, K. S. (2003). Major depression and associated impairment: Same or different genetic and environmental risk factors? *American Journal of Psychiatry*, **160**: 2128–2133.

Foley, D. L., Neale, M. C., & Kendler, K. S. (1996). A longitudinal study of stressful life events assessed at personal interview with an epidemiologic sample of adult twins: The basis of individual variation in event exposure. *Psychological Medicine*, **26**: 1239–1252.

Foley, D. L., Neale, M. C., & Kendler, K. S. (1998). Reliability of a lifetime history of major depression: Implications for heritability and co-morbidity. *Psychological Medicine*, **28**: 857–870.

Freud, S. (1957). Mourning and melancholia. In J. Strachey (Ed. & Trans.), *The standard edition of the complete psychological works of Sigmund Freud* (Vol. 14, pp. 237–260). London: Hogarth Press. (Original work published 1917)

Fulker, D. W. (1988). Path analysis of genetic and cultural transmission in human behavior. In B. S. Weir, E. J. Eisen, M. M. Goodman, & G. Namkoong (Eds.), *Proceedings of the Second International Conference on Quantitative Genetics* (pp. 318–340). Sunderland, MA: Sinauer.

Furukawa, T., & Shibayama, T. (1997). Intra-individual versus extra-individual components of social support. *Psychological Medicine*, **27**: 1183–1191.

Fyer, A. J., Mannuzza, S., Chapman, T. F., Lipsitz, J., Martin, L. Y., & Klein, D. F.

(1996). Panic disorder and social phobia: Effects of comorbidity on familial transmission. *Anxiety*, **2**: 173–178.

Fyer, A. J., Mannuzza, S., Gallops, M. S., Martin, L. Y., Aaronson, C., Gorman, J. M.,
Liebowitz, M. R., & Klein, D. F. (1990). Familial transmission of simple phobias
and fears: A preliminary report. *Archives of General Psychiatry*, **47**: 252–256.

Galton, F. (1875). The history of twins as a criterion of the relative powers of nature
and nurture. *Fraser's Magazine*, **12**: 566–576.

Garcia, T., Sanchez, M., Cox, J. L., Shaw, P. A., Ross, J. B. A., Lehrer, S., & Schachter,
B. (1989). Identification of a variant form of the human estrogen receptor with an
amino acid replacement. *Nucleic Acids Research*, **20**: 8364.

Gerlsma, C., Emmelkamp, P. M. G., & Arrindell, W. A. (1990). Anxiety, depression,
and perception of early parenting: A meta-analysis. *Clinical Psychology Review*,
10: 251–277.

Gilbert, P. (1992). *Depression: The evolution of powerlessness*. New York: Guilford
Press.

Glassman, A. H., Stetner, F., Walsh, B. T., Raizman, P. S., Fleiss, J. L., Cooper, T. B.,
& Covey, L. S. (1988). Heavy smokers, smoking cessation, and clonidine: Results
of a double-blind, randomized trial. *Journal of the American Medical Association*, **259**: 2863–2866.

Goodwin, D. W., Schulsinger, R., Hermansen, L., Guze, S. B., & Winokur, G. (1973).
Alcohol problems in adoptees raised apart from alcoholic biological parents.
Archives of General Psychiatry, **28**: 238–255.

Grant, B. F. (1997). Convergent validity of DSM-III-R and DSM-IV alcohol dependence: Results from the National Longitudinal Alcohol Epidemiologic Survey.
Journal of Substance Abuse, **9**: 89–102.

Grant, B. F., & Dawson, D. A. (1997). Age at onset of alcohol use and its association
with DSM-IV alcohol abuse and dependence: Results from the National Longitudinal Alcohol Epidemiologic Survey. *Journal of Substance Abuse*, **9**: 103–110.

Gray, J. A. (1982). *The neuropsychology of anxiety*. New York: Oxford University Press.

Gynther, L. M., Carey, G., Gottesman, I. I., & Vogler, G. P. (1995). A twin study of
non-alcohol substance abuse. *Psychiatry Research*, **56**: 213–220.

Hagnell, O., Lanke, J., Rorsman, B., & Ojesjo, L. (1982). Are we entering an age of
melancholy? Depressive illnesses in a prospective epidemiological study over 25
years: The Lundby Study, Sweden. *Psychological Medicine*, **12**: 279–289.

Hartl, D. L. (1980). *Principles of population genetics*. Sunderland, MA: Sinauer.

Headey, B., & Wearing, A. (1989). Personality, life events, and subjective well-being:
Toward a dynamic equilibrium model. *Journal of Personality and Social Psychology*, **57**: 731–739.

Heath, A. C., Bucholz, K. K., Madden, P. A. F., Dinwiddie, S. H., Slutske, W. S.,
Bierut, L. J., Statham, D. J., Dunne, M. P., Whitfield, J. B., & Martin, N. G.
(1997). Genetic and environmental contributions to alcohol dependence risk in a
national twin sample: Consistency of findings in women and men. *Psychological
Medicine*, **27**: 1381–1396.

Heath, A. C., Jardine, R., & Martin, N. G. (1989). Interactive effects of genotype and
social environment on alcohol consumption in female twins. *Journal of Studies on
Alcohol*, **60**: 38–48.

Heath, A. C., Kendler, K. S., Eaves, L. J., & Markell, D. (1985). The resolution of
cultural and biological inheritance: Informativeness of different relationships.
Behavior Genetics, **15**: 439–465.

Heath, A. C., & Martin, N. G. (1993). Genetic models for the natural history of smoking: Evidence for a genetic influence on smoking persistence. *Addictive Behaviors*, **18**: 19–34.

Heatherton, T. F., Kozlowski, L. T., Frecker, R. C., & Fagerstrom, K. -O. (1991). The Fagerstrom Test for Nicotine Dependence: A revision of the Fagerstrom Tolerance Questionnaire. *British Journal of Addiction*, **86**: 1119–1127.

Heim, C., & Nemeroff, C. B. (2001). The role of childhood trauma in the neurobiology of mood and anxiety disorders: Preclinical and clinical studies. *Biological Psychiatry*, **49**: 1023–1039.

Heim, C., Newport, D. J., Heit, S., Graham, Y. P., Wilcox, M., Bonsall, R., Miller, A. H., & Nemeroff, C. B. (2000). Pituitary–adrenal and autonomic responses to stress in women after sexual and physical abuse in childhood. *Journal of the American Medical Association*, **284**: 592–597.

Helzer, J. E., Burnam, A., & McEvoy, L. T. (1991). Alcohol abuse and dependence. In L. N. Robins & D. A. Regier (Eds.), *Psychiatric disorders in America: The Epidemiologic Catchment Area study* (pp. 81–115). New York: Free Press.

Henderson, A. S. (1998). Social support: Its present significance for psychiatric epidemiology. In B. P. Dohrenwend (Ed.), *Adversity, stress, and psychopathology* (pp. 390–397). New York: Oxford University Press.

Henry, W., Moffitt, T. E., Caspi, A., Langley, J., & Silva, P. A. (1994). On the "remembrance of things past": A longitudinal evaluation of the retrospective method. *Psychological Assessment*, **6**: 92–101.

Hettema, J. M., Neale, M. C., & Kendler, K. S. (1995). Physical similarity and the equal-environment assumption in twin studies of psychiatric disorders. *Behavior Genetics*, **25**: 327–335.

Hettema, J. M., Neale, M. C., & Kendler, K. S. (2001a). A review and meta-analysis of the genetic epidemiology of anxiety disorders. *American Journal of Psychiatry*, **158**: 1568–1578.

Hettema, J. M., Prescott, C. A., & Kendler, K. S. (2001b). A population-based twin study of generalized anxiety disorder in men and women. *Journal of Nervous and Mental Disease*, **189**: 413–420.

Heun, R., Maier, W., & Muller, H. (2000). Subject and informant variables affecting family history diagnoses of depression and dementia. *Psychiatry Research*, **71**: 175–180.

Hicks, B. M., Krueger, R. F., Iacono, W. G., McGue, M., & Patrick, C. J. (2004). Family transmission and heritability of externalizing disorders: A twin-family study. *Archives of General Psychiatry*, **61**: 922–928.

Hollingshead, A. B. (1957). *Two factor index of social position*. New Haven, CT: Yale University.

Holmes, S. J., & Robins, L. N. (1988). The role of parental disciplinary practices in the development of depression and alcoholism. *Psychiatry*, **51**: 24–36.

Holmes, T. H., & Rahe, R. H. (1967). The Social Readjustment Rating Scale. *Journal of Psychosomatic Research*, **11**: 213–218.

Hope, S., Power, C., & Rodgers, B. (1998). The relationship between parental separation in childhood and problem drinking in adulthood. *Addiction*, **93**: 505–514.

Horn, J. L., Wanberg, K. W., & Foster, F. M. (1987). *Guide to the Alcohol Use Inventory*. Minneapolis, MN: National Computer Systems.

House, J. S., Landis, K. R., & Umberson, D. (1988). Social relationships and health. *Science*, **241**: 540–544.

Hur, Y. M., & Bouchard, T. J., Jr. (1995). Genetic influences on perceptions of childhood family environment: A reared-apart twin study. *Child Development*, **66**: 330–345.

Iacono, W. G., Malone, S. M., & McGue, M. (2003). Substance use disorders, externalizing psychopathology, and P300 event-related potential amplitude. *International Journal of Psychophysiology*, **48**: 147–178.

Jackson, S. W. (1986). *Melancholia and depression: From Hippocratic times to modern times*. New Haven, CT: Yale University Press.

Jacobson, K. C., Prescott, C. A., & Kendler, K. S. (2002). Sex differences in the genetic and environmental influences on the development of antisocial behavior. *Development and Psychopathology*, **14**: 395–416.

James, J. E. (1997). *Understanding caffeine: A Biobehavioral Analysis*. Thousand Oaks, CA: Sage.

Jardine, R., Martin, N. G., & Henderson, A. S. (1984). Genetic covariation between neuroticism and the symptoms of anxiety and depression. *Genetic Epidemiology*, **1**: 89–107.

Jessor, R., & Jessor, S. L. (1977). *Problem behavior and psychosocial development: A longitudinal study of youth*. New York: Academic Press.

John, O. P. (1990). The "big five" factor taxonomy: Dimensions of personality in the natural language and in questionnaires. In L. A. Pervin (Ed.), *Handbook of personality: Theory and research* (pp. 66–100). New York: Guilford Press.

Johnstone, B. M., Leino, E. V., Ager, C. R., Ferrer, H., & Fillmore, K. M. (1996). Determinants of life-course variation in the frequency of alcohol consumption: Meta-analysis of studies from the collaborative alcohol-related longitudinal project. *Journal of Studies on Alcohol*, **57**: 494–506.

Jordan, B. D., Relkin, N. R., Ravdin, L. D., Jacobs, A. R., Bennett, A., & Gandy, S. (1997). Apolipoprotein E ε4 associated with chronic traumatic brain injury in boxing. *Journal of the American Medical Association*, **278**: 136–140.

Kalbfleisch, J. D., & Prentice, R. L. (1980). *The statistical analysis of failure time data*. New York: Wiley.

Kallmann, F. J. (1946). The genetic theory of schizophrenia: An analysis of 691 schizophrenic twin index families. *American Journal of Psychiatry*, **103**: 309–322.

Kaprio, J., Koskenvuo, M., & Rose, R. J. (1990). Change in cohabitation and intrapair similarity of monozygotic (MZ) cotwins for alcohol use, extraversion, and neuroticism. *Behavior Genetics*, **20**: 265–276.

Kaprio, J., Sarna, S., Koskenvuo, M., & Rantasalo, I. (1978). *The Finnish Twin Registry: Baseline characteristics, Section II*. Helsinki, Finland: University of Helsinki Press.

Karkowski, L. M., Prescott, C. A., & Kendler, K. S. (2000). Multivariate assessment of factors influencing illicit substance use in twins from female–female pairs. *American Journal of Medical Genetics (Neuropsychiatric Genetics)*, **96**: 665–670.

Keel, P. K., & Klump, K. L. (2003). Are eating disorders culture-bound syndromes? Implications for conceptualizing their etiology. *Psychological Bulletin*, **129**: 747–769.

Keith, L. G., Papiernik, E., Keith, D. M., & Luke, B. (1995). *Multiple pregnancy, epidemiology, gestation and perinatal outcome*. New York: Parthenon.

Kendler, K. S. (1983). Overview: A current perspective on twin studies of schizophrenia. *American Journal of Psychiatry*, **140**: 1413–1425.

Kendler, K. S. (1996a). Major depression and generalized anxiety disorder: Same genes, (partly) different environments—revisited. *British Journal of Psychiatry*, **168**: 68–75.

Kendler, K. S. (1996b). Parenting: A genetic-epidemiologic perspective. *American Journal of Psychiatry*, **153**: 11–20.

Kendler, K. S. (1997). Social support: A genetic-epidemiologic analysis. *American Journal of Psychiatry*, **154**: 1398–1404.

Kendler, K. S. (2005a). "A gene for . . .": The nature of gene action in psychiatric disorders. *American Journal of Psychiatry*, **162**: 1243–1252.

Kendler, K. S. (2005b). Psychiatric genetics: A methodologic critique. *American Journal of Psychiatry*, **162**: 3–11.

Kendler, K. S., Aggen, S. H., Jacobson, K. C., & Neale, M. C. (2003a). Does the level of family dysfunction moderate the impact of genetic factors on the personality trait of neuroticism? *Psychological Medicine*, **33**: 817–825.

Kendler, K. S., Aggen, S. H., Prescott, C. A., Jacobson, K. C., & Neale, M. C. (2004a). Level of family dysfunction and genetic influences on smoking in women. *Psychological Medicine*, **34**: 1263–1269.

Kendler, K. S., Bulik, C. M., Silberg, J., Hettema, J. M., Myers, J., & Prescott, C. A. (2000c). Childhood sexual abuse and adult psychiatric and substance use disorders in women: An epidemiological and cotwin control analysis. *Archives of General Psychiatry*, **57**: 953–959.

Kendler, K. S., & Eaves, L. J. (1986). Models for the joint effect of genotype and environment on liability to psychiatric illness. *American Journal of Psychiatry*, **143**: 279–289.

Kendler, K. S., Gardner, C. O., Neale, M. C., & Prescott, C. A. (2001a). Genetic risk factors for major depression in men and women: Similar or different heritabilities and same or partly distinct genes? *Psychological Medicine*, **31**: 605–616.

Kendler, K. S., Gardner, C. O., & Prescott, C. A. (1999a). Corrections to 2 prior published articles. *Archives of General Psychiatry*, **57**: 94–95.

Kendler, K. S., Gardner, C. O., & Prescott, C. A. (2001b). Panic syndromes in a population-based sample of male and female twins. *Psychological Medicine*, **31**: 989–1000.

Kendler, K. S., Gardner, C. O., & Prescott, C. A. (2002a). Toward a comprehensive developmental model for major depression in women. *American Journal of Psychiatry*, **159**: 1133–1145.

Kendler, K. S., Gardner, C. O., & Prescott, C. A. (2003b). Personality and the experience of environmental adversity. *Psychological Medicine*, **33**: 1193–1202.

Kendler, K. S., Gardner, C. A., & Prescott, C. A. (2006). Toward a comprehensive developmental model for major depression in men. *American Journal of Psychiatry*, **163**: 115–124.

Kendler, K. S., Gatz, M., Gardner, C., & Pedersen, N. (2006). A Swedish national twin study of lifetime major depression. *American Journal of Psychiatry*, **163**: 109–114.

Kendler, K. S., & Greenspan, R. J. (in press). The nature of genetic influences on behavior: Lessons from "simpler" organisms. *American Journal of Psychiatry*.

Kendler, K. S., Heath, A. C., Martin, N. G., & Eaves, L. J. (1986). Symptoms of anxiety and depression in a volunteer twin population: The etiologic role of genetic and environmental factors. *Archives of General Psychiatry*, **43**: 213–221.

Kendler, K. S., Heath, A. C., Martin, N. G., & Eaves, L. J. (1987). Symptoms of anxiety and symptoms of depression: Same genes, different environments? *Archives of General Psychiatry*, **44**: 451–457.

Kendler, K. S., Heath, A. C., Neale, M. C., Kessler, R. C., & Eaves, L. J. (1992a). A population-based twin study of alcoholism in women. *Journal of the American Medical Association*, **268**: 1877–1882.

Kendler, K. S., Hettema, J. M., Butera, F., Gardner, C. O., & Prescott, C. A. (2003c). Life event dimensions of loss, humiliation, entrapment, and danger in the prediction of onsets of major depression and generalized anxiety. *Archives of General Psychiatry*, **60**: 789–796.

Kendler, K. S., Jacobson, K. C., Prescott, C. A., & Neale, M. C. (2003d). Specificity of genetic and environmental risk factors for use and abuse/dependence of cannabis, cocaine, hallucinogens, sedatives, stimulants, and opiates in male twins. *American Journal of Psychiatry*, **160**: 687–695.

Kendler, K. S., Karkowski, L., Neale, M. C., & Prescott, C. A. (2000a). Illicit psychoactive substance use, heavy use, abuse, and dependence in a US population-based sample of male twins. *Archives of General Psychiatry*, **57**: 261–269.

Kendler, K. S., Karkowski, L., & Prescott, C. A. (1998). Stressful life events and major depression: Risk period, long-term contextual threat and diagnostic specificity. *Journal of Nervous and Mental Disease*, **186**: 661–669.

Kendler, K. S., Karkowski, L. M., & Prescott, C. A. (1999b). Causal relationship between stressful life events and the onset of major depression. *American Journal of Psychiatry*, **156**: 837–841.

Kendler, K. S., Karkowski, L. M., & Prescott, C. A. (1999c). Fears and phobias: Reliability and heritability. *Psychological Medicine*, **29**: 539–553.

Kendler, K. S., Karkowski, L. M., & Prescott, C. A. (1999d). Hallucinogen, opiate, sedative and stimulant use and abuse in a population-based sample of female twins. *Acta Psychiatrica Scandinavica*, **99**: 368–376.

Kendler, K. S., & Karkowski-Shuman, L. (1997). Stressful life events and genetic liability to major depression: Genetic control of exposure to the environment. *Psychological Medicine*, **27**: 539–547.

Kendler, K. S., Kessler, R. C., Neale, M. C., Heath, A. C., & Eaves, L. J. (1993a). The prediction of major depression in women: An integrated etiologic model. *American Journal of Psychiatry*, **150**: 1139–1148.

Kendler, K. S., Kessler, R. C., Walters, E. E., MacLean, C. J., Sham, P. C., Neale, M. C., Heath, A. C., & Eaves, L. J. (1995a). Stressful life events, genetic liability and onset of an episode of major depression in women. *American Journal of Psychiatry*, **152**: 833–842.

Kendler, K. S., Kuhn, J., & Prescott, C. A. (2004b). The interrelationship of neuroticism, sex, and stressful life events in the prediction of episodes of major depression. *American Journal of Psychiatry*, **161**: 631–636.

Kendler, K. S., Kuhn, J. W., & Prescott, C. A. (2004c). Childhood sexual abuse, stressful life events and risk for major depression in women. *Psychological Medicine*, **34**: 1475–1482.

Kendler, K. S., Kuhn, J. W., Vittum, J., Prescott, C. A., & Riley, B. (2005b). The interaction of stressful life events and a serotonin transporter polymorphism in the prediction of episodes of major depression: A replication. *Archives of General Psychiatry*, **62**: 529–535.

Kendler, K. S., MacLean, C. J., Neale, M. C., Kessler, R. C., Heath, A. C., & Eaves, L.

J. (1991a). The genetic epidemiology of bulimia nervosa. *American Journal of Psychiatry*, **148**: 1627–1637.

Kendler, K. S., Myers, J., & Prescott, C. A. (2000b). Parenting and adult mood, anxiety and substance use disorders in female twins: An epidemiological multi-informant, retrospective study. *Psychological Medicine*, **30**: 281–294.

Kendler, K. S., Myers, J., Prescott, C. A., & Neale, M. C. (2001c). The genetic epidemiology of irrational fears and phobias in men. *Archives of General Psychiatry*, **58**: 257–265.

Kendler, K. S., Neale, M. C., Heath, A. C., Kessler, R. C., & Eaves, L. J. (1994a). A twin-family study of alcoholism in women. *American Journal of Psychiatry*, **151**: 707–715.

Kendler, K. S., Neale, M. C., Kessler, R. C., Heath, A. C., & Eaves, L. J. (1992b). A population-based twin study of major depression in women: The impact of varying definitions of illness. *Archives of General Psychiatry*, **49**: 257–266.

Kendler, K. S., Neale, M. C., Kessler, R. C., Heath, A. C., & Eaves, L. J. (1992c). Generalized anxiety disorder in women: A population-based twin study. *Archives of General Psychiatry*, **49**: 267–272.

Kendler, K. S., Neale, M. C., Kessler, R. C., Heath, A. C., & Eaves, L. J. (1992d). The genetic epidemiology of phobias in women: The inter-relationship of agoraphobia, social phobia, situational phobia and simple phobia. *Archives of General Psychiatry*, **49**: 273–281.

Kendler, K. S., Neale, M. C., Kessler, R. C., Heath, A. C., & Eaves, L. J. (1992e). Major depression and generalized anxiety disorder: Same genes, (partly) different environments. *Archives of General Psychiatry*, **49**: 716–722.

Kendler, K. S., Neale, M. C., Kessler, R. C., Heath, A. C., & Eaves, L. J. (1993b). A longitudinal twin study of personality and major depression in women. *Archives of General Psychiatry*, **50**: 853–862.

Kendler, K. S., Neale, M. C., Kessler, R. C., Heath, A. C., & Eaves, L. J. (1993c). A test of the equal environment assumption in twin studies of psychiatric illness. *Behavior Genetics*, **23**: 21–27.

Kendler, K. S., Neale, M. C., Kessler, R. C., Heath, A. C., & Eaves, L. J. (1993d). Panic disorder in women: A population based twin study. *Psychological Medicine*, **23**: 397–406.

Kendler, K. S., Neale, M. C., Kessler, R. C., Heath, A. C., & Eaves, L. J. (1993e). A longitudinal twin study of 1-year prevalence of major depression in women. *Archives of General Psychiatry*, **50**: 843–852.

Kendler, K. S., Neale, M. C., Kessler, R. C., Heath, A. C., & Eaves, L. J. (1993f). Major depression and phobias: The genetic and environmental sources of comorbidity. *Psychological Medicine*, **23**: 361–371.

Kendler, K. S., Neale, M. C., Kessler, R. C., Heath, A. C., & Eaves, L. J. (1993g). A twin study of recent life events and difficulties. *Archives of General Psychiatry*, **50**: 789–796.

Kendler, K. S., Neale, M. C., Kessler, R. C., Heath, A. C., & Eaves, L. J. (1994b). Parental treatment and the equal environment assumption in twin studies of psychiatric illness. *Psychological Medicine*, **24**: 579–590.

Kendler, K. S., Neale, M. C., MacLean, C. J., Heath, A. C., Eaves, L. J., & Kessler, R. C. (1993h). Smoking and major depression: A causal analysis. *Archives of General Psychiatry*, **50**: 36–43.

Kendler, K. S., Neale, M. C., Prescott, C. A., Kessler, R. C., Heath, A. C., Corey, L. A.,

& Eaves, L. J. (1996a). Childhood parental loss and alcoholism in women: A causal analysis using a twin-family design. *Psychological Medicine*, **26**: 79–95.

Kendler, K. S., Neale, M. C., Sullivan P. F., Corey, L. A., Gardner, C. O., & Prescott, C. A. (1999d). A population-based twin study in women of smoking initiation and nicotine dependence. *Psychological Medicine*, **29**: 299–308.

Kendler, K. S., Pedersen, N. L., Neale, M. C., & Mathe, A. A. (1995b). A pilot Swedish twin study of affective illness including hospital- and population-ascertained subsamples: Results of model fitting. *Behavior Genetics*, **25**: 217–232.

Kendler, K. S., Pedersen, N. L., Farahmand, B. Y., & Persson, P.-G. (1996b). The treated incidence of psychotic and affective illness in twins compared to population expectation: A study in the Swedish Twin and Psychiatric Registries. *Psychological Medicine*, **26**: 1135–1144.

Kendler, K. S., & Prescott, C. A. (1998). Cannabis use, abuse and dependence in a population-based sample of female twins. *American Journal of Psychiatry*, **155**: 1016–1022.

Kendler, K. S., & Prescott, C. A. (1999a). A population-based twin study of lifetime major depression in men and women. *Archives of General Psychiatry*, **56**: 39–44.

Kendler, K. S., & Prescott, C. A. (1999b). Caffeine intake, tolerance, and withdrawal in women: A population-based twin study. *American Journal of Psychiatry*, **156**: 223–228.

Kendler, K. S., Prescott, C. A., Jacobson, K., Myers, J., & Neale, J. M. (2002b). The joint analysis of personal interview and family history diagnoses: Evidence for validity of diagnosis and increased heritability estimates. *Psychological Medicine*, **32**: 829–842.

Kendler, K. S., Prescott, C. A., Myers, J., & Neale, M. C. (2003e). The structure of genetic and environmental risk factors for common psychiatric and substance use disorders in men and women. *Archives of General Psychiatry*, **60**: 929–937.

Kendler, K. S., & Robinette, C. D. (1983). Schizophrenia in the National Academy of Sciences–National Research Council Twin Registry: A 16-year update. *American Journal of Psychiatry*, **140**: 1551–1563.

Kendler, K. S., Sheth, K., Gardner, C. O., & Prescott, C. A. (2002c). Childhood parental loss and risk for first-onset major depression and alcohol dependence: The time-decay of risk and sex differences. *Psychological Medicine*, **32**: 1187–1194.

Kendler, K. S., Silberg, J. L., Neale, M. C., Kessler, R. C., Heath, A. C., & Eaves, L. J. (1991b). The family history method: Whose psychiatric history is measured? *American Journal of Psychiatry*, **148**: 1501–1504.

Kessler, R. C. (1997). The effects of stressful life events on depression. *Annual Review of Psychology*, **48**: 191–214.

Kessler, R. C., Berglund, P., Demler, O., Jin, R., Koretz, D., Merikangas, K. R., Rush, A. J., Walters, E. E., & Wang, P. S. (2003). The epidemiology of major depressive disorder: Results from the National Comorbidity Survey Replication (NCS-R). *Journal of the American Medical Association*, **289**: 3095–3105.

Kessler, R. C., Davis, C. G., & Kendler, K. S. (1997). Childhood adversity and adult psychiatric disorder in the US National Comorbidity Survey. *Psychological Medicine*, **27**: 1101–1119.

Kessler, R. C., Kendler, K. S., Heath, A. C., Neale, M. C., & Eaves, L. J. (1992). Social support, depressed mood, and adjustment to stress: A genetic epidemiologic investigation. *Journal of Personality and Social Psychology*, **62**: 257–272.

Kessler, R. C., McGonagle, K. A., Zhao, S., Nelson, C. B., Hughes, M., Eshleman, S.,

Wittchen, H. -U., & Kendler, K. S. (1994). Lifetime and 12-month prevalence of DSM-III-R psychiatric disorders in the United States: Results from the National Comorbidity Survey. *Archives of General Psychiatry*, **51**: 8–19.

King, K. M., & Chassin, L. (2004). Mediating and moderated effects of adolescent behavioral undercontrol and parenting in the prediction of drug use disorders in emerging adulthood. *Psychology of Addictive Behaviors*, **18**: 239–249.

King, R. A., Rotter, J. I., & Motulsky, A. G. (2002). *The genetic basis of common diseases*. New York: Oxford University Press.

Kirk, K. M., Blomberg, S. P., Duffy, D. L., Heath, A. C., Owens, I. P., & Martin, N. G. (2001). Natural selection and quantitative genetics of life-history traits in Western women: A twin study. *International Journal of Organic Evolution*, **55**: 423–435.

Klump, K. L., Holly, A., Iacono, W. G., McGue, M., & Willson, L. E. (2000). Physical similarity and twin resemblance for eating attitudes and behaviors: A test of the equal environments assumption. *Behavior Genetics*, **30**: 51–58.

Klump, K. L., McGue, M., & Iacono, W. G. (2003). Differential heritability of eating attitudes and behaviors in prepubertal versus pubertal twins. *International Journal of Eating Disorders*, **33**: 287–292.

Koob, G. F., & Le Moal, M. (1997). Drug abuse: Hedonic homeostatic dysregulation. *Science*, **278**: 52–57.

Kringlen, E. (1967). *Heredity and environment in the functional psychoses: Case histories*. Oslo, Norway: Universitetsforlaget.

Krueger, R. F. (1999). The structure of common mental disorders. *Archives of General Psychiatry*, **56**: 921–926.

Krueger, R. F., Caspi, A., Moffitt, T. E., & Silva, P. (1998). The structure and stability of common mental disorders (DSM-III-R): A longitudinal-epidemiological study. *Journal of Abnormal Psychology*, **107**: 216–227.

Laird, N., & Olivier, D. (1981). Covariance analysis of censored survival data using log-linear analysis techniques. *Journal of the American Statistical Association*, **76**: 231–240.

Lake, R. I., Eaves, L. J., Maes, H. H., Heath, A. C., & Martin, N. G. (2000). Further evidence against the environmental transmission of individual differences in neuroticism from a collaborative study of 45, 850 twins and relatives on two continents. *Behavior Genetics*, **30**: 223–233.

Lande, R. (1976). The maintenance of genetic variability by mutation in a polygenic character with linked loci. *Genetic Research at Cambridge*, **26**: 221–235.

Larsson, J. O., Larsson, H., & Lichtenstein, P. (2004). Genetic and environmental contributions to stability and change of ADHD symptoms between 8 and 13 years of age: A longitudinal twin study. *Journal of the American Academy of Childhood and Adolescent Psychiatry*, **43**: 1267–1275.

Lendon, C. L., Ashall, F., & Goate, A. M. (1997). Exploring the etiology of Alzheimer disease using molecular genetics. *Journal of the American Medical Association*, **277**: 825–831.

Leon, C. A., & Leon, A. (1998). Panic disorder and parental bonding. *Psychiatric Annals*, **20**: 503–508.

Lessov, C. N., Martin, N. G., Statham, D. J., Todorov, A. A., Slutske, W. S., Bucholz, K. K., Heath, A. C., & Madden, P. A. (2004). Defining nicotine dependence for genetic research: Evidence from Australian twins. *Psychological Medicine*, **34**: 865–879.

Li, M. D., Cheng, R., Ma, J. Z., & Swan, G. E. (2003). A meta-analysis of estimated genetic and environmental effects on smoking behavior in male and female adult twins. *Addiction*, **98**: 23–31.

Lichtenstein, P., Holm, N. V., Verkasalo, P. K., Iliadou, A., Kaprio, J., Koskenvuo, M., Pukkala, E., Skytthe, A., & Hemminki, K. (2000). Environmental and heritable factors in the causation of cancer: Analyses of cohorts of twins from Sweden, Denmark, and Finland. *New England Journal of Medicine*, **343**: 78–85.

Lloyd, C. (1980). Life events and depressive disorder revisited. *Archives of General Psychiatry*, **37**: 525–535.

Loeber, R. (1988). Natural histories of conduct problems, delinquency, and associated substance use: Evidence for developmental progressions. In B. Lahey & A. Kazdin (Eds.), *Advances in clinical child psychology* (Vol. 11, pp. 73–124). New York: Plenum Press.

Loehlin, J. C. (1992). *Genes and environment in personality development.* Newbury Park, CA: Sage.

Loehlin, J. C., & Nichols, R. C. (1976). *Heredity, environment and personality: A study of 850 sets of twins.* Austin: University of Texas Press.

Luepker, R. V., Pallonen, U. E., Murray, D. M., & Pirie, P. L. (1989). Validity of telephone surveys in assessing cigarette smoking in young adults. *American Journal of Public Health*, **79**: 202–204.

Luxenburger, H. (1928). Vorlaufiger Bericht uber psychiatrische Serienuntersuchungen und Zwillingen. *Zeitschrift fur die gesamte Neurologie und Psychiatrie*, **116**: 297–326.

Lykken, D. T., McGue, M., Bouchard, T. J., & Tellegen, A. (1990). Does contact lead to similarity or similarity to contact? *Behavior Genetics*, **20**: 547–561.

Lynch, M., & Walsh, B. (1998). *Genetics and analysis of quantitative traits.* Sunderland, MA: Sinauer.

Lyons, M. J., Eisen, S. A., Goldberg, J., True, W., Lin, N., Meyer, J. M., Toomey, R., Faraone, S. V., Merren, J., & Tsuang, M. T. (1998). A registry-based twin study of depression in men. *Archives of General Psychiatry*, **55**: 468–472.

Lyons, M. J., Goldberg, J., Eisen, S. A., True, W., Tsuang, M. T., Meyer, J. M., & Henderson, W. G. (1993). Do genes influence exposure to trauma? A twin study of combat. *American Journal of Medical Genetics*, **48**: 22–27.

Lyons, M. J., Toomey, R., Meyer, J. M., Green, A. I., Eisen, S. A., Goldberg, J., True, W. R., & Tsuang, M. T. (1997). How do genes influence marijuana use? The role of subjective effects. *Addiction*, **92**: 409–417.

Lyons, M. J., True, W. R., Eisen, S. A., Goldberg, J., Meyer, J. M., Faraone, S. F., Eaves, L. J., & Tsuang, M. T. (1995). Differential heritability of adult and juvenile antisocial traits. *Archives of General Psychiatry*, **52**: 906–915.

Lytton, H. (1977). Do parents create, or respond to, differences in twins? *Developmental Psychology*, **13**: 456–459.

Maccoby, E. E. (1992). The role of parents in the socialization of children: A historical overview. *Developmental Psychology*, **28**: 1006–1017.

Maccoby, E. E., & Martin, J. A. (1983). Socialization in the context of the family: Parent–child interaction. In P. H. Mussen (Series Ed.) & E. M. Hetherington (Vol. Ed.), *Handbook of child psychology: Vol. 4. Socialization, personality, and social development* (4th ed., pp. 1–101). New York: Wiley.

MacGillivray, I. (1986). Epidemiology of twin pregnancy. *Seminars in Perinatology*, **10**: 4–8.

Madden, P. A. F., Heath, A. C., Pedersen, N., Kaprio, J., Koskenvuo, M., & Martin, N. G. (1999). The genetics of smoking persistence in men and women: A multicultural study. *Behavior Genetics*, **29**: 423–431.

Madden, P. A. F., Pedersen, N. L., Kaprio, J., Koskenvuo, M. J., & Martin, N. G. (2004). The epidemiology and genetics of smoking initiation and persistence: Cross-cultural comparisons of twin study results. *Twin Research*, **7**: 82–97.

Maes, H. H., Neale, M. C., Kendler, K. S., Hewitt, J. K., Silberg, J. L., Foley, D. L., Meyer, J. M., Rutter, M., Simonoff, E., Pickles, A., & Eaves, L. J. (1998). Assortative mating for major psychiatric diagnosis in two population-based samples. *Psychological Medicine*, **28**: 1389–1401.

Maes, H. H., Sullivan, P. F., Bulik, C. M., Neale, M. C., Prescott, C. A., Eaves, L. J., & Kendler, K. S. (2004). A twin study of genetic and environmental influences in tobacco initiation, regular tobacco use and nicotine dependence. *Psychological Medicine*, **34**: 1251–1261.

Magee, W. J., Eaton, W. W., Wittchen, H. -U., McGonagle, K. A., & Kessler, R. C. (1996). Agoraphobia, simple phobia, and social phobia in the National Comorbidity Survey. *Archives of General Psychiatry*, **53**: 159–168.

Magnus, K., Diener, E., Fujita, F., & Pavot, W. (1993). Extraversion and neuroticism as predictors of objective life events: A longitudinal analysis. *Journal of Personality and Social Psychology*, **65**: 1046–1053.

Magnusson, D. (1988). *Individual development from an interactional perspective: A longitudinal study*. Hillsdale, NJ: Erlbaum.

Maier, W., Lichtermann, D., Minges, J., Oehrlein, A., & Franke, P. (1993). A controlled family study in panic disorder. *Journal of Psychiatric Research*, **27**: 79–87.

Marks, I. M. (1987). *Fears, phobias, and rituals*. New York: Oxford University Press.

Marks, I. M. (1988). Blood-injury phobia: A review. *American Journal of Psychiatry*, **145**: 1207–1213.

Mather, K. (1966). Variability and selection. *Proceedings of the Royal Society, Series B*, **164**: 328–340.

Mather, K., & Jinks, J. L. (1982). *Biometrical Genetics: The study of continuous variation*. London: Chapman & Hall.

Maughan, B., & Rutter, M. (1997). Retrospective reporting of childhood adversity: Issues in assessing long-term recall. *Journal of Personality Disorders*, **11**: 19–33.

McCrae, R. R., & Costa, P. T., Jr. (1990). *Personality in adulthood*. New York: Guilford Press.

McFarland, R. A. (1957). The role of human factors in accidental trauma. *American Journal of the Medical Sciences*, **234**: 1–26.

McGovern, R. J., Neale, M. C., & Kendler, K. S. (1996). The independence of physical attractiveness and symptoms of depression in a female twin population. *Journal of Psychology*, **130**: 209–219.

McGue, M., & Lykken, D. T. (1992). Genetic influence on risk of divorce. *Psychological Science*, **3**: 368–373.

McGue, M., Pickens, R. W., & Svikis, D. S. (1992). Sex and age effects on the inheritance of alcohol problems: A twin study. *Journal of Abnormal Psychology*, **101**: 3–17.

McGuffin, P., Katz, R., Watkins, S., & Rutherford, J. (1996). A hospital-based twin register of the heritability of DSM-IV unipolar depression. *Archives of General Psychiatry*, **53**: 129–136.

McGuffin, P., Moffitt, T., & Thapar, A. (2002). Personality disorders. In P. McGuffin,

M. J. Owen, & I. I. Gottesman (Eds.), *Psychiatric genetics and genomics* (pp. 183–210). London: Oxford University Press.

Mendlewicz, J., Papadimitriou, G. N., & Wilmotte, J. (1993). Family study of panic disorder: Comparison with generalized anxiety disorder, major depression and normal subjects. *Psychiatric Genetics*, 3: 73–78.

Menninger, K., Ellenberger, H., Pruyser, P., & Mayman, M. (1958). The unitary concept of mental illness. *Bulletin of the Menninger Clinic*, 22: 4–12.

Merikangas, K., Stolar, M., Stevens D. E., Goulet, J., Preisig, M. A., Fenton, B., Zhang, H., O'Malley, S. S., & Rounsaville, B. J. (1998). Familial transmission of substance use disorders. *Archives of General Psychiatry*, 55: 973–979.

Merikangas, K. R., & Gelernter, C. S. (1990). Comorbidity for alcoholism and depression. *Psychiatric Clinics of North America*, 13: 613–632.

Merikangas, K. R., Weissman, M. M., & Pauls, D. L. (1985). Genetic factors in the sex ratio of major depression. *Psychological Medicine*, 15: 63–69.

Merriman, C. (1924). The intellectual resemblance of twins. *Psychological Monographs*, 33: 1–58.

Miles, D. R., & Carey, G. (1997). Genetic and environmental architecture of human aggression. *Journal of Personality and Social Psychology*, 72: 207–217.

Moffitt, T. E. (1993). Adolescence-limited and life-course-persistent antisocial behavior: A developmental taxonomy. *Psychological Review*, 100: 674–701.

Moffitt, T. E., Caspi, A., Rutter, M., & Silva, P. A. (2001). *Sex differences in antisocial behavior: Conduct disorder, delinquency, and violence in the Dunedin Longitudinal Study.* Cambridge, UK: Cambridge University Press.

Monroe, S. M., & Steiner, S. C. (1986). Social support and psychopathology: Interrelations with preexisting disorder, stress, and personality. *Journal of Abnormal Psychology*, 95: 29–39.

Moos, R., & Moos, B. (1986). *Family Environment Scale Manual.* Palo Alto, CA: Consulting Psychologists Press.

Morris-Yates, A., Andrews, G., Howie, P., & Henderson, S. (1990). Twins: A test of the equal environments assumption. *Acta Psychiatrica Scandinavica*, 81: 322–326.

Mullen, P. E., Martin, J. L., Anderson, J. E., Romans, S. E., & Herbison, G. P. (1993). Childhood sexual abuse and mental health in adult life. *British Journal of Psychiatry*, 163: 721–732

Murray, C. J. L., & Lopez, A. D. (1996). Evidence-based health policy: Lessons from the Global Burden of Disease Study. *Science*, 274: 740–743.

Neale, M. C., & Cardon, L. R. (1992). *Methodology for genetic studies of twins and families.* Dordrecht, The Netherlands: Kluwer.

Neale, M. C., Eaves, L. J., & Kendler, K. S. (1994a). The power of the classical twin study to resolve variation in threshold traits. *Behavior Genetics*, 24: 239–258.

Neale, M. C., & Fulker, D. W. (1984). A bivariate path analysis of fear data on twins and their parents. *Acta Genetica Medica et Gemellologia*, 33: 273–286.

Neale, M. C., & Kendler, K. S. (1995). Models of comorbidity for multifactorial disorders. *American Journal of Human Genetics*, 57: 935–953.

Neale, M. C., & Stevenson, J. (1989). Rater bias in the EASI Temperament Scales: A twin study. *Journal of Personality and Social Psychology*, 56: 446–455.

Neale, M. C., Walters, E. E., Eaves, L. J., Kessler, R. C., Heath, A. C., & Kendler, K. S. (1994b). The genetics of blood-injury fears and phobias: A population-based twin study. *American Journal of Medical Genetics*, 54: 326–334.

Nelkin, D., & Lindee, M. S. (1995). *The DNA mystique: The gene as a cultural icon.* New York: Freeman.

Nelson, E. C., Grant, J. D., Bucholz, K. K., Glowinski, A., Madden, P. A. F., Reich, W., & Heath, A. C. (2000). Social phobia in a population-based female adolescent twin sample: Co-morbidity and associated suicide-related symptoms. *Psychological . Medicine*, 30: 797–804.

Nelson, E. C., Heath, A. C., Madden, P. A. F., Cooper, M. L., Dinwiddie, S. H., Bucholz, K. K., Glowinski, A., McLaughlin, T., Dunne, M. P., Statham, D. J., & Martin, N. G. (2002). Association between self-reported childhood sexual abuse and adverse psychosocial outcomes: Results from a twin study. *Archives of General Psychiatry*, 59: 139–145.

Nicoll, J. A. R., Roberts, G. W., & Graham, D. I. (1995). Apolipoprotein E ε4 allele is associated with deposition of amyloid beta-protein following head injury. *Nature Medicine*, 1: 135–137.

Nolen-Hoeksema, S. (1990). *Sex differences in depression.* Palo Alto, CA: Stanford University Press.

Noyes, R., Crowe, R. R., Harris, E. L., Hamra, B. J., McChesney, C. M., & Chaudhry, D. R. (1986). Relationship between panic disorder and agoraphobia. *Archives of General Psychiatry*, 43: 227–232.

O'Connor, T. G., Hetherington, E. M., Reiss, D., & Plomin, R. (1995). A twin-sibling study of observed parent–adolescent interactions. *Child Development*, 66: 812–829.

Ohman, A. (1986). Face the beast and fear the face: Animal and social fears as prototypes for evolutionary analyses of emotion. *Psychophysiology*, 23: 123–145.

Okasha, S. (2002). *Philosophy of science: A very short introduction.* London: Oxford University Press.

Ormel, J., Oldehinkel, A. J., & Brilman, E. I. (2001). The interplay and etiological continuity of neuroticism, difficulties, and life events in the etiology of major and subsyndromal, first and recurrent depressive episodes in later life. *American Journal of Psychiatry*, 158: 885–891.

Ormel, J., & Wohlfarth, T. (1991). How neuroticism, long-term difficulties, and life situation change influence psychological distress: A longitudinal model. *Journal of Personality and Social Psychiatry*, 60: 744–755.

Oslin, D. W., Berrettini, W., Kranzler, H. R., Pettinati, H., Gelernter, J., Volpicelli, J. R., & O'Brien, C. P. (2003). A functional polymorphism of the mu-opioid receptor gene is associated with naltrexone response in alcohol-dependent patients. *Neuropsychopharmacology*, 28: 1546–1552.

Ost, L. G. (1987). Age of onset in different phobias. *Journal of Abnormal Psychology*, 96: 223–229.

Parker, G. (1979). Parental characteristics in relation to depressive disorders. *British Journal of Psychiatry*, 134: 138–147.

Parker, G. (1983). *Parental overprotection: A risk factor in psychosocial development.* New York: Grune & Stratton.

Parker, G. (1989). The Parental Bonding Instrument: Psychometric properties reviewed. *Psychiatric Developments*, 4: 317–335.

Parker, G. (1990). The Parental Bonding Instrument: A decade of research. *British Journal of Medical Psychology*, 52: 1–10.

Parker, G., & Gladstone, G. L. (1996). Parental characteristics as influences on adjustment in adulthood. In G. R. Pierce, B. R. Sarason, & I. G. Sarason (Eds.), *Handbook of social support and the family* (pp. 195–218). New York: Plenum Press.

Parker, G., Tupling, H., & Brown, L. B. (1979). A Parental Bonding Instrument. *British Journal of Medical Psychology*, **52:** 1–10.

Patzer, G. L. (1985). *The physical attractiveness phenomena*. New York: Plenum.

Pauls, D. L., Bucher, K. D., Crowe, R. R., & Noyes, R. (1980). A genetic study of panic disorder pedigrees. *American Journal of Human Genetics*, **32:** 639–644.

Paykel, E. S. (1994). Life events, social support and depression. *Acta Psychiatrica Scandinavica Suppl.*, **377:** 50–58.

Paykel, E. S., Myers, J. K., Dienelt, M. N., Klerman, G. L., Lindenthal, J. J., & Pepper, M. P. (1969). Life events and depression: A controlled study. *Archives of General Psychiatry*, **21:** 754–760.

Pedersen, N. L. (1981). Twin similarity for usage of common drugs. In L. Gedda, P. Parisi, & W. E. Nance (Eds.), *Twin research 3: Epidemiological and clinical studies* (Vol. 69C, pp. 53–59). New York: Liss.

Pedersen, W., & Skrondal, A. (1998). Alcohol consumption debut: Predictors and consequences. *Journal of Studies on Alcohol*, **59:** 32–42.

Perera, F. P. (1997). Environment and cancer: Who are susceptible? *Science*, **278:** 1068–1073.

Perris, C., Arrindell, W. A., & Eisemann, M. (Eds.). (1994). *Parenting and psychopathology*. New York: Wiley.

Perusse, D., Neale, M. C., Heath, A. C., & Eaves, L. J. (1994). Human parental behavior: Evidence for genetic influence and potential implication for gene–culture transmission. *Behavior Genetics*, **24:** 327–335.

Phillips, K., Fulker, D. W., & Rose, R. J. (1987). Path analysis of seven fear factors in adult twin and sibling pairs and their parents. *Genetic Epidemiology*, **4:** 345–355.

Plomin, R., Lichtenstein, P., Pedersen, N., McClearn, G. E., & Nesselroade, J. R. (1990). Genetic influences on life events during the last half of the life span. *Psychology and Aging*, **5:** 25–30.

Plomin, R., McClearn, G. E., Pedersen, N. L., Nesselroade, J. R., & Bergeman, C. S. (1988). Genetic influence on childhood family environment perceived retrospectively from the last half of the life span. *Developmental Psychology*, **24:** 738–745.

Pomerleau, O. F., & Pomerleau, C. S. (1984). Neuroregulators and the reinforcement of smoking: Towards a biobehavioral explanation. *Neuroscience and Biobehavioral Reviews*, **8:** 503–513.

Prescott, C. A., Aggen, S., & Kendler, K. S. (1999). Sex differences in the sources of genetic liability to alcohol abuse and dependence in a population-based sample of U. S. twins. *Alcoholism: Clinical and Experimental Research*, **23:** 1136–1144.

Prescott, C. A., Aggen, S. H., & Kendler, K. S. (2000). Sex-specific genetic influences on the comorbidity of alcoholism and major depression in a population-based sample of US twins. *Archives of General Psychiatry*, **57:** 803–811.

Prescott, C. A., Caldwell, C. B., Carey, G., Vogler, G. P., Trumbetta, S., & Gottesman, I. I. (2005a). The Washington University Twin Study of Alcoholism. *Neuropsychiatric Genetics*, **134:.** 48–55.

Prescott, C. A., Cross, R. J., Kuhn, J. W., Horn, J. L., & Kendler, K. S. (2004). Is risk for alcoholism mediated by individual differences in drinking motivations? *Alcoholism: Clinical and Experimental Research*, **28:** 29–39.

Prescott, C. A., & Kendler, K. S. (1996). Longitudinal stability and change in alcohol consumption among female twins: Contributions of genetics. *Development and Psychopathology*, **8**: 849–866.

Prescott, C. A., & Kendler, K. S. (1999). Age at first drink and risk for alcoholism: A noncausal association. *Alcoholism: Clinical and Experimental Research*, **23**: 101–107.

Prescott, C. A., & Kendler, K. S. (2000). Influence of ascertainment strategy on finding sex differences in genetic estimates from twin studies of alcoholism. *American Journal of Medical Genetics*, **96**: 754–761.

Prescott, C. A., Kessler R. C., Heath, A. C., Neale, M. C., Eaves, L. J., & Kendler, K. S. (1993, October). *Genetic contributions to liability for alcoholism in women moderated by parental diagnosis and parenting style.* Paper presented at the World Congress on Psychiatric Genetics.

Prescott, C. A., Kuhn, J., & Pedersen, N. (2005b). *Twin pair resemblance for lifetime history of psychiatric disorder in the Swedish Twin Registry: A 17-year follow up study of 29, 602 twin pairs.* Manuscript submitted for review.

Prusoff, B. A., Merikangas, K. R., & Weissman, M. M. (1988). Lifetime prevalence and age of onset of psychiatric disorders: Recall 4 years later. *Journal of Psychiatric Research*, **22**: 107–117.

Rachman, S. (1977). The conditioning theory of fear-acquisition: A critical examination. *Behaviour Research and Therapy*, **15**: 375–387.

Reich, T., Van Eerdewegh, P., Rice, J., Mullaney, J., Endicott, J., & Klerman, G. L. (1987). The familial transmission of primary major depressive disorder. *Journal of Psychiatric Research*, **21**: 613–624.

Rice, J. P., Reich, T., Bucholz, K. K., Neuman, R. J., Fishman, R., Rochberg, N., Hesselbrock, V. M., Nurnberger, J. I., Jr., Schuckit, M. A., & Begleiter, H. (1995). Comparison of direct interview and family history diagnoses of alcohol dependence. *Alcoholism: Clinical and Experimental Research*, **19**: 1018–1023.

Rijsdijk, F. V., Sham, P. C., Sterne, A., Purcell, S., McGuffin, P., Farmer, A., Goldberg, D., Mann, A., Cherny, S. S., Webster, M., Ball, D., Eley, T. C., & Plomin, R. (2001). Life events and depression in a community sample of siblings. *Psychological Medicine*, **31**: 401–410.

Robins, L. N., & Helzer, J. E. (1985). *Diagnostic Interview Schedule (DIS): Version III-A.* St. Louis, MO: Washington University School of Medicine.

Robins, L. N., Helzer, J. E., Weissman, M. M., Orvaschel, H., Gruenberg, E., Burke, J. D., & Regier, D. A. (1984). Lifetime prevalence of specific psychiatric disorders in three sites. *Archives of General Psychiatry*, **41**: 949–958.

Robins, L. N., & Regier, D. A. (Eds.). (1991). *Psychiatric disorders in America: The Epidemiological Catchment Area Study.* New York: Free Press.

Robins, L. N., Schoenberg, S. P., Holmes, S. J., Ratcliff, K. S., Benham, A., & Works, J. (1985). Early home environment and retrospective recall: A test for concordance between siblings with and without psychiatric disorder. *American Journal of Orthopsychiatry*, **55**: 27–41.

Rodgers, B. (1996). Reported parental behavior and adult affective symptoms: 1. Associations and moderating factors. *Psychological Medicine*, **26**: 51–61.

Rose, R. J., & Ditto, W. B. (1983). A developmental-genetic analysis of common fears from early adolescence to early adulthood. *Child Development*, **54**: 361–368.

Rose, R. J., Kaprio, J., Williams, C. J., Viken, R., & Obremski, K. (1990). Social con-

372   **References**

tact and sibling similarity: Facts, issues, and red herrings. *Behavior Genetics*, 20: 763–778.

Rose, R. J., Miller, J. Z., Pogue-Geile, M. F., & Cardwell, G. F. (1981). Twin-family studies of common fears and phobias. In L. Gedda, P. Parisi, & W. E. Nance (Eds.), *Twin research 3: Intelligence, personality, and development* (pp. 169–174). New York: Liss.

Rosenberg, C. M. (1969). Determinants of psychiatric illness in young people. *British Journal of Psychiatry*, 115: 907–915.

Rosenthal, D. (1960). Confusion of identity and the frequency of schizophrenia in twins. *Archives of General Psychiatry*, 3: 297–304.

Rowe, D. C., Jacobson, K. C., & Van den Oord, E. J. C. G. (1999). Genetic and environmental influence on vocabulary IQ: Parental education level as moderator. *Child Development*, 70: 1151–1162.

Roy, M. -A., Neale, M. C., Pedersen, N. L., Mathe, A. A., & Kendler, K. S. (1995). A twin study of generalized anxiety disorder and major depression. *Psychological Medicine*, 25: 1037–1049.

Roy, M. -A., Walsh, D., & Kendler, K. S. (1996). Accuracies and inaccuracies of the family history method: A multivariate approach. *Acta Psychiatrica Scandinavica*, 93: 224–234.

Roy, M. -A., Walsh, D., Prescott, C. A., & Kendler, K. S. (1994). Biases in the diagnosis of alcoholism by the family history method. *Alcoholism: Clinical Experimental Research*, 18: 845–851.

Rutter, M., & Redshaw, J. (1991). Annotation: Growing up as a twin: Twin–singleton differences in psychological development. *Journal of Child Psychology and Psychiatry*, 32: 885–895.

Sarason, I. G., Sarason, B. R., & Shearin, E. N. (1986). Social support as an individual difference variable: Its stability, origins, and relational aspects. *Journal of Personality and Social Psychology*, 50: 845–855.

Saudino, K. J., Pedersen, N. L., Lichtenstein, P., McClearn, G. E., & Plomin, R. (1997). Can personality explain genetic influences on life events? *Journal of Personality and Social Psychology*, 72: 196–206.

Scarr, S. (1968). Environmental bias in twin studies. *Eugenics Quarterly*, 15: 34–40.

Schapira, K., Kerr, T. A., & Roth, M. (1970). Phobias and affective illness. *British Journal of Psychiatry*, 117: 25–32.

Scherrer, J. F., True, W. R., Xian, H., Lyons, M. J., Eisen, S. A., Goldberg, J., Lin, N., & Tsuang, M. T. (2000). Evidence for genetic influences common and specific to symptoms of generalized anxiety and panic. *Journal of Affective Disorders*, 57: 25–35.

Schuster, T. L., Kessler, R. C., & Aseltine, R. H., Jr. (1990). Supportive interactions, negative interactions, and depressed mood. *American Journal of Community Psychology*, 18: 423–438.

Seeman, M. V. (1997). Psychopathology in women and men: Focus on female hormones. *American Journal of Psychiatry*, 154: 1641–1647.

Seligman, M. E. P. (1971). Phobias and preparedness. *Behavior Therapy*, 2: 307–320.

Seligman, M. E. P. (1975). *Helplessness: On depression, development, and death*. San Francisco: Freeman.

Siemens, H. (1924). *Die Zwillingspathologie*. Berlin, Germany: Springer.

Sigvardsson, S., Bohman, M., & Cloninger, C. R. (1996). Replication of the Stock-holm Adoption Study of alcoholism: Confirmatory cross-fostering analysis. *Archives of General Psychiatry*, **53**: 681–687.

Simonoff, E., Pickles, A., Hewitt, J., Silberg, J., Rutter, M., Loeber, R., Meyer, J., Neale, M., & Eaves, L. (1995). Multiple raters of disruptive child behavior: Using a genetic strategy to examine shared views and bias. *Behavior Genetics*, **25**: 311–326.

Skre, I., Onstad, S., Torgersen, S., Lygren, S., & Kringlen, E. (1993). A twin study of DSM-III-R anxiety disorders. *Acta Psychiatrica Scandinavica*, **88**: 85–92.

Slattery, M. L., Hunt, S. C., French, T. K., Ford, M. H., & Williams, R. R. (1989). Validity of cigarette smoking habits in three epidemiologic studies in Utah. *Preventive Medicine*, **18**: 11–19.

Slutske, W. S., Cronk, N. J., Sher, K. J., Madden, P. A. F., Bucholz, K. K., & Heath, A. C. (2002a). Genes, environment, and individual differences in alcohol expectancies among female adolescents and young adults. *Psychology of Addictive Behaviors*, **16**: 308–317.

Slutske, W. S., Heath, A. C., Madden, P. A. F., Bucholz, K. K., Dunne, M. P., Statham, D. J., & Martin, N. G. (1997). Modeling genetic and environmental influences in the etiology of conduct disorder: A study of 2, 682 adult twin pairs. *Journal of Abnormal Psychology*, **106**: 266–279.

Slutske, W. S., Heath, A. C., Madden, P. A. F., Bucholz, K. K., Statham, D. J., & Martin, N. G. (2002b). Personality and the genetic risk for alcohol dependence. *Journal of Abnormal Psychology*, **111**: 124–133.

Snieder, H., MacGregor, A. J., & Spector, T. D. (1998). Genes control the cessation of a woman's reproductive life: A twin study of hysterectomy and age at menopause. *Journal of Clinical Endocrinology and Metabolism*, **83**: 1875–1880.

Spence, J. E., Corey, L. A., Nance, W. E., Marazita, M. L., Kendler, K. S., & Schieken, R. M. (1988). Molecular analysis of twin zygosity using VNTR DNA probes. *American Journal of Human Genetics*, **43**(3): A159.

Spitzer, R. L., Endicott, J., & Robins, E. (1975). *Research diagnostic criteria for a selected group of functional disorders*. New York: New York Psychiatric Institute.

Spitzer, R. L., Williams, J. B., & Gibbon, M. (1987). *Structured Clinical Interview for DSM-III-R*. New York: New York State Psychiatric Institute Biometrics Research Department.

Srisurapanont, M., & Jarusuraisin, N. (2005). Naltrexone for the treatment of alcoholism: A meta-analysis of randomized controlled trials. *International Journal of Neuropsychopharmacology*, **26**: 1–14.

Steiger, J. H. (1990). Structural model evaluation and modification: An interval estimation approach. *Multivariate Behavioral Research*, **25**: 173–180.

Stein, M. B., Koverola, C., Hanna, C., Torchia, M. G., & McClarty, B. (1997). Hippocampal volume in women victimized by childhood sexual abuse. *Psychological Medicine*, **27**: 951–959.

Stevenson, J., Batten, N., & Cherner, M. (1992). Fears and fearfulness in children and adolescents: A genetic analysis of twin data. *Journal of Child Psychology and Psychiatry*, **33**: 977–985.

Substance Abuse and Mental Health Services Administration. (1997). *National Household Survey on Drug Abuse: Population Estimates 1996*. Washington, DC: U.S. Department of Health and Human Services.

Sullivan, P. F., & Kendler, K. S. (1998). The genetic epidemiology of smoking. *Nicotine and Tobacco Research*, 1: S51–S57.

Sullivan, P. F., Neale, M. C., & Kendler, K. S. (2000). The genetic epidemiology of major depression: Review and meta-analysis. *American Journal of Psychiatry*, 157: 1552–1562.

Sundet, J. M., Skre, I., Okkenhaug, J. J., & Tambs, K. (2003). Genetic and environmental causes of the interrelationships between self-reported fears: A study of a non-clinical sample of Norwegian identical twins and their families. *Scandinavian Journal of Psychology*, 44: 97–106.

Szasz, T. S. (1984). *The myth of mental illness: Foundations of a theory of personal conduct*. New York: Harper & Row.

Tennant, C. (1988). Parental loss in childhood: Its effect in adult life. *Archives of General Psychiatry*, 45: 1045–1050.

Tennant, C., Hurry, J., & Bebbington, P. (1982). The relation of childhood separation experiences to adult depressive and anxiety states. *British Journal of Psychiatry*, 141: 475–482.

Tennant, C., Smith, A., Bebbington, P., & Hurry, J. (1981). Parental loss in childhood: Relationship to adult psychiatric impairment and contact with psychiatric services. *Archives of General Psychiatry*, 38: 309–314.

Thapar, A., & McGuffin, P. (1996). Genetic influences on life events in childhood. *Psychological Medicine*, 26: 813–820.

Thapar, A., & Scourfield, J. (2002). Childhood disorders. In P. McGuffin, M. J. Owen, & I. I. Gottesman (Eds.), *Psychiatric genetics and genomics* (pp. 147–180). London: Oxford University Press.

Thoits, P. A. (1983). Dimensions of life events that influence psychological distress: An evaluation and synthesis of the literature. In H. B. Kaplan (Ed.), *Psychosocial stress: Trends in theory and research* (pp. 33–102). New York: Academic Press.

Thomasson, H. R., Edenberg, H. J., Crabb, D. W., Mai, X. -L., Jerome, R. E., Li, T. -K., Wang, S. -P., Lin, Y. -T., Lu, R. -B., & Yin, S. -J. (1991). Alcohol and aldehyde dehydrogenase genotypes and alcoholism in Chinese men. *American Journal of Human Genetics*, 48: 677–681.

Tienari, P. (1991). Interaction between genetic vulnerability and family environment: The Finnish adoptive family study of schizophrenia. *Acta Psychiatrica Scandinavica*, 84: 460–465.

Tillmann, W. A., & Hobbs, G. E. (1949). The accident-prone automobile driver: A study of the psychiatric and social background. *American Journal of Psychiatry*, 106: 321–331.

Torgersen, S. (1979). The nature and origin of common phobic fears. *British Journal of Psychiatry*, 134: 343–351.

Torgersen, S. (1983). Genetic factors in anxiety disorders. *Archives of General Psychiatry*, 40: 1085–1089.

True, W. R., Xian, H., Scherrer, J. F., Madden, P. A., Bucholz, K. K., Heath, A. C., Eisen, S. A., Lyons, M. J., Goldberg, J., & Tsuang, M. (1999). Common genetic vulnerability for nicotine and alcohol dependence in men. *Archives of General Psychiatry*, 56: 655–661.

Tsuang, M. T., & Faraone, S. V. (1990). *The genetics of mood disorders*. Baltimore: Johns Hopkins University Press.

Tsuang, M. T., Lyons, M. J., Eisen, S. A., Goldberg, J., True, W., Lin, N., Meyer, J. M., Toomey, R., Faraone, S. V., & Eaves, L. (1996). Genetic influences on DSM-

III-R drug abuse and dependence: A study of 3, 372 twin pairs. *American Journal of Medical Genetics*, **67**: 473–477.

Tsuang, M. T., Lyons, M. J., Meyer, J. M., Doyle, T., Eisen, S. A., Goldberg, J., True, W., Lin, N., Toomey, R., & Eaves, L. (1998). Co-occurence of abuse of different drugs in men. *Archives of General Psychiatry*, **55**: 967–972.

Turkheimer, E., Haley, A., Waldron, M., D'Onofrio, B., & Gottesman, I. I. (2003). Socioeconomic status modifies heritability of IQ in young children. *Psychology Science*, **14**: 623–628.

Tyas, S. L., & Pederson, L. L. (1998). Psychosocial factors related to adolescent smoking: A critical review of the literature. *Tobacco Control*, 7: 409–420.

Uhl, G. R., Liu, Q. R., Walther, D., Hess, J., & Naiman, D. (2001). Polysubstance abuse–vulnerability genes: Genome scans for association, using 1, 004 subjects and 1, 494 single-nucleotide polymorphisms. *American Journal of Human Genetics*, **69**: 1290–1300.

Urberg, K. A., Shyu, S. -J., & Liang, J. (1990). Peer influence in adolescent cigarette smoking. *Addictive Behaviors*, **15**: 247–255.

Vaillant, G. E. (1983). *The natural history of alcoholism: Causes, patterns, and paths to recovery*. Cambridge, MA: Harvard University Press.

van den Berg, S. M., Posthuma, D., & Boomsma, D. I. (2004). A longitudinal genetic study of vocabulary knowledge in adults. *Twin Research*, 7: 284–291.

van den Bree, M. B. M., Johnson, E. O., Neale, M. C., & Pickens, R. W. (1998). Genetic and environmental influences on drug use and abuse/dependence in male and female twins. *Drug and Alcohol Dependence*, **52**: 231–241.

Van Eerdewegh, P. (1982). *Statistical selection in multivariate systems with applications in quantitative genetics*. Unpublished doctoral dissertation, Washington University.

Van Os, J., & Jones, P. B. (1999). Early risk factors and adult person–environment relationships in affective disorder. *Psychological Medicine*, **29**: 1055–1067.

Vierikko, E., Pulkkinen, L., Kaprio, J., & Rose, R. J. (2004). Genetic and environmental influences on the relationship between aggression and hyperactivity–impulsivity as rated by teachers and parents. *Twin Research*, 7: 261–274.

Viken, R. J., Johnson, J. K., Kaprio, J., & Rose, R. J. (2002). Genetic and environmental contributions to variation in alcohol expectancies and to the covariation between expectancies and related phenotypes. *Behavior Genetics*, **32**: 488.

Vythilingam, M., Heim, C., Newport, J., Miller, A. H., Anderson, E., Bronen, R., Brummer, M., Staib, L., Vermetten, E., Charney, D. S., Nemeroff, C. B., & Bremner, J. D. (2002). Childhood trauma associated with smaller hippocampal volume in women with major depression. *American Journal of Psychiatry*, **159**: 2072–2080.

Wade, T., Neale, M. C., Lake, R. I., & Martin, N. G. (1999). A genetic analysis of the eating and attitudes associated with bulimia nervosa: Dealing with the problem of ascertainment in twin studies. *Behavior Genetics*, **29**: 1–10.

Wade, T. D., & Kendler, K. S. (2000). Absence of interactions between social support and stressful life events in the prediction of major depression and depressive symptomatology in women. *Psychological Medicine*, **30**: 965–974.

Wahlsten, D. (1990). Insensitivity of the analysis of variance to heredity–environment interaction. *Behavior and Brain Science*, **13**: 109–161.

Watson, J. B., & Rayner, B. (1920). Conditioned emotional reactions. *Journal of Experimental Psychology*, 3: 1–14.

Wells, J. E., & Horwood, L. J. (2004). How accurate is recall of key symptoms of depression? A comparison of recall and longitudinal reports. *Psychological Medicine*, **34**: 1001–1011.

Werner, E. (1987). Vulnerability and resiliency in children at risk for delinquency: A longitudinal study from birth to young adulthood. In J. Burchard, & S. Burchard (Eds.), *Prevention of delinquent behavior* (pp. 16–43). Newbury Park, CA: Sage.

Werner, E. E., & Johnson, J. L. (2004). The role of caring adults in the lives of children of alcoholics. *Substance Use and Misuse*, **39**: 699–720.

Werner, E. W., & Smith, R. S. (1989). *Vulnerable but invincible: A longitudinal study of resilient children and youth*. New York: Adams Bannister Cox.

Windle, M. (1992). Temperament and social support in adolescence: Interrelations with depressive symptoms and delinquent behaviors. *Journal of Youth and Adolescence*, **21**: 1–21.

Winokur, G., Cadoret, R. J., Dorzab, J., & Baker, M. (1971). Depressive disease: A genetic study. *Archives of General Psychiatry*, **24**: 135–144.

Xian, H., Scherrer, J. F., Eisen, S. A., True, W. R., Heath, A. C., Goldberg, J., Lyons, M. J., & Tsuang, M. T. (2000). Self-reported zygosity and the equal-environments assumption for psychiatric disorders in the Vietnam Era Twin Registry. *Behavior Genetics*, **30**: 303–310.

Zerbin-Rudin, E., & Kendler, K. S. (1996). Ernst Rudin and his genealogic-demographic department in Munich: An introduction to their family studies of schizophrenia. *American Journal of Medical Genetics*, **67**: 332–337.

Zuckerman, M. (1972). Drug use as one manifestation of a "sensation-seeking trait. " In W. Keup (Ed.), *Drug abuse: Current concepts and research* (pp. 154–163). Springfield, IL: Thomas.

Zuckerman, M. (1994). *Behavioral expressions and biosocial bases of sensation seeking*. Cambridge, MA: Cambridge University Press.

Publications from the VATSPSUD

1990

Silberg, J. L., Heath, A. C., Kessler, R. C., Neale, M. C., Meyer, J. M., Eaves, L. J., & Kendler, K. S. (1990). Genetic and environmental effects of self-reported depressive symptoms in a general population twin sample. *Journal of Psychiatric Research*, **24**: 197–212.

1991

Kendler, K. S., Kessler, R. C., Heath, A. C., Neale, M. C., & Eaves, L. J. (1991). Coping: A genetic epidemiological investigation. *Psychological Medicine*, **21**: 337–346.

Kendler, K. S., MacLean, C. J., Neale, M. C., Kessler, R. C., Heath, A. C., & Eaves, L. J. (1991). The genetic epidemiology of bulimia nervosa. *American Journal of Psychiatry*, **148**: 1627–1637.

Kendler, K. S., Silberg, J. L., Neale, M. C., Kessler, R. C., Heath, A. C., & Eaves, L. J. (1991). The family history method: Whose psychiatric history is measured? *American Journal of Psychiatry*, **148**: 1501–1504.

Silberg, J. L., Meyer, J. M., Eaves, L. J., Neale, M. C., Hewitt, J. K., Heath, A. C., & Kendler, K. S. (1991). The effect of bias on the estimates of the genetic and environmental influences on ratings of depressive symptoms. *International Journal of Methods in Psychiatric Research*, **1**: 59–67.

1992

Kendler, K. S., Heath, A. C., Neale, M. C., Kessler, R. C., & Eaves, L. J. (1992). A population-based twin study of alcoholism in women. *Journal of the American Medical Association*, **268**: 1877–1882.

Kendler, K. S., Neale, M. C., Kessler, R. C., Heath, A. C., & Eaves, L. J. (1992). Childhood parental loss and adult psychopathology in women: A twin study perspective. *Archives of General Psychiatry*, **49**: 109–116.

Kendler, K. S., Neale, M. C., Kessler, R. C., Heath, A. C., & Eaves, L. J. (1992). Familial influences on the clinical characteristics of major depression. *Acta Psychiatrica Scandinavica*, **86**: 371–378.

Kendler, K. S., Neale, M. C., Kessler, R. C., Heath, A. C., & Eaves, L. J. (1992). Generalized anxiety disorder in women: A population-based twin study. *Archives of General Psychiatry*, **49**: 267–272.

Kendler, K. S., Neale, M. C., Kessler, R. C., Heath, A. C., & Eaves, L. J. (1992). The genetic epidemiology of phobias in women: The inter-relationship of agoraphobia, social phobia, situational phobia and simple phobia. *Archives of General Psychiatry*, **49**: 273–281.

Kendler, K. S., Neale, M. C., Kessler, R. C., Heath, A. C., & Eaves, L. J. (1992). Major depression and generalized anxiety disorder: Same genes (partly) different environments? *Archives of General Psychiatry*, **49**: 716–722.

Kendler, K. S., Neale, M. C., Kessler, R. C., Heath, A. C., & Eaves, L. J. (1992). A population-based twin study of major depression in women: The impact of varying definitions of illness. *Archives of General Psychiatry*, **49**: 257–266.

Kendler, K. S., Silberg, J. L., Neale, M. C., Kessler, R. C., Heath, A. C., & Eaves, L. J. (1992). Genetic and environmental factors in the aetiology of menstrual, premenstrual and neurotic symptoms: A population-based twin study. *Psychological Medicine*, **22**: 85–100.

Kessler, R. C., Kendler, K. S., Heath, A. C., Neale, M. C., & Eaves, L. J. (1992). Social support, depressed mood and adjustment to stress: A genetic epidemiologic investigation. *Journal of Personality and Social Psychology*, **62**: 257–272.

Walters, E. E., Neale, M. C., Eaves, L. J., Heath, A. C., Kessler, R. C., & Kendler, K. S. (1992). Bulimia nervosa and major depression: A study of common genetic and environmental factors. *Psychological Medicine*, **22**: 617–622.

1993

Heath, A. C., Neale, M. C., Hewitt, J. K., Eaves, L. J., Kessler, R. C., & Kendler, K. S. (1993). Testing hypotheses about direction of causation using cross-sectional family data. *Behavior Genetics*, **23**: 29–50.

Kendler, K. S., Heath, A. C., Neale, A. C., Kessler, R. C., & Eaves, L. J. (1993). Alcoholism and major depression in women: A twin study of the causes of comorbidity. *Archives of General Psychiatry*, **50**: 690–698.

Kendler, K. S., Kessler, R. C., Neale, M. C., Heath, A. C., & Eaves, L. J. (1993). The prediction of major depression in women: Toward an integrated etiologic mode. *American Journal of Psychiatry*, **50**: 1139–1148.

Kendler, K. S., Neale, M. C., Kessler, R. C., Heath, A. C., & Eaves, L. J. (1993). The lifetime history of major depression in women: Reliability of diagnosis and heritability. *Archives of General Psychiatry*, **50**: 863–870.

Kendler, K. S., Neale, M. C., Kessler, R. C., Heath, A. C., & Eaves, L. J. (1993). A longitudinal twin study of 1-year prevalence of major depression in women. *Archives of General Psychiatry*, **50**: 843–852.

Kendler, K. S., Neale, M. C., Kessler, R. C., Heath, A. C., & Eaves, L. J. (1993). A longitudinal twin study of personality and major depression in women. *Archives of General Psychiatry*, **50**: 853–862.

Kendler, K. S., Neale, M. C., Kessler, R. C., Heath, A. C., & Eaves, L. J. (1993). Major depression and phobias: The genetic and environmental sources of comorbidity. *Psychological Medicine*, **23**: 361–371.

Kendler, K. S., Neale, M. C., Kessler, R. C., Heath, A. C., Eaves, L. J. (1993). Panic disorder in women: A population-based twin study. *Psychological Medicine*, **23**: 397–406.

Kendler, K. S., Neale, M. C., Kessler, R. C., Heath, A. C., & Eaves, L. J. (1993). A test of the equal environment assumption in twin studies of psychiatric illness. *Behavior Genetics*, **23**: 21–27.

Kendler, K. S., Neale, M. C., Kessler, R. C., Heath, A. C., & Eaves, L. J. (1993). A twin study of recent life events and difficulties. *Archives of General Psychiatry*, : 789–796.

Kendler, K. S., Neale, M. C., MacLean, C. M., Heath, A. C., Eaves, L. J., & Kessler, R. C. (1993). Smoking and major depression: A causal analysis. *Archives of General Psychiatry*, **50**: 36–43.

Walters, E. E., Neale, M. C., Eaves, L. J., Heath, A. C., Kessler, R. C., & Kendler, K. S. (1993). Bulimia nervosa: A population-based study of purgers vs. non-purgers. *International Journal of Eating Disorders*, **13**: 265–272.

1994

Kendler, K. S., Neale, M. C., Heath, A. C., Kessler, R. C., & Eaves, L. J. (1994). A twin-family study of alcoholism in women. *American Journal of Psychiatry*, **151**: 707–715.

Kendler, K. S., Neale, M. C., Kessler, R. C., Heath, A. C., & Eaves, L. J. (1994–1995). The clinical characteristics of familial generalized anxiety disorder. *Anxiety*, **1**: 186–191.

Kendler, K. S., Neale, M. C., Kessler, R. C., Heath, A. C., & Eaves, L. J. (1994). The clinical characteristics of major depression as indices of the familial risk to illness. *British Journal of Psychiatry*, **165**: 66–72.

Kendler, K. S., Neale, M. C., Kessler, R. C., Heath, A. C., & Eaves, L. J. (1994). Parental treatment and the equal environment assumption in twin studies of psychiatric illness. *Psychological Medicine*, **24**: 579–590.

Kendler, K. S., Walters, E. E., Truett, K. R., Heath, A. C., Neale, M. C., Martin, N. G., & Eaves, L. J. (1994). Sources of individual differences in depressive symptoms: An analysis of two samples of twins and their families. *American Journal of Psychiatry*, **151**: 1605–1614.

Kessler, R. C., Kendler, K. S., Heath, A. C., Neale, M. C., & Eaves, L. J. (1994). Perceived support and adjustment to stress in a general population sample of female twins. *Psychological Medicine*, **24**: 317–334.

Neale, M. C., Eaves, L. J., Heath, A. C., Kessler, R. C., & Kendler, K. S. (1994). Multiple regression with data collected from relatives: Testing assumptions of the model. *Multivariate Behavioral Research*, **29**: 33–61.

Neale, M. C., Eaves, L. J., & Kendler, K. S. (1994). The power of the classical twin study to resolve variation in threshold traits. *Behavior Genetics*, **24**: 239–258.

Neale, M. C., Walters, E. E., Eaves, L. J., Kessler, R. C., Heath, A. C., & Kendler, K. S. (1994). Genetics of blood–injury fears and phobias: A population-based twin study. *American Journal of Medical Genetics (Neuropsychiatric Genetics)*, **54**: 326–334.

Neale, M. C., Walters, E. E., Eaves, L. J., Maes, H. H., & Kendler, K. S. (1994). Multivariate genetic analysis of twin-family data on fears: Mx models. *Behavior Genetics*, 24: 119–139.

Neale, M. C., Walters, E. E., Heath, A. C., Kessler, R. C., Perusse, D., Eaves, L. J., & Kendler, K. S. (1994). Depression and parental bonding: Cause, consequence, or genetic covariance? *Genetic Epidemiology*, 11: 503–522.

Sham, P. C., Walters, E. E., Neale, M. C., Heath, A. C., MacLean, C. J., & Kendler, K. S. (1994). Logistic regression analysis of twin data: Estimation of parameters of the multifactorial liability threshold model. *Behavior Genetics*, 24: 229–238.

Truett, K. R., Eaves, L. J., Walters, E. E., Heath, A. C., Hewitt, J. K., Meyer, J. M., Silberg, J. L., Neale, M. C., Martin, N. G., & Kendler, K. S. (1994). A model system for analysis of family resemblance in extended kinships of twins. *Behavior Genetics*, 24: 35–49.

1995

Hettema, J. M., Neale, M. C., & Kendler, K. S. (1995). Physical similarity and the equal environment assumption in twin studies of psychiatric disorders. *Behavior Genetics*, 25: 327–335.

Kendler, K. S. (1995). Adversity, stress and psychopathology: A psychiatric genetic perspective. *International Journal of Methods in Psychiatric Research*, 5: 163–170.

Kendler, K. S. (1995). Is seeking treatment for depression predicted by a history of depression in relatives? Implications for family studies of affective disorder. *Psychological Medicine*, 25: 807–814.

Kendler, K. S. (1995). Methods of proband ascertainment in psychiatric genetics: An historical and epidemiologic perspective. *International Journal of Methods in Psychiatric Research*, 4: 111–121.

Kendler, K. S., Kessler, R. C., Walters, E. E., MacLean, C. J., Neale, M. C., Heath, A. C., & Eaves, L. J. (1995). Stressful life events, genetic liability and onset of an episode of major depression in women: Evidence for genetic control of sensitivity to the environment. *American Journal of Psychiatry*, 152: 833–842.

Kendler, K. S., Martin, N. G., Heath, A. C., & Eaves, L. J. (1995). Self-report psychiatric symptoms in twins and their nontwin relatives: Are twins different? *American Journal of Medical Genetics (Neuropsychiatric Genetics)*, 60: 588–591.

Kendler, K. S., & Roy, M. -A. (1995). Validity of a diagnosis of lifetime major depression by personal interview versus family history. *American Journal of Psychiatry*, 152: 1608–1614.

Kendler, K. S., Walters, E. E., Neale, M. C., Kessler, R. C., Heath, A. C., & Eaves, L. J. (1995). The structure of the genetic and environmental risk factors for six major psychiatric disorders in women: Phobia, generalized anxiety disorder, panic disorder, bulimia, major depression and alcoholism. *Archives of General Psychiatry*, 52: 374–883.

Kendler, K. S., Walters, E. E., Truett, K., Heath, A. C., Neale, M. C., Martin, N. G., & Eaves, L. J. (1995). A twin-family study of self-report symptoms of depression, panic-phobia, and somatization. *Behavior Genetics*, 25: 499–515.

Neale, M. C., & Kendler, K. S. (1995). Models of comorbidity for multifactorial disorders. *American Journal of Human Genetics*, 57: 935–953.

Prescott, C. A., & Kendler, K. S. (1995). Genetic and environmental influences on alcohol and tobacco dependence among women. In J. B. Fertig & A. P. Allen (Eds.), *Alcohol and tobacco: From basic science to clinical practice* (National Institute on Alcohol Abuse and Alcoholism Research Monograph No. 30; NIH Publication No. 95-3931, pp. 59–87). Bethesda, MD: National Institutes of Health.

Roy, M. -A., Neale, M. C., & Kendler, K. S. (1995). The genetic epidemiology of self-esteem. *British Journal of Psychiatry*, **166**: 813–820.

Walters, E. E., & Kendler, K. S. (1995). Anorexia nervosa and anorexic-like syndromes in a population-based female twin sample. *American Journal of Psychiatry*, **152**: 64–71.

1996

Fanous, A. H., Walsh, D., & Kendler, K. S. (1996). Do endogenous features in depression predict the risk of psychiatric illness in relatives? *Acta Psychiatrica Scandinavica*, **94**: 56–59.

Foley, D. L., & Kendler, K. S. (1996). A longitudinal study of stressful life events assessed at personal interview with an epidemiologic sample of adult twins: The basis of individual variation in event exposure. *Psychological Medicine*, **26**: 1239–1252.

Kendler, K. S. (1996). Major depression and generalized anxiety disorder: Same genes (partly) different environments—revisited. *British Journal of Psychiatry*, **168**(suppl. 30): 68–75.

Kendler, K. S. (1996). Parenting: A genetic-epidemiologic perspective. *American Journal of Psychiatry*, **153**: 11–20.

Kendler, K. S., Eaves, L. J., Walters, E. E., Neale, M. C., Heath, A. C., & Kessler, R. C. (1996). The identification and validation of distinct depressive syndromes in a population-based sample of female twins. *Archives of General Psychiatry*, **53**: 391–399.

Kendler, K. S., Neale, M. C., Prescott, C. A., Kessler, R. C., Heath, A. C., Corey, L. A., & Eaves, L. J. (1996). Childhood parental loss and alcoholism in women: A causal analysis using a twin-family design. *Psychological Medicine*, **26**: 79–85.

McGovern, R. J., Neale, M. C., & Kendler, K. S. (1996). The independence of physical attractiveness and symptoms of depression in a female twin population. *Journal of Psychology*, **130**: 209–219.

Prescott, C. A., & Kendler, K. S. (1996). Longitudinal stability and change in alcohol consumption among female twins: Contributions of genetics. *Development and Psychopathology*, **8**: 849–866.

1997

Karkowski, L, & Kendler, K. S. (1997). An examination of the genetic relationship between bipolar and unipolar illness in a epidemiologic sample. *Psychiatric Genetics*, **7**: 159–163.

Kendler, K. S. (1997). The diagnostic validity of melancholic major depression in a population-based sample of female twins. *Archives of General Psychiatry*, **54**: 299–304.

Kendler, K. S. (1997). Social support: A genetic epidemiologic analysis. *American Journal of Psychiatry*, **154**: 1309–1404.

Kendler, K. S., Gardner, C. O., & Prescott, C. A. (1997). Religion, psychopathology and substance use and abuse: A multimeasure, genetic–epidemiologic study. *American Journal of Psychiatry*, **154**: 322–329.

Kendler, K. S., & Karkowski-Shuman, L. (1997). Stressful life events and genetic liability to major depression: Genetic control of exposure to the environment? *Psychological Medicine*, **27**: 539–547.

Kendler, K. S., Sham, P. C., & MacLean, C. J. (1997). The determinants of parenting: An epidemiologic, multi-informant study. *Psychological Medicine*, **27**: 549–563.

Kendler, K. S., Walters, E. E., & Kessler, R. C. (1997). The prediction of length of major depressive episodes: Results from an epidemiologic sample of female twins. *Psychological Medicine*, **27**: 107–117.

Prescott, C. A., Neale, M. C., Corey, L. A., & Kendler, K. S. (1997). Predictors of problem drinking and alcohol dependence in a population-based sample of female twins. *Journal of Studies on Alcohol*, **58**: 167–181.

1998

Bulik, C. M., Sullivan, P. F., & Kendler, K. S. (1998). Heritability and reliability of binge-eating and bulimia nervosa. *Biological Psychiatry*, **44**: 1210–1218.

Foley, D. L., Neale, M. C., & Kendler, K. S. (1998). Reliability of a lifetime history of major depression: Implications for heritability and comorbidity. *Psychological Medicine*, **28**: 857–870.

Kendler, K. S. (1998). Major depression and the environment: A psychiatric genetic perspective. *Pharmacopsychiatry*, **31**: 5–9.

Kendler, K. S., & Gardner, C. O. (1998). The boundaries of major depression: An evaluation of DSM-IV criteria. *American Journal of Psychiatry*, **15**: 172–177.

Kendler, K. S., & Gardner, C. O. (1998). Twin studies of adult psychiatric and substance dependence disorders: Childhood and adolescence? *Psychological Medicine*, **28**: 625–633.

Kendler, K. S., Gardner, C. O., & Prescott, C. A. (1998). A population-based twin study of self-esteem and gender. *Psychological Medicine*, **28**: 1403–1409.

Kendler, K. S., Karkowski, L. M., & Neale, M. C. (1998). A longitudinal population-based twin study of retrospectively reported premenstrual symptoms and lifetime major depression. *American Journal of Psychiatry*, **155**: 1234–1240.

Kendler, K. S., Karkowski, L. M., & Prescott, C. A. (1998). Stressful life events and major depression: Risk period, long-term contextual threat and diagnostic specificity. *Journal of Nervous and Mental Disease*, **186**: 661–669.

Kendler, K. S., & Prescott, C. A. (1998). Cannabis use, abuse and dependence in a population-based sample of female twins. *American Journal of Psychiatry*, **155**: 1016–1022.

O'Neill, F., & Kendler, K. S. (1998). Longitudinal study of interpersonal dependency in female twins. *British Journal of Psychiatry*, **155**: 172–177.

1999

Kendler, K. S., Gardner, C. O., & Prescott, C. A. (1999). Clarifying the relationship between religiosity and psychiatric illness: The impact of covariates and the specificity of buffering effects. *Twins Research*, **2**: 137–144.

Kendler, K. S., Gardner, C. O., & Prescott, C. A. (1999). The clinical characteristics of major depression that predict risk of depression in relatives. *Archives of General Psychiatry*, **56**: 322–327.

Kendler, K. S., Karkowski, L. M., Corey, L. A., Prescott, C. A., & Neale, M. C. (1999). Genetic and environmental risk factors in the aetiology of drug initiation and subsequent misuse in women. *British Journal of Psychiatry*, **175**: 351–358.

Kendler, K. S., Karkowski, L. M., & Prescott, C. A. (1999). The causal relationship between stressful life events and the onset of major depression. *American Journal of Psychiatry*, **156**: 837–841.

Kendler, K. S., Karkowski, L. M., & Prescott, C. A. (1999). Fears and phobias: Reliability and heritability. *Psychological Medicine*, **29**: 539–553.

Kendler, K. S., Karkowski, L. M., & Prescott, C. A. (1999). Hallucinogen, opiate, sedative and stimulant use and abuse in a population-based sample of female twins. *Acta Psychiatrica Scandinavica*, **99**: 368–376.

Kendler, K. S., Neale, M. C., Sullivan, P. F., Corey, L. A., Gardner, C. O., & Prescott, C. A. (1999). A population-based twin study in women of smoking initiation and nicotine dependence. *Psychological Medicine*, **29**: 299–308.

Kendler, K. S., & Prescott, C. A. (1999). Caffeine intake, tolerance and withdrawal in women: A population-based twin study. *American Journal of Psychiatry*, **156**: 223–228.

Kendler, K. S., & Prescott, C. A. (1999). A population-based twin study of lifetime major depression in men and women. *Archives of General Psychiatry*, **56**: 39–44.

Prescott, C. A., Aggen, S. H., & Kendler, K. S. (1999). Sex differences in the sources of genetic liability to alcohol abuse and dependence in a population-based sample of US twins. *Alcohol Clinical Experimental Research*, **23**: 1136–1144.

Prescott, C. A., & Kendler, K. S. (1999). Age at first drink and risk for alcoholism: A noncausal association. *Alcoholism: Clinical and Experimental Research*, **23**: 101–107.

Prescott, C. A., & Kendler, K. S. (1999). Genetic and environmental contributions to alcohol abuse and dependence in a population-based sample of male twins. *American Journal of Psychiatry*, **156**: 34–40.

Roberts, S. B., & Kendler, K. S. (1999). Neuroticism and self-esteem as indices of the vulnerability to major depression in women. *Psychological Medicine*, **29**: 1101–1109.

2000

Bulik, C. M., Sullivan, P. F., & Kendler, K. S. (2000). An empirical study of the classification of eating disorders. *American Journal of Psychiatry*, **157**: 886–895.

Foley, D. L., Neale, M. C., & Kendler, K. S. (2000). Does intra-uterine growth discordance predict differential risk for adult psychiatric disorder in population-based monozygotic twins? *Psychiatric Genetics*, **10**: 1–8.

Jacobson, K. C., Prescott, C. A., & Kendler, K. S. (2000). Genetic and environmental influences on juvenile antisocial behavior assessed on two occasions. *Psychological Medicine*, **30**: 1315–1325.

Jacobson, K. S., Prescott, C. A., Neale, M. C., & Kendler, K. S. (2000). Cohort differences in genetic and environmental influences on retrospective reports of conduct disorder among adult male twins. *Psychological Medicine*, **30**: 775–787.

Jonnal, A. H., Gardner, C. O., Prescott, C. A., & Kendler, K. S. (2000). Obsessive and compulsive symptoms in a general population sample of female twins. *Neuropsychiatric Genetics*, **96**: 791–796.

Kendler, K. S., Bulik, C. M., Silberg, J., Hettema, J. M., Myers, J., & Prescott, C. A.

(2000). Childhood sexual abuse and adult psychiatric and substance use disorders in women: An epidemiological and co-twin control analysis. *Archives of General Psychiatry*, **57**: 953–959.

Kendler, K. S., Karkowski, L. M., & Gardner, C. O. (2000). Stressful life events and previous episodes in the etiology of major depression in women: An evaluation of the kindling hypothesis. *American Journal of Psychiatry*, **157**: 1243–1251.

Kendler, K. S., Karkowski, L. M., Neale, M. C., & Prescott, C. A. (2000). Illicit psychoactive substance use, heavy use, abuse and dependence in a US population-based sample of male twins. *Archives of General Psychiatry*, **57**: 261–269.

Kendler, K. S., Myers, J. M., & Neale, M. C. (2000). A multidimensional twin study of mental health in women. *American Journal of Psychiatry*, **157**: 506–513.

Kendler, K. S., Myers, J. M., & Prescott, C. A. (2000). Parenting and adult mood, anxiety and substance use disorders in female twins: An epidemiological multi-informant, retrospective study. *Psychological Medicine*, **30**: 281–294.

Prescott, C. A., Aggen, S. H., & Kendler, K. S. (2000). Sex-specific genetic influences on the comorbidity of alcoholism and MD. *Archives of General Psychiatry*, **57**: 803–811.

Prescott, C. A., & Kendler, K. S. (2000). The influence of ascertainment strategy on finding sex differences in genetic estimates from twin studies of alcoholism. *Neuropsychiatric Genetics*, **96**: 754–761.

Sullivan, P. F., Neale, M. C., & Kendler, K. S. (2000). Genetic epidemiology of MD: Review and meta-analysis. *American Journal of Psychiatry*, **157**: 1553–1562.

Wade, T. D., Bulik, C. M., & Kendler, K. S. (2000). Reliability of lifetime history of bulimia nervosa: A comparison with major depression. *British Journal of Psychiatry*, **177**: 72–76.

Wade, T. D., Bulik, C. M., Neale, M., & Kendler, K. S. (2000). Anorexia nervosa and major depression: Shared genetic and environmental risk factors. *American Journal of Psychiatry*, **157**: 469–471.

Wade, T. D., Bulik, C. M., Sullivan, P. F., Neale, M. C., & Kendler, K. S. (2000). The relationship between risk factors for binge eating and bulimia nervosa: A population-based female twin study. *Health Psychology*, **19**: 115–123.

Wade, T. W., & Kendler, K. S. (2000). Absence of interactions between social support and stressful life events in the prediction of major depression and depressive symptomatology in women. *Psychological Medicine*, **30**: 965–974.

Wade, T. D., & Kendler, K. S. (2000). The genetic epidemiology of parental discipline. *Psychological Medicine*, **30**: 1303–1313.

Wade, T. D., & Kendler, K. S. (2000). The relationship between social support and major depression: Cross-sectional, longitudinal and genetic perspectives. *Journal of Nervous and Mental Disease*, **188**: 251–258.

2001

Bulik, C. M., Prescott, C. A., & Kendler, K. S. (2001). Features of childhood sexual abuse and the development of the psychiatric and substance use disorders. *British Journal of Psychiatry*, **179**: 444–449.

Bulik, C. M., Wade, T. D., & Kendler, K. S. (2001). Characteristics of monozygotic twins discordant for bulimia nervosa. *International Journal of Eating Disorders*, **29**: 1–10.

Bullers, S., & Prescott, C. A. (2001). An exploration of the independent contributions of genetics, shared environment, specific environments, and adult roles and statuses on perceived control. *Sociological Inquiry*, **71:** 145–163.

Foley, D. L., Neale, M. C., & Kendler, K. S. (2001). Genetic and environmental risk factors for depression assessed by subject-rated symptom checklist versus structured clinical interview. *Psychological Medicine*, **31:** 1413–1423.

Foley, D. L., Neale, M. C., & Kendler, K. S. (2001). Pregnancy and perinatal complications with risks for common psychiatric disorder in a population-based sample of female twins. *American Journal of Medical Genetics*, **105:** 426–431.

Goldstein, R. B., Prescott, C. A., & Kendler, K. S. (2001). Genetic and environmental factors in conduct problems and adult antisocial behavior among adult female twins. *Journal of Nervous and Mental Disease*, **189:** 201–209.

Hettema, J., Prescott, C. A., & Kendler, K. S. (2001). A population-based twin study of generalized anxiety disorder in men and women. *Journal of Nervous and Mental Disease*, **189:** 413–420.

Kendler, K. S., & Aggen, S. H. (2001). Time, memory and the heritability of major depression. *Psychological Medicine*, **31:** 923–928.

Kendler, K. S., & Gardner, C. O. (2001). Monozygotic twins discordant for major depression: A preliminary exploration role of environmental experiences in the Aetiology and course of illness. *Psychological Medicine*, **31:** 411–423.

Kendler, K. S., Gardner, C. O., Neale, M. C., & Prescott, C. A. (2001). Genetic risk factors for major depression in men and women: Similar or different heritabilities and same or partly different genes? *Psychological Medicine*, **31:** 605–616.

Kendler, K. S., Gardner, C. O., & Prescott, C. A. (2001). Are there sex differences in the reliability of a lifetime history of major depression and its predictors? *Psychological Medicine*, **31:** 617–625.

Kendler, K. S., Gardner, C. O., & Prescott, C. A. (2001). Panic syndromes in a population-based sample of male and female twins. *Psychological Medicine*, **31:** 989–1000.

Kendler, K. S., Myers, J. M., Prescott, C. A., & Neale, M. C. (2001). The genetic epidemiology of irrational fears and phobias in men. *Archives of General Psychiatry*, **58:** 257–265.

Kendler, K. S., Thornton, L. M., & Gardner, C. O. (2001). Genetic risk, number of previous depressive episodes and stressful life events in predicting onset of major depression. *American Journal of Psychiatry*, **158:** 582–586.

Kendler, K. S., Thornton, L. M., & Prescott, C. A. (2001). Gender differences in the rates of exposure to stressful life events and sensitivity to their depressogenic effects. *American Journal of Psychiatry*, **158:** 587–593.

Prescott, C. A., & Kendler, K. S. (2001). Associations between marital status and alcohol consumption in a longitudinal study of female twins. *Journal of Studies on Alcohol*, **62:** 589–601.

Wade, T. D., Bulik, C. M., & Kendler, K. S. (2001). An investigation of the quality of the parental relationship as a risk factor for sub-clinical bulimia nervosa. *International Journal of Eating Disorders*, **30:** 389–400.

Wade, T. D., & Kendler, K. S. (2001). Parent, child, and social correlates of parental discipline style: A retrospective, multi-informant investigation with female twins. *Social Psychiatry and Psychiatric Epidemiology*, **36:** 177–185.

2002

Agrawal, A., Jacobson, K. C., Prescott, C. A., & Kendler, K. S. (2002). A twin study of sex differences in social support: Analysis of quantitative and qualitative sex differences in social support. *Psychological Medicine*, **32**: 1155–1164.

Bulik, C. M., Sullivan, P. F., & Kendler, K. S. (2002). Medical and psychiatric morbidity in obese women with and without binge-eating. *International Journal of Eating Disorders*, **32**: 72–78.

Jacobson, K. C., Prescott, C. A., & Kendler, K. S. (2002). Sex differences in the genetic and environmental influences on the development of antisocial behavior. *Development and Psychopathology*, **14**: 395–416.

Kendler, K. S. (2002). The etiology of phobias: An evaluation of the stress–diathesis model. *Archives of General Psychiatry*, **59**: 242–248.

Kendler, K. S. (2002). Psychiatric genetics: An intellectual journey. *Clinical Neuroscience Research*, **2**: 110–119.

Kendler, K. S., Gardner, C. O., & Prescott, C. A. (2002). Toward a comprehensive developmental model for major depression in women. *American Journal of Psychiatry*, **159**: 1133–1145.

Kendler, K. S., Jacobson, K. C., Myers, J., & Prescott, C. A. (2002). Sex differences in genetic and environmental risk factors for irrational fears and phobias. *Psychological Medicine*, **32**: 209–217.

Kendler, K. S., Prescott, C. A., Jacobson, K., Myers, J., & Neale, M. C. (2002). The joint analysis of personal interview and family history diagnosis: Evidence for validity of diagnosis and increased heritability estimates. *Psychological Medicine*, **32**: 828–842.

Khan, A. A., Gardner, C. O., Prescott, C. A., & & Kendler, K. S. (2002). Gender differences in the symptoms of major depression in opposite sex dizygotic twin pairs. *American Journal of Psychiatry*, **159**: 1427–1429.

Sullivan, P. F., Prescott, C. A., & Kendler, K. S. (2002). The subtypes of major depression: A latent class analysis. *Journal of Affective Disorders*, **68**: 273–274.

2003

Bulik, C. M., Sullivan, P. F., & Kendler, K. S. (2003). Genetic and environmental contributions to obesity and binge-eating. *International Journal of Eating Disorder*, **33**: 293–298.

Foley, D. L., Neale, M. C., Gardner, C. O., Pickles, A., Prescott, C. A., & Kendler, K. S. (2003). Major depression and associated impairment: Same or different genetic and environmental risk factors? *American Journal of Psychiatry*, **160**: 2128–2133.

Hettema, J. M., Prescott, C. A., & Kendler, K. S. (2003). The effects of anxiety and substance use and conduct disorders on risk for major depression. *Psychological Medicine*, **33**: 1423–1432.

Kendler, K. S., Aggen, S. H., Jacobson, K. C., & Neale, M. C. (2003). Does the level of family dysfunction moderate the impact of genetic factors on the personality trait of neuroticism? *Psychological Medicine*, **33**: 817–825.

Kendler, K. S., Gardner, C. O., & Prescott, C. A. (2003). Personality and the experience of environmental adversity. *Psychological Medicine*, **33**: 1193–1202.

Kendler, K. S., Hettema, J., Butera F., Gardner, C. O., & Prescott, C. A. (2003). Life event dimensions of loss, humiliation, entrapment and danger in the prediction of onsets of major depression and generalized anxiety. *Archives of General Psychiatry*, **60**: 789–796.

Kendler, K. S., Jacobson, K. C., Prescott, C. A., & Neale, M. C. (2003). The specificity of genetic and environmental risk factors in men for the illicit use and abuse/dependence of cannabis, cocaine, hallucinogens, sedatives, stimulants and opiates. *American Journal of Psychiatry*, **160**: 687–695.

Kendler, K. S., Liu, X. Q., Gardner, C. O., McCullough, M. E., Larson, D., & Prescott, C. A. (2003). The dimensions of religiosity and their relationship to lifetime psychiatric and substance use disorders. *American Journal of Psychiatry*, **160**: 196–250.

Kendler, K. S., Prescott, C. A., Myers, J., & Neale, M. C. (2003). The structure of genetic and environmental risk factors for common psychiatric and substance use disorders in men and women. *Archives of General Psychiatry*, **60**: 929–937.

Kendler, K. S., Sheth, K., Gardner, C. O., & Prescott, C. A. (2003). Childhood parental loss and risk for major depression and alcohol dependence: The time-decay of risk and sex differences. *Psychological Medicine*, **32**: 1187–1194.

Sanathara, V., Gardner, C. O., Prescott, C. A., & Kendler, K. S. (2003). Interpersonal dependence and major depression: Etiologic inter-relationship and gender differences. *Psychological Medicine*, **33**: 927–931.

Sullivan, P. F., Kovalenko, P., York, T. P., Prescott, C. A., & Kendler, K. S. (2003). Fatigue in a community sample of twins. *Psychological Medicine*, **33**: 263–281.

2004

Agrawal, A, Jacobson, K. C., Gardner, C. O., Prescott, C. A., & Kendler, K. S. (2004). A population based twin study of sex differences in depressive symptoms. *Twin Research*, **7**: 176–181.

Agrawal, A., Jacobson, K. C., Gardner, C. O., Prescott, C. A., & Kendler, K. S. (2004). A twin study of personality and illicit drug use and abuse/dependence. *Twin Research*, **7**: 72–81.

Agrawal, A., Neale, M. C., Prescott, C. A., & Kendler, K. S. (2004). Cannabis and other illicit drugs: Comorbid use and abuse/dependence in males and females. *Behavior Genetics*, **34**: 217–228.

Agrawal, A., Neale, M. C., Prescott, C. A., & Kendler, K. S. (2004). A twin study of early cannabis use and subsequent use and abuse/dependence of other illicit drugs. *Psychological Medicine*, **34**: 1227–1237.

Agrawal, A., Prescott, C. A., & Kendler, K. S. (2004). Forms of cannabis and cocaine: A twin study. *American Journal of Medical Genetics*, **129B**: 125–128.

Bolinskey, P. K., Neale, M. C., Jacobson, K. C., Prescott, C. A., & Kendler, K. S. (2004). Sources of individual differences in stressful life event exposure in male and female twins. *Twin Research*. , **7**: 33–38.

Fanous, A. H., Prescott, C. A., & Kendler, K. S. (2004). The prediction of thoughts of death or self-harm in population-based sample of female twins. *Psychological Medicine*. , **34**: 301–312.

Hettema, J. M., Prescott, C. A., & Kendler, K. S. (2004) Genetic and environmental sources of covariation between generalized anxiety disorder and neuroticism. *American Journal of Psychiatry*. , **161**: 1581–1587.

Kendler, K. S., Aggen, S. H., Prescott, C. A., Jacobson, K. C., & Neale, M. C. (2004).

Level of family dysfunction and genetic influences on smoking in women. *Psychological Medicine*, **34**: 1263–1269.

Kendler, K. S., Kuhn, J., & Prescott, C. A. (2004). Childhood sexual abuse, stressful life events and risk for major depression in women. *Psychological Medicine*, **34**: 1475–1482.

Kendler, K. S., Kuhn, J., & Prescott, C. A. (2004). The inter-relationship of neuroticism, sex and stressful life events in the predictions of episodes of major depression. *American Journal of Psychiatry*, **161**: 631–636.

Maes, H. H., Sullivan, P. F., Bulik, C. M., Neale, M. C., Prescott, C. A., Eaves, L. J., & Kendler, K. S. (2004). A twin study of genetic and environmental influences on tobacco initiation, regular tobacco use and nicotine dependence. *Psychological Medicine*, **34**: 1251–1261.

Mazzeo, S. E., Slof, R. M., Tozzi, F., Kendler, K. S., & Bulik, C. M. (2004). Characteristics of men with persistent thinness. *Obesity Research*, **12**: 1367–1369.

Prescott, C. A., Cross, R. J., Kuhn, J. W., Horn, J. L., & Kendler, K. S. (2004). Is risk for alcoholism mediated by individual differences in drinking motivations? *Alcohol Clinical Experimental Research*, **28**: 29–39.

Wade, T. D., Bulik, C. M., Prescott, C. A., & Kendler, K. S. (2004). Sex influences on shared risk factors for bulimia nervosa and other psychiatric disorders. *Archives of General Psychiatry*, **61**: 251–256.

2005

Aggen, S., Neale, M. C., & Kendler, K. S. (2005). DSM-III-R Criteria for major depression: An evaluation using latent-trait item response models. *Psychological Medicine*, **35**: 475–487.

Agrawal, A., Gardner, C. O., Prescott, C. A., & Kendler, K. S. (2005). The differential impact of risk factors on illicit drug involvement in females. *Social Psychiatry and Psychiatric Epidemiology*, **40**: 454–466.

Agrawal, A., Neale, M. C., Jacobson, K. C., Prescott, C. A., & Kendler, K. S. (2005). Illicit drug use and abuse/dependence: Modeling of two-stage variables using the CCC approach. *Addictive Behaviors*, **30**: 1043–1048.

Furberg, H., Sullivan, P. F., Maes, H., Prescott, C. A., Lerman, C., Bulik, C., et al. (2005). The types of regular cigarette smokers: A latent class analysis. *Nicotine and Tobacco Research*, 7(3): 351–360.

Hettema, J. M., Prescott, C. A., Myers, J. M., Neale, M. C., & Kendler, K. S. (2005). The structure of genetic and environmental risk factors for anxiety disorders in men and women. *Archives of General Psychiatry*, **62**: 182–189.

Kendler, K. S., Gardner, C. O., Jacobson, K. C., Neale, M. C., & Prescott, C. A. (2005). Genetic and environmental influences in illicit drug use and tobacco use across birth cohorts. *Psychological Medicine*, **35**: 1–8.

Kendler, K. S., Kuhn, J. W., Vittum, J., Prescott, C. A., & Riley, B. (2005). The interaction of stressful life events and a serotonin transporter polymorphism in the prediction of episodes of major depression. *Archives of General Psychiatry*, **62**: 529–535.

Kendler, K. S., Myers, J., & Prescott, C. A. (2005). Sex differences in the relationship between social support and risk for major depression: A longitudinal study of opposite-sex twin pairs. *American Journal of Psychiatry*, **162**: 250–256.

Khan, A. A., Jacobson, K. C., Gardner, C. O., Prescott, C. A., & Kendler, K. S. (2005). Personality and comorbidity of common psychiatric disorders. *British Journal of Psychiatry*, **186**: 190–196.

Kubarych, T. S., Aggen, S. H., Hettema, J. M., Kendler, K. S., & Neale, M. C. (2005). Endorsement frequencies and factor structure of DSM-III-R and DSM-IV generalized anxiety disorder symptoms in women: Implications for future research, classification, clinical practice and comorbidity. *International Journal of Methods in Psychiatric Research*, **14**: 69–81.

Schmitt, J. E., Prescott, C. A., Gardner, C. O., Neale, M. C., & Kendler, K. S. (2005). The differential heritability of regular tobacco use based on method of administration. *Twin Research and Human Genetics*, **8**: 60–62.

2006

Hettema, J. M., Kuhn, J. W., Prescott, C. A., & Kendler, K. S. (2006). The impact of generalized anxiety disorder and stressful life events on risk for major depressive epiodes. *Psychological Medicine*, **36**: 789–795.

Kendler, K. S., Gardner, C. O., & Prescott, C. A. (2006). Toward a comprehensive developmental model for major depression in men. *American Journal of Psychiatry*, **163**(1): 115–124.

Author Index

Subject Index